A Century of Progress in
Head and Neck Cancer

A Century of Progress in
Head and Neck Cancer

Editor

Jatin P Shah

Associate Editors

Dennis Kraus
Ashok Shaha

Editorial Committee

David W Eisele, Ralph Gilbert, Patrick J Gullane,
Ehab Hanna, Randal S Weber

JAYPEE BROTHERS MEDICAL PUBLISHERS (P) LTD

Philadelphia • New Delhi • London • Panama

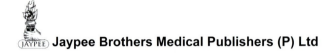

Jaypee Brothers Medical Publishers (P) Ltd

Headquarters

Jaypee Brothers Medical Publishers (P) Ltd
4838/24, Ansari Road, Daryaganj
New Delhi 110 002, India
Phone: +91-11-43574357
Fax: +91-11-43574314
Email: jaypee@jaypeebrothers.com

Overseas Offices

J.P. Medical Ltd
83, Victoria Street, London
SW1H 0HW (UK)
Phone: +44-2031708910
Fax: +02-03-0086180
Email: info@jpmedpub.com

Jaypee-Highlights.
Medical Publishers Inc
City of Knowledge, Bld. 237
Clayton, Panama City, Panama
Phone: +1 507-301-0496
Fax: +1 507-301-0499
Email: cservice@jphmedical.com

Jaypee Medical Inc.
The Bourse
111 South Independence Mall East
Suite 835, Philadelphia,
PA 19106, USA
Phone: +1 267-519-9789
Email: jpmed.us@gmail.com

Jaypee Brothers
Medical Publishers (P) Ltd
17/1-B Babar Road, Block-B
Shaymali, Mohammadpur
Dhaka-1207, Bangladesh
Mobile: +08801912003485
Email: jaypeedhaka@gmail.com

Jaypee Brothers
Medical Publishers (P) Ltd
Shorakhute, Kathmandu
Nepal
Phone: +00977-9841528578
Email: jaypee.nepal@gmail.com

Website: www.jaypeebrothers.com
Website: www.jaypeedigital.com

Inquiries for bulk sales may be solicited at: jaypee@jaypeebrothers.com

A Century of Progress in Head and Neck Cancer

First Edition: **2014**

ISBN 978-93-5152-312-3

Printed at: Replika Press Pvt. Ltd.

Dedication

This compilation of commentaries on seminal articles of the 20th century is dedicated to those men and women whose groundbreaking work in the past century, shifted existing paradigms of the times and brought our specialty, to what it is today. We are grateful for their ingenious work, innovation and contributions to advance the specialty of Head and Neck Surgery and Oncology. Their accomplishments are a stimulus for us all, to move our specialty forward in the 21st century.

Editors, Contributors and Commentators

Preface

Cancer of the Head and Neck has been a major challenge to the medical profession, over past several centuries, since it not only costs life to those afflicted with the disease, but also causes a devastating impact on the form and function of the unfortunate individuals who suffer from this human tragedy. However, in the past century, significant progress is made in improving the cure rates for this disease, and improving the quality of life of the patients suffering from head and neck cancer. Scores of publications in the literature are a testament to the continuing advances and the specialty. These range from advances in surgical techniques, to application and integration of radiotherapy, and continuing evolution of chemotherapy with introduction of newer drugs in the past four decades. Coupled with therapeutic advances are major strides in understanding the pathobiology of head and neck cancer and advances in basic research in genetics and molecular biology. To summarize all the advances would need dozens of volumes of books. Clearly that is not possible, and is not the intent of this publication. The editors, *Contributors* and *Commentators* in this book have strived to highlight major advances in this specialty, which contributed to paradigm shifts in their opinion in the past century.

The process of selecting 100 best contributions to the literature in the past century was a laborious and difficult task. However, in order to maintain balance between various topics, an initial allocation of publications to be selected per each topic was made to cover all aspects of the specialty. Five prominent leaders *(Contributors)* per each topic from around the globe were then approached to submit a list of the best ten published articles in their opinion, on their topic in the past century. From those who responded, a list of over 2100 articles were received. The Editorial Committee then went to work and selected ten best articles from this list per topic, for a total of 200 publications. The Associate Editors and the Editor then selected 100 best articles from this list, to include in this publication.

Contemporary leaders *(Commentators)*, with special expertise in the selected topics, in the Specialty of Head and Neck Surgery and Oncology were then requested to write a "Commentary" on each of the selected articles, describing the importance and impact of the article/contribution to the literature, and how it helped to make progress in the diagnosis, management and outcomes from cancer of the head and neck. This compilation is thus a collaborative effort of dozens of colleagues and experts in recognizing the individuals and their contributions responsible for progress in Head and Neck cancer in the past century.

The abstracts of each of the selected articles in this publication are reproduced verbatim, from the original publication, followed by the Commentary. The Editorial committee hopes that, the contents of this volume will stimulate future generations of physicians, scientists and educators, in continuing their efforts for growth and advances in our specialty, and build upon the accomplishments of the past century.

Jatin P Shah

Acknowledgments

The Editors wish to acknowledge the generous support from

Jaypee Brothers Medical Publishers (P) Ltd.,

who provided complimentary copies of this book to
all the attendees at the 5th World Congress of the

International Federation of Head and Neck Oncologic Societies,

and the Annual Meeting of the

American Head and Neck Society

Celebrating the Centennial of the

**Head and Neck Program at
Memorial Sloan-Kettering Cancer Center**

in New York

July 26–30, 2014

The Editors also wish to acknowledge the arduous work done by the editorial staff of the Head and Neck Service in the Department of Surgery at Memorial Sloan-Kettering Cancer Center. Benjamin Hegel and Raia Mohammed deserve special mention, for their commitment to this project from the outset, in communicating with dozens of *Contributors, Commentators,* and publishers to secure the required materials. They were fully engaged in the compilation phase of this work, in the design of the cover, and finally, in editing and final manuscript assembly. But for their dedication and commitment, this work would not have been possible. The final editing done by George Monemvasitis and Alexandra MacDonald is much appreciated. We are grateful to all of them for bringing this project to fruition.

Contributors

David H Abramson USA

Peter E Andersen USA

Patrick J Bradley UK

Murray F Brennan USA

Joseph Califano USA

Claudio R Cernea Brazil

Pankaj Chaturvedi India

Ezra Cohen USA

Jack Coleman USA

David W Eisele USA

Dan M Fliss Israel

Arlene A Forestiere USA

Jeremy L Freeman Canada

Patrick J Gullane Canada

Ehab Hanna USA

Keith Heller USA

Gopal Iyer Singapore

Jonas T Johnson USA

Robert Baatenburg de Jong Netherlands

Luiz P Kowalski Brazil

Nancy Y Lee USA

Jean-Louis LeFebvre France

William M Lydiatt USA

Ernest L Mazzaferri USA

Jesus E Medina USA

Randall P Morton New Zealand

Jeffrey N Myers USA

Piero Nicolai Italy

Carsten Palme Australia

David G Pfister USA

Vincent van der Poorten Belgium

Gregory W Randolph USA

Alexis Rapidis Greece

Alan Richards USA

Clarence Sasaki USA

Crispian Scully UK

Jatin P Shah USA

Donald P Shedd USA

Man Hei Shiu Hong Kong

Peter M Som USA

David S Soutar UK

Elliot W Strong USA

Samaan Warankulsuriya UK

Randal S Weber USA

Gregory S Weinstein USA

William I Wei Hong Kong

Ernie A Weymuller USA

Commentators

Peter E Andersen USA

K Kian Ang USA

Stephan Ariyan USA

Manjit S Bains USA

Philip L Bailin USA

Jacques Bernier Switzerland

Jay Boyle USA

Carol R Bradford USA

Patrick J Bradley UK

Lenine G Brandão Brazil

Daniel Branovan USA

Murray F Brennan USA

David M Brizel USA

Atul Budukh India

Joseph Califano USA

Thomas E Carey USA

Diane Carlson USA

Pankaj Chaturvedi India

Shie-Lee Cheah Singapore

Amy Y Chen USA

Herbert Chen USA

Claudio R Cernea Brazil

Peter G Cordeiro USA

June Corry Australia

Fernando L Dias Brazil

Joseph J Disa USA

David W Eisele USA

Willard E Fee, Jr USA

Robert L Ferris USA

Dan M Fliss Israel

Arlene A Forastiere USA

Jeremy L Freeman Canada

Matthew G Fury USA

Neal Futran USA

Ian Ganly USA

Javier Gavilán Spain

Ziv Gil Israel

Ralph Gilbert Canada

Lawrence E Ginsberg USA

Michael Gleeson UK

Jennifer Grandis USA

Vincent Gregoire Belgium

Patrick J Gullane Canada

Paul M Harari USA

Louis B Harrison USA

Frans JM Hilgers Netherlands

Jonas T Johnson USA

Merril S Kies USA

Jan Klozar Czech Republic

Paul P Knegt Netherlands

Wayne Koch USA

Luiz P Kowalski Brazil

Dennis H Kraus USA

Nancy Y Lee USA

Anne WM Lee China

C René Leemans Netherlands

Jean-Louis LeFebvre France

John P Leonetti USA

William M Lydiatt USA

Brian P Marr USA

Jesus E Medina USA

Christopher McHenry USA

Marcus M Monroe USA

Eric J Moore USA

Randall P Morton New Zealand

Sara E Murray USA

Eugene N Myers USA

Jeffrey N Myers USA

David Myssiorek USA

Steven A Newman USA

Kerry D Olsen USA

Brian O'Sullivan Canada

Donato Pacione USA

David G Pfister USA

Marshall R Posner USA

Gregory W Randolph USA

Guillermo Raspall Spain

John A "Drew" Ridge USA

James W Rocco USA

Chandranath Sen USA

Jatin P Shah USA

Ashok R Shaha USA

Donald P Shedd USA

Carl E Silver USA

Bhuvanesh Singh USA

Carl H Snyderman USA

Yoke-Lim Soong Singapore

Elliot W Strong USA

Erich M Sturgis USA

Harvey M Tucker USA

Ivan Tham Singapore

R Michael Tuttle USA

Mark L Urken USA

Michiel WM van den Brekel Netherlands

Vincent van der Poorten Belgium

Isaäc van der Waal Netherlands

Allison T Vidimos USA

Bhadrasain Vikram USA

Mark K Wax USA

Randal S Weber USA

Joseph Wee Singapore

Ernest A Weymuller USA

Richard J Wong USA

Martha A Zeiger USA

Contents

19. Quality of Life   307

Chapter 1

Epidemiology

THE ROLE OF ALCOHOL AND TOBACCO IN MULTIPLE PRIMARY CANCERS OF THE UPPER DIGESTIVE SYSTEM, LARYNX AND LUNG: A PROSPECTIVE STUDY

David Schottenfeld, Rebecca C Gantt, Ernest L Wynder

A 5-year prospective study was conducted on 733 patients admitted to Memorial Sloan-Kettering Cancer Center with a single primary epidermoid carcinoma of the oral cavity, pharynx or larynx, diagnosed between 1965 and 1968. The survival in women at 5 years following diagnosed of the index cancer was significantly better than in men. The average annual incidence for second primary carcinomas of the respiratory and upper digestive systems was 18.2 per 1,000 in men and 15.4 per 1,000 in women. The women were distinguished from the men by their less intensive exposure to tobacco and alcohol previous to the index cancer. The risk of developing a second primary cancer enhanced significantly by more intensive, combined exposures to tobacco and alcohol prior to the index cancer. Within the first 5 years after the clinical presentation of the index cancer, the development of any new neoplastic process previously initiated in the exposed tissues was unaffected by altered smoking and drinking habits after the index cancer.

Of the 433 deaths occurring at 5 years in the study population, two-thirds were attributed to metastases or the complications of treatment of a single or multiple primary cancer of the oral cavity, pharynx or larynx, 1.5% to a new primary cancer of the lung or esophagus and 1.4% to a new primary cancer of an organ outside of the respiratory and upper digestive tracts. The significant excesses in cancer mortality in men and women were particularly evident between 45–64 years of age and were distributed throughout all levels of exposure to tobacco and alcohol. The underlying cause in 30.7% was due to diseases other than cancer.

Future follow-up will enable us to determine the risk of new primary cancers and intercurrent nonneoplastic diseases in patients who continue to smoke and/or drink, and whether these risks, as suggested by our retrospective study, are enhanced as a result of previous radiation therapy.

Schottenfeld D, Gantt RC, Wynder EL. The role of alcohol and tobacco in multiple primary cancers of the upper digestive system, larynx and lung: a prospective study. Prev Med.1974;3:277-293.

Commentary by: *Luiz P Kowalski*

Billroth in 1860 was the first to register simultaneous tumors that occurred in a single patient. In 1932, Warren and Gates included their own experience with 1,078 autopsies among which 40 new cases of multiple malignant tumors were diagnosed. They proposed criteria for the diagnosis of multiple primary tumors which are still being used today: (a) confirmation of malignancy in both tumors, (b) each tumor must be distinct, and (c) it is necessary to exclude the possibility that one tumor is a metastasis of the other. More than two decades later, in 1953, Slaughter et al. introduced the "condemned mucosa" hypothesis, aiming to explain the high incidence of multiple primary tumors in patients with carcinomas, and introduced the concept of "field cancerization". They showed that the epithelium around the tumor had microscopic findings that could be associated with the chronic exposure of the same environmental factors (mainly smoke components and alcohol consumption), and thus more susceptible to malignant transformation. The existence of microscopic multicentric foci of preneoplastic changes was further documented.

The first tumor diagnosed has been defined as the primary or index tumor. Most authors also emphasized that the diagnosis of multiple primary tumors should be based on clinical and pathological data and that the possibility of locally recurrent carcinoma must be excluded. Considering the time of diagnosis, multiple tumors can be classified into (1) synchronous (diagnosed simultaneously or within 6 months after the diagnosis of the index tumor); or (2) metachronous (diagnosed after a time interval of 6 months).

Most studies prior to the 1970s were retrospective and have just addressed the issue of how frequently multiple primary cancers occur. Less attention was directed to the measure of excess risk of multiple cancers. In 1970, Berg et al. published a retrospective series of 9,415 patients with upper respiratory and digestive tract cancers treated at MSKCC. During 23,802 patient-years of observation, 518 new cancers were diagnosed; most were situated in other head and neck sites. Wynder et al. reviewed 1,025 patients with single and 104 patients with multiple squamous cell carcinoma of the head and neck mucosa treated at MSKCC from 1965 to 1988. The group of patients with multiple primary cancers tended to smoke more cigarettes than the group with single primary tumors. Drinking pattern was not associated with the risk of multiple cancers in this study.

The landmark study from Shottenfeld et al. reported a series of 733 patients with single primary head and neck epidermoid carcinoma treated at MSKCC from 1965 to 1968. Data on tobacco and alcohol consumption were collected at the time of diagnosis of the index cancer. A total of 53 cases (7.3%) of second primary cancers were diagnosed from 3 years to 6 years of follow-up, and most were located in the upper aerodigestive tract mucosa. The annual incidence in women was 15.4/1,000, and in men it was 18.2/1,000.

There were no significant demographic differences in the risk of second primary cancers according to gender, race, religion, foreign birth, or education. The risk of a second primary cancer was associated to the index tumor site (higher in supraglottic cancer than in glottic in men, and tongue than glottis in women). There was no significant association of multiple primary cancers and the type and quantity of tobacco consumption previous to the diagnosis of the index cancer. The greater consumption of alcoholic beverages was associated with the risk of multiple primary tumors. The age when drinking began and the duration of drinking did not influence such risk. The risk of developing multiple primary cancers was higher in the group of patients with combined exposures to tobacco and alcohol prior to the index cancer. On the other hand, the risk of multiple primaries was not affected by altered smoking and drinking habits after the index cancer diagnosis (64% of the patients with multiple primaries and 65% of those with single primaries stopped smoking or remained nonsmokers after the treatment of the index tumor).

The results of this well-designed prospective study confirmed that multiple primary cancers are concentrated in the mucosa of the upper aerodigestive tract and can occur several years after the treatment of the index tumor. It became evident that surveillance using clinical and image methods for early detection of recurrences and second primary tumors should be strongly recommended. The study also pointed to the role for combined tobacco and alcohol consumption prior to the treatment of the index tumor as determinants of the high risk of developing further squamous carcinomas.

Further evidence of microscopic premalignant epithelial changes in macroscopic mucosa of patients with head and neck squamous carcinomas was also demonstrated in other studies. Califano et al. used cytogenetic analysis and microsatellite instability investigation and identified sequential losses and possible sites of tumor suppressor genes cumulatively during tumor progression from normal epithelium to dysplasia, *in situ* carcinoma, and invasive carcinoma. The genetic alterations identified in *in situ* carcinoma are present in invasive carcinomas, to which are added additional ones. The different genetic alterations of the same chromosomes distributed irregularly in different sites of the mucous epithelium support the thesis of "field cancerization" and the polyclonal origin of the multiple head and neck squamous cell carcinomas.

The risk factors for multiple primary tumors had been extensively investigated. Most showed that the risk continues even many years after the treatment of the index tumor. Age under 66 years, prior to, and continuation of the habit of smoking and alcohol consumption, and early stage index tumors (associated with longer survival) were among the risk factors for multiple primary tumors. Numerous studies reported genetic abnormalities associated with the risk of developing multiple primary tumors, among them, *p53* overexpression and polymorphisms of *p21* and glutathione S-transferase.

The understanding of risk factors and biology of precancerous lesions was followed by numerous chemoprevention trials that unfortunately, due to toxicity, cost or failure in demonstrating reduction on multiple primary tumors incidence, did not substantially impact clinical practice. The current standard of care is close follow-up, aiming for early diagnosis of precancerous or early tumors. The role of routine triple endoscopy (laryngoscopy, broncho-scopy, and esophagoscopy) was felt to be useful in earlier reports than in the most recent publications. The most recent publications favor the use fluore-scence spectroscopy, microendoscopy and PET-CT.

INCIDENCE RATES OF ORAL CANCER AND NATURAL HISTORY OF ORAL PRECANCEROUS LESIONS IN A 10-YEAR FOLLOW-UP STUDY OF INDIAN VILLAGERS

Prakash C Gupta, Fali S Mehta, Dinesh K Daftary, et al.

Motivated by many reports that oral cancer is one of the most frequently encountered cancers in India, a large scale epidemiologic survey of oral cancer and precancer was initiated in 1966 by the Basic Dental Research Unit of the Tata Institute of Fundamental Research, Bombay, headed by Dr Fali S Mehta.

As most of the previous reports were based upon figures obtained from hospital records, pathology departments, cancer hospitals of selected population groups, the need was felt for a house-to-house survey with the main emphasis on oral precancer with a preventive aspect in mind.

Gupta PC, Mehta FS, Daftary DK, et al. Incidence rates of oral cancer and natural history of oral precancerous lesions in a 10-year follow-up study of Indian villagers. Community Dent Oral Epidemiol. 1980;8:283-333.

Commentary by: *Jay Boyle*

The paper by Gupta and Mehta et al. is an important paper because it comprehensively describes the findings of an enormous oral cancer community screening program accomplished with 10 years of follow-up in an endemic population in India. The most important contribution to the field of head and neck oncology is that this study demonstrated the feasibility of oral cancer screening programs, which directly led to a randomized controlled trial of oral cancer screening that showed decreased mortality of oral cancer in populations screened versus those not screened (Sankaranarayanan and Ramadas in the *Lancet* 2005). Also, this paper provides a glimpse into the natural history of oral precancer in India, and it clearly links tobacco abuse, oral precancer and oral cancer in a continuum. The study points out the critical need for health education, tobacco cessation efforts, and anti-tobacco legislation in developing nations.

Oral cancer rates in India are among the highest in the world, with up to 45 cases per 100,000, and oral cancer is the leading cause of cancer death in males in India. With well over a billion inhabitants, the burden of oral cancer in India is tremendous. The hypothesis that trained health care workers could effectively screen large populations at risk was an important question at the time of the study. From 1966–1969, 50,000 rural subjects were screened for oral cancer and precancer by trained health workers going door to door in villages of several different provinces of India. The subjects were then followed for an average of more than 7 years, and the natural history of the observed precancerous lesions and the associated tobacco habits were assessed. This study overcame obvious logistics and data collection challenges and provides a cross sectional and then a longitudinal look at oral precancer and tobacco habits in India. The limitations of this study include the data reliability, since so many observers were used. Also, the broad applicability of these findings to worldwide populations is unclear due to the relative ethnic homogeneity of the population and the prevalence of tobacco habits that are rare in the Western world.

The heterogeneity of tobacco habits practiced is intriguing. The important findings include that all tobacco habits lead to clinical precancerous oral leukoplakia, and the highest risk patients for oral cancer are those who chew tobacco. Tobacco abuse habits in this population include oral tobacco chewing with areca nut, smoking of small, locally made cigarettes called bidi, reverse smoking with the lighted end in the mouth, cigarette smoking, and clay pipe smoking. All are still practiced today.

Oral precancerous lesions were seen most frequently in tobacco chewers. They tended to be reversible with cessation but had the highest rate of transformation to cancer. The overall rate of transformation of oral leukoplakia to oral cancer was about 7%, or 1% per year of follow-up. Importantly, over the entire follow-up period, no oral cancers were identified in subjects without clinical precancerous lesions. Dysplastic lesions were at higher risk than hyperkeratotic lesions.

Interestingly, the clinical lesions observed were subcategorized as preleukoplakia, leukoplakia, nodular leukoplakia, ulcerated leukoplakia, leukoedema, lichen planus leukokeratosis nicotina palate, and atrophy. It remains challenging to adequately categorize, characterize, and differentiate these many variants.

The study demonstrates the tremendous commitment by the investigators to use the resources at hand to address an important public health problem and to gather critical data regarding the natural history of precancerous lesions and the scope and nature of tobacco abuse habits in the community. These data were used as a foundation for the subsequent randomized intervention trial of Sankaranarayanan and Ramadas, published in the *Lancet* in 2005, which proved that oral cancer screening in the community down-staged the oral cancers identified and improved survival from oral cancer. This progress could not have been made without the dedicated efforts of Gupta, Mehta, and the hundreds of health care workers screening villagers in the 1960s. Finally, this paper is a cornerstone for health education and tobacco cessation and legislation programs in India.

THE CAUSES OF CANCER: QUANTITATIVE ESTIMATES OF AVOIDABLE RISKS OF CANCER IN THE UNITED STATES TODAY

Richard Doll, Richard Peto

Evidence that the various common types of cancer are largely avoidable disease is reviewed. Life-style and other environmental factors are divided into a dozen categories, and for each category the evidence relating those particular factors to cancer onset rates is summarized where possible, an estimates are based chiefly on evidence from epidemiology, as the available evidence from animal and other laboratory studies cannot provide reliable human risk assessments. By far the largest reliably known percentage is the 30% if current–US cancer deaths that are due to tobacco, although it is possible that some nutritional factor(s) may eventually be found to be of comparable importance. The percentage of US cancer deaths that are due to tobacco is still increasing, and must be expected to continue to increase for some years yet due to the delayed effects of the adoption of cigarettes in earlier decades.

Treads in mortality and in onset rates for many separate types of cancer are studied in detail in appendixes to this paper. Biases in the available data on registration of new cases produce apparent trends in cancer incidence which are spurious. Biases also produce spurious trends in cancer death certification rates, especially among old people. In (and before) middle age, where the biases are smaller, there appear to be a few real increases and few real decreases in mortality from some particular types of cancer, but there is no evidence of any generalized increase other than that due to tobacco. Moderate increases or decreases due to some new agent(s)–might of course be overlooked in such large-scale analyses. But, such analyses do suggest that, are currently common are not peculiarly modern diseases and are likely to depend chiefly on some long-established factor(s). (A prospective study utilizing both questionnaires and stored blood and other biological materials might help elucidate these factors).

The proportion of current US cancer deaths attributed to occupational factors is provisionally estimated as 4% (lung cancer being the major contributor to this). This is far smaller than has recently been suggested by various US Government agencies. The matter could be resolved directly by a "case-control" study of lung cancer two or three times larger than the recently completed US National Bladder Cancer Study but similar to it in methodology and unit costs; there are also other reasons for such a study.

Doll R, Peto R. The causes of cancer: quantitative estimates of avoidable risks of cancer in the United States today. J Natl Cancer Inst. 1981;66:1191-1308.

Commentary by: *Amy Y Chen*

This paper was among the first to examine the epidemiology of cancer. Avoidable risk factors for cancer are discussed in this paper. The purpose of this dated paper is to review the established evidence and current research relating to each of several groups of ways of avoiding cancer and to estimate the percentage reduction in today's age-standardized US cancer death rates.

The first evidence for avoidable risk factors for cancer was proposed by the World Health Organization in 1964. "The categories of cancer that are thus influenced, directly or indirectly, by extrinsic factors include many tumors of the skin and mouth, the respiratory, gastrointestinal and urinary tracts, . . . which collectively, account for more than three quarters of human cancers. . . . Therefore, . . . the majority of human cancer is potentially preventable". Therefore, the purpose of this report is to review the evidence and research pertaining to various ways of avoiding cancer (cancer prevention) and to estimate the percent reduction of death rates that might occur with cancer prevention.

- *The paper presents the evidence for the avoidability of cancer:*
    - Differences in cancer incidence among different settled communities.
    - Differences between migrants from a community and those who remain.
    - Variations with time in cancer incidence rates within particular communities.
    - Actual identification of many specific causes or preventive factors. One has to exercise caution before stating causation. However, usually data reflect a "modifiable" risk factor, e.g., colon cancer and meat consumption.
- The authors state that in 1970 about 75–80% of the cases of cancer in both sexes might have been avoidable. Tobacco is the largest risk factor. The authors estimate that the percentage would increase each year because of the steady increase of tobacco-induced lung cancer. It is the hope of the authors that this percentage may decrease with avoidance of risk factors (such as tobacco).
- *Attribution of risk:* The authors admit that gauging cancer trends is difficult, because an increase in incidence rates may be a result of improved detection. How does one know that the increase is due to "real" cancers and not just better detection? Some ways to detect whether there is an actual increase is to study the effects of risk factors on cultured cells, on cells of living animals, and on the behavior of cultured cells. The authors state that short-term tests may miss the relation of risk and causation because of a long latency period. These tests also overlook the very important determinants of human behavior on cancer.
- *Use of epidemiological observations:* Because of the problems of extrapolating cancer development in the lab to humans, the authors discuss the importance of using epidemiologic observations rather than laboratory data. The advantages of using epidemiological data are the ability to account for human behavior, the ability to study large populations of people, and the ability to measure an effect on humans (rather than cells). The disadvantages include the inability to measure an effect if there is a long latency period, lack of generalizability, and bias.

- *Avoidable causes*:
  - The single most important avoidable cause is tobacco. In 1978, between 75,000 and 90,000 of the deaths certified as lung cancer were caused by tobacco. About 12,000 deaths due to lung cancer were NOT caused by tobacco. There were an additional 40,000 deaths due to other tobacco-related cancers (instead of 155,000). In the authors' view, the difference of 110,000 represents a fairly reliable estimate of the number of US deaths from these four types of cancer caused by smoking in 1978.
  - Alcohol is also an important cause, and it "interacts" with tobacco as an important avoidable risk factor. Cancers related to alcohol consumption account for 7% of male and 3% of female cancer deaths.
  - Diet has been a very frustrating risk factor to study. The data are sparse.
  - Reproductive and sexual behaviors are also described as risk factors for cancer, e.g., cancer of the cervix.
  - Occupation was first described as a risk factor from Pott in 1775 when he linked chimney sweepers to cancer of the scrotum. This has been further studied and discussed in the OSHA paper of 1978.
  - Pollution in our air, water, and food can contribute to cancer deaths. Air pollution is probably the best-described avoidable environmental factor.
  - Other factors mentioned are industrial products such as asbestos, geophysical factors such as ionizing radiation, and infection.

In conclusion, this paper was one of the early papers to describe the rationale behind the discipline of cancer prevention and control. The authors report an exhaustive account of the statistics behind their risk adjusted mortality rates and also the epidemiological science behind the attribution of risk to carcinogens. It is especially interesting to note how in our age of HPV-related oropharynx cancer, that sexual behavior and viruses are once again at the forefront of cancer research. This risk factor of HPV could only have been discovered by broad population-based research, the type that these authors proposed more than 30 years ago.

ALCOHOL DRINKING IN NEVER USERS OF TOBACCO, CIGARETTE SMOKING IN NEVER DRINKERS, AND THE RISK OF HEAD AND NECK CANCER: POOLED ANALYSIS IN THE INTERNATIONAL HEAD AND NECK CANCER EPIDEMIOLOGY CONSORTIUM

Mia Hashibe, Paul Brennan, Simone Benhamou, et al.

Background: At least 75% of head and neck cancers are attributable to a combination of cigarette smoking and alcohol drinking. A precise understanding of the independent association of these factors in the absence of the other with the risk of head and neck cancer is needed to elucidate mechanisms of head and neck carcinogenesis and to assess the efficacy of interventions aimed at controlling either risk factor.

Methods: We examined the extent to which head and neck cancer is associated with cigarette smoking among never drinkers and with alcohol drinking among never users of tobacco. We pooled individual-level data from 15 case-control studies that included 10,244 head and neck cancer case subjects and 15,227 control subjects, of whom 1,072 case subjects and 5,775 control subjects were never users of tobacco and 1,598 case subjects and 4,051 control subjects were never drinkers of alcohol. Odds ratios (ORs) and 95% confidence intervals (CIs) were estimated using unconditional logistic regression models. All statistical tests were two-sided.

Results: Among never drinkers, cigarette smoking was associated with an increased risk of head and neck cancer (OR for ever versus never smoking = 2.13, 95% CI = 1.52 to 2.98), and there were clear dose-response relationships for the frequency, duration, and number of pack-years of cigarette smoking. Approximately 24% (95% CI = 16% to 31%) of head and neck cancer cases among nondrinkers in this study would have been prevented if these individuals had not smoked cigarettes. Among never users of tobacco, alcohol consumption was associated with an increased risk of head and neck cancer only when alcohol was consumed at high frequency (OR for three or more drinks per day versus never drinking = 2.04, 95% CI = 1.29 to 3.21). The association with high frequency alcohol intake was limited to cancers of the oropharynx/hypopharynx and larynx.

Conclusions: Our results represent the most precise estimates available of the independent association of each of the two main risk factors of head and neck cancer and they exemplify the strengths of large-scale consortia in cancer epidemiology.

Hashibe M, Brennan P, Benhamou S, et al. Alcohol drinking in never users of tobacco, cigarette smoking in never drinkers, and the risk of head and neck cancer: pooled analysis in the International Head and Neck Cancer Epidemiology Consortium. J Natl Cancer Inst. 2007;99:777-789.

Commentary by: *Pankaj Chaturvedi, Atul Budukh*

As per GLOBOCAN 2008, there are 634,760 new cases of lip, oral cavity, nasopharynx, other pharynx, and larynx cancers annually, and more than 356,705 deaths worldwide. Tobacco and alcohol use are the most important risk factors for oral cavity, oropharynx, hypopharynx and larynx cancers. Greater than 70% of these cases are attributable to a combination of cigarette smoking and alcohol drinking. An independent association of cigarette smoking alone and alcohol drinking alone was difficult to study, as these two habits are strongly associated with each other. Previous studies to determine an independent association among cigarette smoking, alcohol drinking, and the risk of head and neck cancer were imprecise and based on small sample sizes.

A precise understanding of the independent association of each of these factors in the absence of the other with the risk of head and neck cancer was needed. It was a difficult task to recruit the cases and controls of never drinkers who smoked and vice versa. The study was made possible by the International Head and Neck Cancer Epidemiology (INHANCE) consortium in collaboration with several research groups working on molecular epidemiology studies of head and neck cancer.

The study was conducted by pooled individual level data from 15 case control studies. There were 1,072 case subjects and 5,775 control subjects who were never users of tobacco and 1,598 case subjects and 4,051 control subjects who were never drinkers of alcohol. Strengths of the study included that the cases and controls were from different locations in Europe, North America, South/Central America, and the international, multicenter group, and the sample was of good size (2,670 cases and 9,826 controls). The case percentages of never drinkers from the total sample were 11.5%, 33.2%, 15.4%, and 39.9%, and the control percentages were 27.7%, 36.3%, 15%, and 21%, respectively, from Europe, North America, South/Central America, and from the international multicenter study. The case percentages of never users of tobacco were 18.8%, 47.4%, 14.5%, and 19.4%, and the control percentages were 44.4%, 29.8%, 12.4%, and 19.4%, respectively. The cases and controls were included from the period of 1984 to 2006.

This study has made great contributions to the epidemiology of head and neck cancers in reporting the risk of cigarette smoking alone among never drinkers [OR, 2.13 (95% CI, 1.52 to 2.98)]. There were clear dose response relationships for the frequency and number of pack years of cigarette smoking. After excluding the cases from India (a large proportion of never drinker cases and controls were from India), the association was 2.21 [95% CI, 1.54 to 3.18). One strength of the study was that it reported the association of cigarette smoking among never drinkers by sub site of head and neck cancer. The risk of laryngeal cancer was strongly associated with cigarette smoking among never drinkers [OR, 6.84 (95% CI, 4.25 to 11.01)]; however, the risk of oral cavity cancer [OR: 1.35 (95% CI, 0.90 to 2.01)] was not as strong. This study confirmed cigarette smoking as a risk factor among never drinkers, and the highest risk was for laryngeal cancer.

This study reported that there was no association between never users of tobacco and never users of alcohol and the risk of head and neck cancer [OR, 1.18 (95% CI, 0.93 to 1.50)]. However, never users of tobacco who consumed three or more alcoholic drinks per day had approximately double the risk of developing a head and neck cancer over never drinkers [OR, 2.04 (95% CI, 1.29 to 3.31)]. The association was also reported for subsites of head and neck cancer. Increased risk was observed for pharyngeal cancer in subjects who drank one or two drinks per day [OR, 1.66 (95% CI, 1.18 to 2.34)], whereas for laryngeal cancer, an increased risk was observed for drinking five or more drinks per day [OR, 2.98 (95% CI, 1.72 to 5.17)]. This study confirmed that among never users of tobacco, a high frequency of alcohol consumption was associated with an increased risk of cancer of the oropharynx/hypopharynx and larynx only.

As per Scopus, this study has been cited in 157 research and review articles. This study has made a great contribution to the prevention of head and neck cancers. This study showed that if never drinkers had not smoked cigarettes, approximately one quarter of the head and neck cancers from this group would have been prevented. The results reported by this study will be of a great support to health policy makers, anti-tobacco activists, epidemiologist, and to cancer control centers for the prevention of head and neck cancers.

Chapter 2

Pathology, Molecular Biology and Genetics

THICKNESS, CROSS-SECTIONAL AREAS AND DEPTH OF INVASION IN THE PROGNOSIS OF CUTANEOUS MELANOMA

Alexander Breslow

Cutaneous melanoma is a most unpredictable lesion. The marked variation in prognosis is probably a function of many variables, one of which is the size of the tumor. Though there is a roughly inverse relationship between the diameter of the lesion and survival, very small lesions have recurred or metastasized. One possible reason for the lack of reliability of tumor size in estimating prognosis may be that studies to date have considered size in only two dimensions and have neglected tumor volume. Two melanomas can have the same diameter but differ greatly in thickness because of variation in either depth of invasion or degree of protrusion from the surface of the skin or both. A recent study has shown that prognosis correlates well with staging of the depth of invasion, but there have been no studies relating survival to tumor volume.

To measure tumor volume it is necessary to know the surface area of the tumor, but in this retrospective study we only know the maximal diameters of the lesions. By measuring the maximal thickness of the lesions we can calculate the maximal cross-sectional area, which should be roughly proportional to the volume of the tumor. The depth of invasion was also studied using the criteria for staging of Clark et al.

Breslow A. Thickness, cross-sectional areas and depth of invasion in the prognosis of cutaneous melanoma. Ann Surg. 1970;172:902-908.

Commentary by: *John A* "Drew" *Ridge*

Breslow's landmark monograph on the prognosis of primary cutaneous melanoma represents an important and instructive work. Published in the *Annals of Surgery,* its findings form the basis of the current TNM staging system for the primary tumor, helped to guide surgical management of the disease in the era of prophylactic lymphadenectomy, and led to important insights into the behavior of squamous cancers of the oral cavity, which continue to influence our treatment today. The paper, showing little resemblance to contemporary academic publications, stands as a model of simplicity, exposition, and honesty in medical prose. All cancer surgeons should read it.

Melanoma is an aggressive malignancy. Though screening may be accomplished through physical examination alone, many patients present with life-threatening lesions. By comparison to most other solid tumors, a remarkably small primary tumor burden is associated with the development of nodal metastases and distant spread. In the mid-20th century the disease seemed unpredictable, but "tumor size" seemed important. Lesions of larger diameter seemed to have a worse prognosis than smaller cancers—though many patients with seemingly small lesions developed regional and distant recurrences.

After Wallace Clark proposed a staging system based upon histologic depth of invasion, Breslow sought to predict recurrence risk in terms of tumor volume. A retrospective review of slides permitted the measurement of the greatest tumor diameter, but not the cross-sectional area, of the pigmented lesion. Hence, he was forced to combine the (readily measured) depth of the tumor with its diameter to define its "maximal cross-sectional area," which he considered proportional to the volume of the primary site. Ninety-eight patients were studied. None had presented with satellite nodules or metastases. The 5-year follow-up was 92%. Patients who died of other causes within 5 years, who died of unknown cause, or who were lost to follow-up were excluded. Breslow considered lesion diameter, maximal thickness (< 0.76 mm., 0.76–1.50 mm., etc. up to > 3.00 mm.), and cross sectional area [sic] (in mm.²). Findings were analyzed with attention to Clark's levels. While "...The incidence of recurrent or metastatic disease appears to be a function of all three variables and was 100% for lesions over 30 mm. wide or over 5 mm. thick and almost 100% for lesions over 40 mm.² in maximal cross-sectional area". It proved possible to identify patients with good prognosis despite their Clark level. The difference was significant at 0.05. The manuscript is distinguished by intellectually honesty; Breslow's initial hypothesis proved wanting but was discussed as the rationale for the analysis.

Subsequently, large databases were interrogated. The Breslow thickness proved the single most important predicative indicator. While subsequent research that survival was a "smooth" function of tumor depth, permitting use of integer depth (rather than fractions of mm.), the importance of tumor depth to staging and prognosis for melanoma has endured for more than 40 years, and "microstaging" with an ocular micrometer remains the basis of the clinical and pathologic staging system for cutaneous melanoma. Findings correlate nicely with Breslow's groupings, which prove more robust than other features such as ulceration and anatomic subsites (ear, face, neck and scalp) for head and neck melanoma.

When comprehensive cervical lymphadenectomy was employed for staging of the N0 neck in oral cancer, all patients experienced undue morbidity. As attention turned to selective approaches to the neck for patients with oral cavity malignancies, the primary tumor stage (reflecting only greatest lesion diameter) proved to be a poor predictor of nodal metastases and prognosis. During the 1980s, influenced by Breslow and the head and neck melanoma experience, attention focused on tumor thickness as a prognostic indicator. In 1986, two groups reported that the thickness of the primary tumor was a more potent prognostic factor and predictor of nodal metastases than tumor diameter for lesions of the floor of the tongue and of the floor of the mouth. Findings were confirmed for other oral cavity subsites and for the lip as well. Tumor thickness has proven far more important than lesion diameter with respect to the development of nodal metastases for lesions of the oral cavity, and its estimation has proven important in recommendations for observation of the neck, selective neck dissection, and sentinel lymphadenectomy.

However, squamous cancers of the oral cavity are not melanomas. Excisional biopsy for "microstaging" of oral cancers is impractical and justifiably discouraged. Imaging studies, while promising, are not sufficiently robust to assess depth of early lesions. In addition, it has proven difficult to reproduce proposed prognostic "break points" from different subsites, centers, and clinical series. As a result, though tumor thickness plays an important part in preoperative planning for most head and neck surgeons, it has yet to be incorporated into the AJCC staging system for lip and oral cavity cancers. Lesion diameter, easily measured, holds sway despite its poor correlation with risk of nodal metastases and prognosis.

Alexander Breslow's observation on melanoma, that tumor thickness is a more important predictor of metastases and recurrence than histologic depth of invasion or lesion diameter, dominates staging and management of that disease. Its influence extends beyond cutaneous malignancy to inform modern treatment planning for cancers of the oral cavity. In addition, the work stands as an exemplar of intellectual honesty. Breslow's report reveals the intellectual roots of his conclusions. "Thickness, cross-sectional areas and depth of invasion in the prognosis of invasive melanoma" is an important publication and well worth study.

OCCURRENCE OF *p53* GENE DELETIONS AND HUMAN PAPILLOMA VIRUS INFECTION IN HUMAN HEAD AND NECK CANCER

David G Brachman, Deborah Graves, Everett Vokes, et al.

Little is known regarding the molecular genetic events in head and neck carcinoma. Epidemiological evidence suggests that both alcohol and tobacco use are related to the development of these neoplasms, and viral infections have also been postulated to play a role in some tumors. Loss of p53 tumor suppressor gene function has been found in many malignancies and can occur through either gene mutation or by interaction with the E6 protein of oncogenic human papilloma viruses (HPV). Because the mucosal surfaces of the head and neck are exposed to mutagens and HPVs, we studied DNA derived from 30 stage I–IV squamous cell carcinomas of the head and neck (9 primary tumors and 21 early passage cell lines) for p53 gene mutations as well as for the presence of oncogenic HPV DNA. Exons 2 through 11 of the p53 gene were examined using single, strand conformation polymorphism analysis followed by direct genomic sequencing of all variants. HPV detection was done using polymerase chain reaction amplification with HPV E6 region type specific primers as well as L1 region degenerate ("consensus") primers; HPV type was determined by restriction fragment length polymorphism analysis of the amplified fragment as well as by Southern blotting of genomic DNA. Sixteen of 30 tumors (53%) had p53 mutations and oncogenic HPV DNA was detected in 3 of 30 (10%) tumors, none of which had p53 mutations. The p53 mutational spectrum observed was characterized by equal frequencies of transversions (6 of 16), transitions (5 of 16), and deletions (5 of 16). This distribution of mutations differs from the spectrum of p53 mutation reported in esophageal (P = 0.05) and lung (P = 0.02) cancers, two other tobacco associated neoplasms. A previously undescribed clustering of 3 mutations at codon 205 was also observed. A trend toward a shorter time to tumor recurrence after treatment was noted for those patients with tumors exhibiting p53 gene mutations, and no relationship between p53 mutations and tumor stage or node status was noted. Alteration in p53 gene function appears common in head and neck cancer, and the mutational spectrum observed may reflect the role of different mutagens or mutagenic processes than those responsible for the p53 mutations in lung and esophageal neoplasms.

Brachman DG, Graves D, Vokes E, et al. Occurrence of p53 gene deletions and human papilloma virus infection in human head and neck cancer. Cancer Res. 1992;52:4832-4836.

Commentary by: *Wayne Koch*

Over two decades ago, in September 1992, this article appeared in *Cancer Research*, in the noteworthy *Advances in Brief* section, as the first report demonstrating mutations in *p53* in fresh specimens of head and neck cancer (HNC). While this manuscript was very much a product of its time, coming in the wake of a deluge of reports on the importance of *p53* mutation in human cancers, it is remarkable to read it in light of subsequent research and make note of just how much the authors got right.

Even now, more than 20 years after the explosion of molecular biology research in human cancer, there are no more important factors that have been found to play a role in HNC than mutation of *p53* and the presence of oncogenic human papillomavirus type 16 (HPV-16). Despite high-throughput platforms to screen for genetic and epigenetic alterations in large cohorts of HNC, innovations in tumor DNA sequencing that allow for investigation of the entire coding region of the tumor genome, and sophisticated analysis of interaction of numerous molecular targets in complex functional pathways, *p53* mutational status, and HPV-16 status together with EGFR overexpression remain as pre-eminent molecular entities in HNC and the only ones rigorously identified to have prognostic significance.

The early 90s were a heady time for cancer biology investigation. Scharf and colleagues had shown that the polymerase chain reaction could clone DNA sequences just a few years earlier, opening the door to investigation of the sequence of specific genes and identification of tumor-related mutations. Attention had been drawn to *p53* protein in the early 80s because of its association with simian virus T antigen and ability to transform normal mouse fibroblasts. Three years before the Brachman paper, Vogelstein and colleagues had shown that *p53* was altered in a variety of tumor cells, particularly colon cancer. Subsequently, *p53* was found to be mutated in carcinomas from lung, bladder, breast, cervix, brain, bladder, as well as sarcomas and melanoma. All these reports appeared just prior to this Brachman article.

Exploration of *p53* alteration in HNC had also begun before the Brachman article appeared. Earlier in the year, Reiss and colleagues at Yale had reported mutations to be present in human squamous cell carcinoma cell lines and Coltrera's report of increased immunohistochemical staining of *p53* in HNC samples appeared shortly after Brachman's landmark article. Still, it was the Brachman group that first reported *p53* mutations in a cohort of 9 primary HNC tumors and 21 early passage cell lines.

The Brachman article is not remarkable only for being the first to report *p53* mutations in HNC, but also for drawing attention to the inverse association between *p53* mutation and HPV-16. The HPV-16 story was a decade older than that of *p53*, having been explored by the Scandanavian investigators Syrjanen and Pyrhonen; they showed that HPV antigens were present in laryngeal and oral cavity lesions in the early 80s. In 1986, Milde and Loning demonstrated the HPV DNA by *in situ* hybridization in 4 oral carcinomas. It took 7 years for Werness and associates to demonstrate the association of HPV-16 and-18 E6 protein binding to *p53* protein in human anogenital cancers and show the correlation of that event with transforming activity of these viruses. With this background, the stage was set for Brachman's work.

The cohort sample size that constituted the Brachman study was modest (n = 30) but included, importantly, some primary tumor samples. In order to amplify DNA from cases with scant samples available, short-term tissue culture methods were used. Later improvements in tissue microdissection and PCR made this step unnecessary in subsequent studies. It is worth noting that all subjects that were included were smokers and drinkers, a fact that may account for the paucity of HPV-related tumors. Mutations in *p53* were first evaluated using the single strand conformation polymorphism (SSCP) technique, which may have missed a few altered cases, followed by direct genomic DNA sequencing of the common coding portion of the gene for all variants. HPV-16 detection was similarly rigorous and up to date using *PCR* for *E6* and *L1* genes and confirming positive results using Southern blot analysis.

Several key results were reported, which have remarkably stood the test of time and have now been confirmed by much larger cohort studies. First, the Brachman group found *p53* mutations in 53% of the tumors. This proportion is roughly the same as that reported by Poeta, et al. in a multi-institutional, cooperative group study involving a cohort 15 times larger. When the entire *p53* gene is sequenced, the capture of mutations increases modestly, approaching 60%. Second, the Brachman article correctly points out that HPV-16 presence is inversely correlated with *p53* mutation. This observation had been made in uterine cervix cancer prior to the Brachman report, and the Brachman observation is based on only 3 cases with HPV DNA present. Therefore, while provocative, the observation that *p53* mutation is not present, interpreted as unnecessary, when oncogenic HPV is present is far from confirmed here. It would require another decade and careful analysis of larger cohorts that included more oropharyngeal cases and nonsmokers to arrive at the current understanding of two distinct pathways to HNC: one involving exposure to carcinogens in cigarette smoke and demonstrating *p53* mutation and the other involving longstanding transformation of tumor cells by oncogenic HPV. Furthermore, the Brachman cohort suggested the preponderance of HPV-16 tumors arising in the oropharynx. Here the numbers are small, and this association was noted in the manuscript, but somewhat obscured by a single HPV-18 positive hard palate lesion, which may have been due to technical problems, and 3 oropharynx cancers lacking HPV. The latter may be attributable in part to the fact that all subjects included had been smokers. Still, the statement that "the possibility that patients with oncogenic HPV-mediated *p53* abrogation of function represent a distinct clinical subset of head and neck cancer is under investigation in our laboratory" is nearly prescient, testifying to the remarkable insight of this group of investigators.

Finally, despite the small cohort size and brief follow-up period, Brachman and coauthors correctly noted a trend toward shorter disease-free interval for patients whose tumors had *p53* mutation. A larger number of cases with mutation recurred (73% vs 46% for wild-type [WT]*p53*), although this did not reach statistical significance. Recurrences occurred at a median interval of 6 months after treatment among those cases with mutation compared with 17.4 months among those with WT *p53*. Subsequent reports about the prognostic significance of *p53* alteration have been mixed, making conclusions hard to draw amidst small sample size, under-powering rigorous multivariate analysis, and mixed methodology, often involving immunohistochemical staining for *p53* protein, which may mistakenly score *p53* status. It was not until the Poeta report of a large cohort from the cooperative groups that the concept of disruptive mutation of *p53*, affecting the critical DNA binding function of the protein, was carefully analyzed and the prognostic implication of TP53 alteration was more convincingly established.

In the intervening decades, many other molecular markers have been investigated in HNC, perhaps most notably the epithelial growth factor receptor (EGFR) and *p16*. While these alterations are common, they have disappointed hopes that they may serve as either prognostic markers or effective treatment targets, perhaps because of their high prevalence in HNC and because of the complexity of molecular pathways at work in these tumors, providing many means for cells to avoid intervention. Other individual HNC tumor-specific genetic alterations are few. Even the tour-de-force sequencing of the HNC cancer genome by two groups in recent years failed to demonstrate major new tumor alterations, the most notable being NOTCH-1 mutation, present in about 15% (a third to a quarter as common as *p53* mutation) of tested samples.

In conclusion, the landmark paper by Brachman and colleagues at the University of Chicago demonstrates what can be accomplished by a group of investigators who stay current with events in other specialty areas within clinical translational oncology, who have both the clinical and laboratory resources to quickly follow leads in the literature, and who have the clinical and molecular expertise to evaluate and interpret their results in light of the best information available. Small cohorts (30 cases seems to be a minimum required to begin to reach the approximate accurate result for prominent population-wide features such as *p53* alteration) can produce provocative and surprisingly accurate observations in this setting, observations that then require years of tedious tumor and clinical outcome data collection and rigorous laboratory analysis to confirm. TP53 and HPV-16 were "low-hanging fruit" and nothing like them has followed. It remains to be seen what breakthrough similar to PCR will be required to usher translational cancer research into the next era.

MOLECULAR ASSESSMENT OF HISTOPATHOLOGICAL STAGING IN SQUAMOUS-CELL CARCINOMA OF THE HEAD AND NECK

Joseph A Brennan, Li Mao, Ralph H Hruban, et al.

Background: Surgical oncologists rely heavily on the histopathological assessment of surgical margins to ensure total excision of the tumor in patients with head and neck cancer. However, current techniques may not detect small numbers of cancer cells at the margins of resection or in cervical lymph nodes.

Methods: We used molecular techniques to determine whether clonal populations of infiltrating tumor cells harboring mutations of the p53 gene could be detected in histopathologically negative surgical margins and cervical lymph nodes of patients with squamous-cell carcinoma of the head and neck.

Results: We identified 25 patients with primary squamous cell carcinoma of the head and neck containing a p53 mutation who appeared to have had complete tumor resection on the basis of a negative histopathological assessment. In 13 of these 25 patients, molecular analysis was positive for a p53 mutation in at least one tumor margin. In 5 of 13 patients with positive margins by this method (38 percent), the carcinoma has recurred locally, as compared with none of 12 patients with negative margins (P = 0.02 by the log-rank test). Furthermore, molecular analysis identified neoplastic cells in 6 of 28 lymph nodes (21 percent) that were initially negative by histopathological assessment.

Conclusions: Among specimens initially believed to be negative on light microscopy, a substantial percentage of the surgical margins and lymph nodes from patients with squamous-cell carcinoma of the head and neck contained p53 mutations specific for the primary tumor. Patients with these positive margins appear to have a substantially increased risk of local recurrence. Molecular analysis of surgical margins and lymph nodes can augment standard histopathological assessment and may improve the prediction of local tumor recurrence.

Brennan JA, Mao L, Hruban RH, et al. Molecular assessment of histopathological staging in squamous cell carcinoma of the head and neck. N Engl J Med. 1995;332:429-435.

Commentary by: *James W Rocco*

Head and neck oncologists know well that the single most important prognostic factor after surgical therapy of head and neck squamous cell carcinoma is complete removal of the primary tumor with a cuff of normal tissue referred to as "the margin". Margin status can be assessed intra-operatively through frozen tissue sections at the tumor-tissue interface after close consultation between the resecting surgeon and pathologist. However, final margin status is only determined on histopathologic analysis of the permanent paraffin-fixed tissue that more closely preserves tissue and cellular architecture. Despite experienced surgeons' and pathologists' best efforts, tumor recurrence can still be high after a negative margin surgical excision.

In this innovative report, Brennan and the group at Johns Hopkins applied for the first time the use of "molecular" staging to assess the adequacy of histopathologic surgical margins. To accomplish this goal, they assessed the mutational status of the *p53* tumor suppressor gene in both the primary tumor and surgical margins. Known as the guardian of the genome, the *p53* gene had already been shown to be mutated in approximately 50% of head and neck squamous cell carcinomas, making it a reasonable candidate marker for this analysis. Critical to their molecular staging efforts was the novel application of existing molecular techniques to create the capability to detect one mutant cancer cell among a large number of normal cells.

The authors developed a polymerase chain reaction (PCR)-based strategy that could detect one mutant cancer cell among 10,000 normal cells using genetic alterations in *p53* as their maker of dysplasia. As a first step, the authors determined the *p53* mutational status of the primary tumor. Next, in tumors with mutant *p53*, DNA was extracted from stored surgical margins and lymph nodes and exons 5-9 of the *p53* gene were amplified by the PCR. The authors analyzed 25 patients with a *p53* mutation in their primary tumor and negative margins by histopathologic assessment (light microscopy to look for premalignant cells). In 13 of these 25 patients, at least one margin was positive based on the molecular assessment (52%), and 5 of these 13 patients went on to have local recurrence (38%). None of the patients with negative molecular margins recurred. Based on these results, the authors maintained that patients with positive molecular margins have a significantly increased risk of local recurrence despite negative margins by histopathologic assessment. In addition, by applying the same molecular technique to lymph nodes from N0 neck dissections, the authors identified tumor cells in 6 of 28 lymph nodes that were also negative by histopathologic criteria. This resulted in the upstaging of 21% of patients formerly considered to have N0 necks by histopathologic analysis. These results established for the first time that molecular staging can identify previously undetectable tumor cells in surgical margins and lymph nodes initially thought to be clear of disease by traditional histopathologic analysis.

The introduction of molecular techniques with exquisite sensitivity to predict surgical margin status was an important innovation for several reasons. First, the authors addressed a critical issue in that local recurrence rates range from 10% to 30% among patients with clear histopathologic margins. They correctly hypothesized that unidentified microscopic disease is present in the area surrounding the resected primary tumor in the form of occult neoplastic tumor cells. They directly tested whether the molecular detection of these occult tumor cells would better assess surgical margin status, predict outcome, and guide subsequent therapy more accurately. Second, by applying the same molecular staging technology to nodal specimens from stored neck dissection specimens, they accurately predicted nodal status at a level of sensitivity likely to assess the true risk of recurrence and the subsequent need for adjuvant therapy.

The impact of this seminal report cannot be overstated. Molecular staging-the ability to detect microscopic disease based on the analysis of *p53* mutational status in tumor DNA-promoted many subsequent advances in the field of head and neck oncology.

First and foremost, the paper verified that treatment failures result from residual microscopic disease, previously undetectable by conventional histopathologic analysis. At the time this paper came out, this was a stimulating new advance, and like all influential manuscripts, generated significant excitement in the head and neck oncology community. It was the subject of four separate letters to the *New England Journal of Medicine*, all which praised the authors for this landmark work. As one letter commented regarding the significance of the manuscript, the recurrence rate in this study among patients with histopathologic negative margins, but positive by PCR, who were treated with surgical resection and postoperative radiation therapy is similar to that of patients with histologically positive margins who are also treated with radiation therapy, though this is not surprising considering that in both of these clinical situations residual cancer remains.

Second, this paper solidified the critical role that the *p53* gene plays in the pathogenesis of head and neck squamous cell carcinoma. We now know that the *p53* gene or other regulatory elements of the *p53* pathway are disrupted in almost all known cancers. As a consequence of this manuscript, robust discussions and subsequent investigations, the issue of the appropriateness of *p53* as a marker was also challenged. While *p53* was just used as a prognostic marker in this study, it has become apparent that *p53* also plays a critical role in tumor response to different therapies, and hence is now considered a predictive biomarker as well. Stimulated by this study, additional investigations by the same group have established that a subset of *p53* altered tumors, termed "disruptive" *p53* mutations, have significantly worse clinical outcome.

Third, this study highlighted a limitation of molecular staging that stimulated searches for alternative approaches. The *p53* DNA sequence mutations needed for this approach are only present in about half of head and neck squamous cell cancers, so only about 50% of patients would be eligible for the molecular staging strategy as described. The obvious success of molecular staging in this report provided the impetus to develop alternative approaches that use markers for tumor cells that can be applied to all tumors, such as tumor-specific promoter hypermethylation or mitochondrial DNA mutations. Without this initial landmark study, these subsequent, exciting developments would not be as far along as they are today.

Fourth, the study helped to define the complications for molecular staging posed by field cancerization. The authors were concerned about issues related to field cancerization, because their prior studies had shown that the tissue surrounding head and neck tumors, often normal by histopathologic analysis, could share the same *p53* mutation as the primary tumor. The resulting challenge is quite obvious: if negative histopathologic margins are found surrounding a tumor, distinguishing rare occult tumor cells likely to recur versus field cancerization with the same *p53* mutation is currently impossible. This landmark publication stimulated sometimes heated conversations about these challenges. One could have hoped that these challenges would have been met in the nearly 20 years since this publication, making analysis of molecular margins more widespread. Yet such disappointment is common; even with our current understanding of field cancerization and cancer stem cells and major technical advances like next generation sequencing, few molecular approaches have been successfully transferred from the bench to the bedside despite the scientific insights they offer.

Finally, the approach described in this paper laid the groundwork for subsequent studies trying to predict the presence of microscopic metastatic disease in the N0 setting for oral cancer. Several of these approaches have entered the clinical arena where intraoperative PCR based on established DNA markers are being applied to sentinel lymph nodes to predict the need for neck dissection.

This paper applied nascent molecular biological techniques to support the surgeon's sense that tumor margin status is the most important predictor of treatment outcome and survival in head and neck cancer after surgical therapy. It solidified the surgeon's intuition that recurrence is a consequence of disease being left behind, whether at the tumor margins or in lymph nodes. It demonstrated that histopathologic margin status is not absolute, and that molecular approaches can significantly improve the sensitivity of tumor detection. The ideas and techniques presented and developed introduced the notion of molecular staging. As a consequence, we are witnessing the entry of next generation sequencing into the clinical arena and the flourishing of ideas like cancer stem cell populations and intratumor heterogeneity.

FREQUENT MICROSATELLITE ALTERATIONS AT CHROMOSOMES 9p21 AND 3p14 IN ORAL PREMALIGNANT LESIONS AND THEIR VALUE IN CANCER RISK ASSESSMENT

Li Mao, Jin S Lee, You H Fan, et al.

To better understand genetic alterations in oral premalignant lesions, we examined 84 oral leukoplakia samples from 37 patients who had been enrolled in a chemoprevention trial. The samples were analyzed for two microsatellite markers located at chromosomes 9p21 and 3p14. Loss of heterozygosity (LOH) at either or both loci was identified in 19 of the 37 (51%) patients. Of these 19 patients, seven (37%) have developed head and neck squamous cell carcinoma (HNSCC) while only one of 18 (6%) of patients without LOH developed HNSCC. Our data suggest that clonal genetic alterations are common in oral premalignant lesions; that multiple genetic alterations are common in oral premalignant lesion; that multiple genetic alterations have already occurred in oral premalignant lesions, allowing at least a focal clonal expansion; and that losses of the 9p21 and 3p14 regions may be related to early processes of tumorigenesis in HNSCC. These genetic alterations in premalignant tissues may serve as markers for cancer risk assessment.

Mao L, Lee JS, Fan YH, et al. Frequent microsatellite alterations at chromosomes 9p21 and 3p14 in oral premalignant lesions and their value in cancer risk assessment. Nat Med. 1996;2:682-685.

Commentary by: *Jeffrey N Myers, Marcus M Monroe*

Oral premalignant lesions (OPLs), including leukoplakia and erythroplakia, are well-known precursors of oral squamous cell carcinoma. Based on preclinical and early clinical evidence that retinoids could reverse changes of leukoplakia, a series of studies were conducted in the 1980s and early 1990s to examine the effectiveness of chemoprevention with 13-cis retinoic acid in this at-risk population. The first study, published in 1986, demonstrated that 13-cis retinoic acid caused clinical and histologic resolution of OPLs. Based on these results, subsequent studies were performed demonstrating initial promise in the prevention of OPL progression to carcinoma as well as the development of second primary malignancies in head and neck cancer patients. However, long-term follow-up of these trials demonstrated significant relapse rates following treatment cessation, along with drug toxicity that dampened the initial enthusiasm for these chemoprophylaxis regimens. It was recognized that additional work would be needed to understand the molecular progression of oral cancer in order to more accurately define the at-risk population and develop tailored prevention strategies.

Around the same time that these studies were ongoing, increasing evidence was being presented that genetic alterations could contribute to carcinogenesis. In the early to mid-1980s, it was observed in retinoblastoma and Wilms tumors that loss of heterozygosity (LOH) at certain chromosomal regions was a common event and likely a contributing factor in tumorigenesis. Following this discovery, early reports demonstrated that LOH at multiple sites was a frequent occurrence in head and neck cancer.

In a translational study attached to the 13-cis retinoic acid chemoprevention trial, Mao et al. examined the risk of oral cancer development based upon loss of genetic material at 3p14 and 9p21, two loci previously reported to be frequently altered in head and neck cancer. Through microsatellite analysis, they demonstrated that LOH at either one or both loci was a common event in OPL specimens, occurring in half of the patients studied. Furthermore, when the 37 patients were followed for a median of 63 months (range, 5–94), the risk of subsequent cancer development was significantly higher in those specimens containing LOH at 3p14 and/or 9p21 (37% versus 6%). This study demonstrated that loss of genetic material at 3p and 9p were not only common but also early, and likely important, events in oral cancer development. In addition, this study highlighted the fact that these genetic alterations could serve an important role as biomarkers for cancer risk assessment.

Following this first step towards molecular risk assessment in head and neck cancer, subsequent work would validate LOH at 3p and 9p as a biomarker for cancer risk assessment not only in OPL but also for risk of second primaries in patients with a history of oral cancer. Additional genetic alterations with prognostic and predictive utility, such as *p53* mutational status, have since been defined, expanding our understanding of key early events in oral carcinogenesis.

Because of this work, current chemoprevention trials are now able to focus their efforts on the population most at risk for cancer development. Ongoing studies addressing the role of molecularly targeted agents such as erlotinib and vandetanib in oral cancer prevention have set LOH at 3p and 9p as entry criteria, thereby defining a population most likely to benefit.

Despite a well-documented risk of malignant transformation, the optimal management strategy for patients with OPLs continues to lack consensus. In large part this stems from a still-incomplete knowledge of the molecular blueprint of oral cancer. Significant early contributions towards our understanding of the molecular underpinnings of oral cancer were made by Mao et al. As recent technological advances continue to provide more and more insight into the genetic basis of head and neck cancer, it is hoped that we will one day have the ability to identify patients most at risk for oral cancer development and apply tailored prevention strategies.

GENETIC PROGRESSION MODEL FOR HEAD AND NECK CANCER: IMPLICATIONS FOR FIELD CANCERIZATION

Joseph Califano, Peter van der Riet, William Westra, et al.

A genetic progression model of head and neck squamous cell carcinoma has not yet been elucidated, and the genetic basis for "field cancerization" of the aerodigestive tract has also remained obscure. Eighty-seven lesions of the head and neck, including preinvasive lesions and benign lesions associated with carcinogen exposure, were tested using microsatellite analysis for allelic loss at 10 major chromosomal loci which have been defined previously. The spectrum of chromosomal loss progressively increased at each histopathological step from benign hyperplasia to dysplasia to carcinoma in situ to invasive cancer. Adjacent areas of tissue with different histopathological appearance shared common genetic changes, but the more histopathologically advanced areas exhibited additional genetic alterations. Abnormal mucosal cells surrounding preinvasive and microinvasive lesions shared common genetic alterations with those lesions and thus appear to arise from a single progenitor clone. Based on these findings, the local clinical phenomenon of field cancerization seems to involve the expansion and migration of clonally related preneoplastic cells.

Califano J, van der Riet P, Westra W, et al. Genetic progression model for head and neck cancer: implications for field cancerization. *Cancer Res.* 1996;56:2488-2492.

Commentary by: *Bhuvanesh Singh*

That oncogenesis is a multistep process, has been accepted for decades. This was brought to the forefront for head and neck cancers by the landmark clinicopathologic study by Slaughter and colleagues published in 1953. The presence of histopathologic abnormalities surrounding oral cancers combined with clinical observations, such as increased rates of second primary cancers in patients with head and neck cancers, led Slaughter to propose the concept of *"field-cancerization"*, the underlying mechanisms of which remain to be defined. While a genetic basis for carcinogenesis was postulated by Theodore Boveri in the early 1900s, the identification of the Philadelphia chromosome (reciprocal translocation between 9 and 22) in chronic myeloid leukemia established this as a causal relationship.

The accumulated evidence suggests that rather than a specific, sequential accrual of cancer-causing abnormalities, genetic aberrations develop randomly, with those providing survival advantages selected in a Darwinian-like manner in individual cells. As critical genetic aberrations accumulate, mucosal keratinocytes progress through distinct histopathologic stages from premalignant to *in situ*, and ultimately to invasive head and neck cancers. Many other cancers show clinicopathologic evidence of progression, including those of the colon, breast, esophagus, and bladder. In their seminal work, Feron and Vogelstein utilized contemporary analytic tools to show that a progressive accumulation of genetic abnormalities underlies progression of benign adenomas to colon carcinomas. While they suggested that the accumulation of genetic events was most important, a genetic model of colon cancer progression was developed, linking individual genetic events to different clinicopathologic stages of progression based on relative frequency of occurrence. This work provided valuable insight into the basis for oncogenic progression and established a framework for the genetic modeling of other cancer types.

David Sidransky's laboratory published several papers that suggested that like colon cancer, genetic progression was also the basis for the development of head and neck cancers. In one report, they found the presence of *p53* mutation in 19% of non-invasive lesions and 43% of invasive lesions. In another report, they found abnormalities at 9p occurred equally in preinvasive (71%) and invasive (72%) lesions. These data, combined with results from allotype analysis of a series of head and neck cancers, and the paradigms established by Vogelstein's work set the stage for the development of a genetic progression model for head and neck cancer, which was reported in the article by Califano and colleagues—the subject of this review.

Following the approach used by Vogelstein and colleagues, 10 distinct genetic loci, commonly aberrant in head and neck cancer and contained in a minimal area of loss of a putative tumor suppressor, were analyzed in a cohort of 87 preinvasive head and neck lesions from 83 patients. Overall, 34 cases of benign squamous hyperplasia, 31 of dysplasia, and 21 of carcinoma *in situ* were assessed and compared to previously published results on invasive head and neck cancers. Similar to the findings in colorectal cancers, a progressive increase in accumulation of genetic abnormalities was seen in hyperplasia (0.7 +/– 1.3), dysplasia (2.7 +/– 1.5), carcinoma *in situ* (3.3 +/– 2.0), and invasive cancers (3.6 +/– 2.2). By analyzing the frequency of abnormality at each locus, a genetic progression model was developed. In this model, loss of 9p was associated with progression from normal mucosa to benign hyperplasia; 3p and 17p to dysplasia; 11q, 13q, and 14q to *in situ* carcinoma; and 6p, 8, and 4q to invasive cancer. The progression model was validated by analysis of 5 cases with histopatho-logically distinct areas of intralesional progression, which demonstrated genetic evidence for clonal progression.

These findings from Califano and colleagues provided a framework around which our understanding of the genetic basis for head and neck cancer has grown. Application of genome wide analyses, including comparative genomic hybridization, expression, and methylation arrays have added to the progression model and identified candidate genes at individual loci associated with progression. The current head and neck cancer progression model includes well over 30 different genes and loci, the exact functional relevance of which remains to be defined. Moreover, subsequent reports confirm that there is continued genetic progression, even after the development of invasive cancers, which is associated with tumor differentiation, invasion, and metastasis. The numbers of genetic events present in current progression models far outnumber the mathematical predictions of 8–10 genetic aberrations required for progression to invasive head and neck cancer. The challenge for modern genetic analysis is to differentiate consequential genetic aberrations from the background/ bystander events that are accompanying cancer progression.

The authors suggest that their model may have several clinical implications, including margin prediction, molecular cancer screening of saliva and serum, prognostication, as well as identification of genetic targets for therapeutic intervention. Many of the authors' predictions have proven accurate. Screening of saliva and serum for tumor markers have been shown to detect presence of head and neck cancers. Molecular margins (i.e. assessment for genetic abnormalities in histopathologically normal tumor resection margins), better predictors of local recurrence, were shown to be better predictors of recurrence. In addition, many genetic markers have been shown to be associated with disease progression and clinical outcome. However, while we have learned a great deal about the genetic basis for head and neck cancer progression, the promise of routine clinical use for genetic-based detection and treatment remains elusive. Global screening strategies have identified targetable genetic abnormalities in several tumors (i.e. EGFR in lung cancer), but no such aberrations have been identified in head and neck cancers. The key limitation is that while global screening tools allow cataloguing of genetic abnormalities, they do not provide functional or biological relevance. As this challenge is realized, we can expect better clinical translation of genetic findings, allowing us to achieve the possibilities envisaged by Califano et al. in his seminal work.

LEVELS OF TGF-α AND EGFR PROTEIN IN HEAD AND NECK SQUAMOUS CELL CARCINOMA AND PATIENT SURVIVAL

Jennifer Rubin Grandis, Mona F Melhem, William E Gooding, et al.

Background: The most accurate predictor of disease recurrence in patients treated for head and neck squamous cell carcinoma is, at present, the extent of regional lymph node metastasis. Since elevated levels of epidermal growth factor receptor (EGFR) and of its ligand, transforming growth factor-α (TGF-α), have been detected in primary tumors of patients with head and neck squamous cell carcinoma, we determined whether tumor levels of these proteins were of prognostic importance.

Methods: Monoclonal antibodies specific for EGFR and TGF-α were used for immunohistochemical detection of each protein in tissue sections of primary tumors from 91 patients who were treated by surgical resection. Levels of immunoreactive EGFR and TGF-α were quantified by use of a computerized image analysis system and were normalized to appropriate standards. The logrank test and proportional hazards regression analysis were used to calculate the probability that EGFR and TGF-α levels were associated with disease-free survival (i.e., patients do not die of their disease). All P values were two-sided.

Results: When tumor levels of EGFR or TGF-α were analyzed as continuous variables, disease-free survival and cause-specific survival were reduced among patients with higher levels of EGFR (both P = .0001) or TGF-α (both P = .0001) In a multivariate analysis, tumor site, tumor level of EGFR, and tumor level of TGF-α were statistically significant predictors of disease-free survival; in a similar analysis, regional lymph node stage and tumor levels of EGFR and of TGF-α were significant predictors of cause-specific survival.

Conclusion: Quantitation of EGFR and TGF-α protein levels in primary head and neck squamous cell carcinomas may be useful in identifying subgroups of patients at high risk of tumor recurrence and in guiding therapy.

Rubin Grandis J, Melhem MF, Gooding WE, et al. Levels of TGF-α and EGFR protein in head and neck squamous cell carcinoma and patient survival. J Natl Cancer Inst. 1998;90:824-832.

Commentary by: *K Kian Ang**

A polypeptide that accelerates eyelid opening and incisor eruption in newborn mice was identified by Cohen in 1962. This polypeptide was subsequently found to stimulate proliferation and keratinization of mouse epidermis *in vivo* and the growth of chick embryo epidermis *in vitro* and, thereby, referred to as the epidermal growth factor (EGF). Its specific receptor, EGFR, was identified more than a decade later by the same group along with the demonstration that its tyrosine-specific phosphorylation activated intracellular signal transduction. EGFR was then characterized as a 170-kDa transmembrane receptor tyrosine kinase (RTK) of the ERBB family, which is essential for normal development. Its chromosomal location (*7p12–p22*), cDNA and amino-acid sequence, and genomic structure were

**Dr Ang passed away on June 19, 2013.

subsequently identified along with its ligands. EGFR activation initiates multiple layers of signaling diversity and amplification, which play roles in governing cellular biological responses.

The findings that many squamous cell carcinoma cell lines express a high level of EGFR and that perturbation of EGFR signaling might play a role in cell transformation spurred the interest to address the biological significance of tumor EGFR expression. Three early correlative studies in head and neck carcinoma focused on patients with laryngeal cancer treated with radiotherapy or surgery, which showed that recurrent tumors expressed a higher level of EGFR than tumors that did not recur and that tumors with higher expression of EGFR or one of its ligands, transforming growth factor alpha (TGF-α), relapsed more frequently than those expressing a lower level of EGFR or TGF-α.

Interestingly, these three reports with consistent findings attracted relatively little clinical attention until Grandis and colleagues published robust confirmatory data featured in this centennial commemoration book. The latter group measured TGF-α and EGFR expression of primary tumors by immunohistochemical assay and correlated the results with clinical, pathologic, and outcome parameters. The study population consisted of 91 patients with various tumor sites and stages treated by surgical resection, followed by adjuvant radiotherapy or chemotherapy in 72 patients. They found that the expression level of TGF-α (both P=0.0001) or EGFR (both P=0.0001) was the strongest predictor of disease-free survival and cause-specific survival. In addition, TGF-α (P=0.0001) and EGFR levels also had a significant impact on the recurrence of the index tumor (P=0.001). In multivariate analyses, tumor site and level of TGF-α or EGFR expression were found to be significant predictors of disease-free survival, and the combination of higher TGF-α or EGFR levels plus lymph node stage was the strongest predictor of death from disease. This study also showed that the reproducibility of the TGF-α assay was more problematic than the EGFR assay.

The publication of the work of Grandis et al. in a prominent journal along with the growing general understanding of the role of RTKs in regulating cellular behavior during the mid-1990s galvanized many other studies, which yielded firm validation of the prognostic significance of EGFR expression and also generated additional biological insights. For example, a study using specimens of a well-defined group of patients with locally advanced head and neck carcinoma enrolled into a phase III trial of the Radiation Therapy Oncology Group and treated uniformly with radiation alone showed that the poorer overall survival rate of patients with high EGFR-expressing tumors was attributable to the failure of radiotherapy to eradicate primary tumor and/or nodal disease rather than to the difference in the incidence of distant metastasis. These observations along with other emerging data suggested that EGFR overexpressing tumors were more resistant to radiation.

Collectively, the findings summarized above provided compelling scientific rationale for attempting to improve tumor control by targeting the perturbed EGFR signaling pathway using either antibodies (e.g., cetuximab) or small molecule tyrosine kinase inhibitors (e.g., gefitinib or erlotinib). Preclinical data indeed showed that cetuximab enhanced tumor response to single-dose or fractionated radiation in tumor cell lines and in xenograft models quantified using apoptosis, regrowth delay and tumor control as endpoints. Therefore, a phase III clinical trial was launched to address whether adding cetuximab to radiotherapy can increase local-regional control of locally advanced head and neck carcinoma in humans, thereby improving overall survival. This pivotal trial, highlighted elsewhere in this centennial book, validated the proof-of-concept that modulating a perturbed RTK signaling pathway can selectively sensitize tumors to radiotherapy and, consequently, truly improve the therapeutic index. The work of Grandis and colleagues thus contributed to identifying a new biomarker and to encouraging many investigators to conduct integrated translational research that established a novel, less toxic treatment option for the management of patients with locally advanced head and neck carcinoma. Consequently, it is fitting to feature this publication as a seminal paper in this centennial commemorative book.

MUTATIONS IN *SDHD*, A MITOCHONDRIAL COMPLEX II GENE, IN HEREDITARY PARAGANGLIOMA

Bora E Baysal, Robert E Ferrell, Joan E Willett-Brozick, et al.

Hereditary paraganglioma (PGL) is characterized by the development of benign, vascularized tumors in the head and neck. The most common tumor site is the carotid body (CB), a chemoreceptive organ that senses oxygen levels in the blood. Analysis of families carrying the PGL1 gene, described here, revealed germ line mutations in the SDHD gene on chromosome 11q23. SDHD encodes a mitochondrial respiratory chain protein—then small subunit of cytochrome b in succinate-ubiquinone oxidoreductase (cybS). In contrast to expectations based on the inheritance pattern of PGL, the SDHD gene showed no evidence of imprinting. These findings indicate that mitochondria play an important role in the pathogenesis of certain tumors and that cybS plays a role in normal CB physiology.

Baysal BE, Ferrell RE, Willett-Brozick JE, et al. Mutations in SDHD, a mitochondrial complex II gene, in hereditary paraganglioma. Science. 2000;287:848-851.

Commentary by: *David Myssiorek*

A genetic disposition to paragangliomas was suspected as early as 1933 by both Chase, who described sisters with carotid paragangliomas, and Goekoop, who reported familial jugular paragangliomas. Subsequent studies by many authors reported familial transmission of these tumors in multiple locations in the head and neck. Eventually, a Mendelian pattern of inheritance was discovered. Van der Mey finally described a parent of origin inheritance in many pedigrees secondary to genomic imprinting. These events prompted a search for a gene responsible for paragangliomas.

In 2000, Baysal et al. discovered the gene *PGL 1* coding for familial or hereditary paragangliomas. Estimates of the prevalence of familial paragangliomas range from 10% to 50%, depending on where the data was recorded. In 1994, Heutink et al. had localized the gene to chromosome 11q23 based on studies of Dutch pedigrees. The chromosomal region that was localized covered an 11 megabase region. Following this, the Dutch group refined the region to a 2 megabase length. From a gene mapping perspective, this group had been off the target, which was subsequently defined by Baysal et al. in this manuscript through painstaking work in Pittsburgh. The gene *PGL 1* was found to be a mutation of the succinate dehydrogenase D subunit (SDHD). Following this, mutations of SDH subunits B and C were discovered in Europe based on this refinement of the PGL locus.

Prior to this discovery, familial paragangliomas were suspected by history and physical findings. A familial presentation, bilateral or multiple paragangliomas, earlier onset of symptoms, and in some cases vagal paragangliomas were the criteria used to determine if someone possessed a familial paraganglioma. An index of suspicion allowed physicians to evaluate family members with the various tools available for screening

(MRI, Octreotide scintigraphy, angiography). However, these methods would require every member of every family to be tested. Firm knowledge about who is carrying the genotype would allow streamlined testing, decreased exposure to X-rays, and saving of resources.

The primary significance of this paper is that since the gene had been localized, it could now be identified in prospective patients with paraganglioma. The testing of the phenotypically positive patient would prompt the investigation of family members vertically and horizontally within their pedigree. The detection of carriers earlier has definite implications. The surveillance of select potential paraganglioma patients would allow for early detection of lesions at a much smaller size. Since early penetrance is one of the hallmarks of familial paragangliomas, eventually some form of treatment is necessary in many of these patients. Early detection translates to earlier treatment of lesions.

Usually, small paragangliomas remain asymptomatic. Symptoms from these tumors are eventually due to cranial nerve involvement (cranial nerves VII, IX, X, XI, XII) later in the disease process. Vagal paragangliomas uniformly result in vagal nerve paralysis, unless the lesions are small. When operated, carotid paragangliomas larger than 4.5 cm in diameter have a marked increase in the complication rate. The morbidity of operations for these lesions would be diminished and the blood loss would be less. The rehabilitation of these patients after surgery for large lesions may require swallowing therapy, vocal therapy (including vocal medialization procedures), facial reanimation, and palatal procedures for incompetency.

Many familial paraganglioma patients have multiple paragangliomas, and a positive genotype would spur a search for second lesions as well. Furthermore, since these lesions may show up metachronously, the need for lifetime surveillance would be predicted. Patients with sporadic paragangliomas would not require family evaluations, prolonged follow-up, and costly surveillance with radionuclide imaging, MRI, or CT scanning.

After Baysal et al. delineated the SDHD mutation, abnormalities in SDHB and SDHC were detected. In particular, the SDHB mutation bore an association with malignancy and pheochromocytomas. The significance of this cannot be overstated. The possibility of malignancy in a paraganglioma necessitates careful observation during surgical procedures, such as the evaluation of lymph nodes. The continued surveillance of blood pressure (potential for pheochromocytoma) and for metastasis would be needed. Benign paragangliomas cannot be distinguished from malignant versions. It is possible for a histopathologically benign paraganglioma to actually be malignant (judged by *subsequent* metastasis). Family members of SDHB carriers with hypertension should strongly be suspected of pheochromocytoma.

A secondary contribution of this paper was not evident right away. In 1930, Warburg had published his theory on mitochondria as a source of cancer. He postulated that cancer cells do not utilize oxygen to produce ATP. Rather, they depended on glycolysis, an inefficient way of producing ATP. However, no paper had ever revealed a mitochondrial genetic defect as a root cause of neoplasm. The Baysal paper showed a genetic defect in the oxygen sensing and signaling pathway that resulted in neoplasia. Although the SDHD mutation was responsible for mostly benign tumors, the subsequent discovery of SDHB mutation revealed a strong association with malignant varieties of paragangliomas. Effectively, this was the first evidence of a mitochondrial defect linked to cancer.

Since that time, according to Scopus, almost 700 references citing the article have appeared. Many of these articles deal with cancers associated with mitochondria. Warburg's original hypothesis was revived. Articles concerning the other SDH subunits flourished, and the discovery of pedigrees with malignant varieties of paragangliomas were reported.

THE MUTATIONAL LANDSCAPE OF HEAD AND NECK SQUAMOUS CELL CARCINOMA

Nicolas Stransky, Ann Marie Egloff, Aaron D Tward, et al.

Head and neck squamous cell carcinoma (HNSCC) is a common, morbid, and frequently lethal malignancy. To uncover its mutational spectrum, we analyzed whole-exome sequencing data from 74 tumor-normal pairs. The majority exhibited a mutational profile consistent with tobacco exposure; human papilloma virus was detectable by sequencing of DNA from infected tumors. In addition to identifying previously known HNSCC genes (TP53, CDKN2A, PTEN, PIK3CA, and HRAS), the analysis revealed many genes not previously implicated in this malignancy. At least 30% of case harbored mutations in genes that regulate squamous differentiation (e.g. NOTCH1, IRF6, and TP63), implicating its dysregulation as a major driver of HNSCC carcinogenesis. More generally, the results indicate the ability of large-scale sequencing to reveal fundamental tumorigenic mechanisms.

Stransky N, Egloff AM, Tward AD, et al. The mutational landscape of head and neck squamous cell carcinoma. Science. 2011;6046:1157-1160

Commentary by: *Joseph Califano*

The articles simultaneously published by Agrawal et al. (1) and Stransky et al. (2) in the August 26, 2011, issue of *Science* represent a critical inflection point in the study of head and neck cancer. Both of these manuscripts represent the first efforts for high throughput sequencing of exomic, coding region DNA in primary head and neck squamous cell carcinoma, and provided new information on coding mutations in genes critical to head and neck cancer development. The nature of the investigation, the investigators, and the biologic insights gained by the definitive nature of these studies formally ushered in a new era of investigation into head and neck cancer biology.

There are a total of 69 investigators cited as authors in these two studies, demonstrating that high throughput, resource intense, whole genomic investigation requires large teams of investigators with highly specific skill sets working in a coordinated fashion. The advent of team-based investigation applied to large-scale "omic" analyses that comprehensively describe whole genomic status is now reported in essentially all tumor systems, and will define significant advances in the next decade or two for cancer biology. This effort has perhaps reached its ultimate expression in the current National Cancer Institute effort to define The Cancer Genome Atlas (TCGA) by defining large, whole genome genetic, epigenetic, and expression datasets for all major cancer types, including hundreds of head and neck cancers.

The definition of individual gene mutations in these studies is striking for two reasons: (1) novel gene targets were discovered that may be targeted therapeutically, (2) on the other hand, these gene-specific mutation frequencies were relatively low (< 20%). While these studies defined novel mutational targets in head and neck cancer, including *NOTCH* genes and other genes that may potentially be targeted therapeutically, the relatively low frequency and noted heterogeneity of mutated genes raises significant challenges for therapeutic application. This trend is noted in many other solid tumors, and as a result, a call for "individualized" therapy, treating patients with specific targeted agents based on unique and diverse patterns of gene mutations, has been advanced. However, this is anticipated to be a highly challenging endeavor due to the high cost of targeted drug development and the need for clinical trial validation within smaller subsets of patients that have specific alterations susceptible to targeting by specific drugs.

Of note, both studies reported highly similar findings, including similar mutation targets, activating and inactivating mutations in *NOTCH* genes, and a decreased mutational burden in human papillomavirus-related head and neck cancers. This lends support to these findings, and sets the stage for investigation into the mechanisms of these genes as drivers of carcinogenesis by a broader set of investigators. Perhaps the most interesting findings from these studies are related to what they do not describe. The additional mutational load (in excess of previously described, mutated genes, including TP53) is unexpectedly low. The phenotypic changes present in head and neck cancer are associated with dysregulation of thousands of critical pathways, yet precious few genes are mutated in comparison to the profound changes seen in cellular pathways. How can these changes be affected with so little mutational load?

The answer, of course, is that these studies examine a very small portion of the alterations that lead to the full phenotypic expression of head and neck cancer. Exome sequencing performed in these studies examines only the coding region of DNA, and regions between exons may have sequence alterations that affect mRNA splicing and therefore coding. Mutations in regulatory regions, including enhancers, promoters, and other regulatory regions may affect gene expression dramatically in the absence of exon mutation. Gross chromosomal structural alteration, highly prevalent in head and neck cancer, may result in novel fusion genes and altered gene expression by chromosomal loss or amplification. Epigenetic alterations, those that affect the noncoding structure and composition of DNA, are more profound and numerous than mutations in terms of number of genes altered. Noncoding RNA alterations in microRNA and other noncoding RNA species are also a rapidly growing class of changes that participate in carcinogenesis.

Finally, the study of cancer biology is transitioning into a field that no longer focuses on single gene alterations in isolation. Rather, multiple genetic, epigenetic, and expression perturbations are viewed within the context of regulatory and effector networks of molecules that coordinate to affect a variety of cellular processes. This network-based viewpoint is a tool to integrate seemingly disparate DNA and RNA alterations within functional groups. Network based analysis is expected to become the dominant perspective from which cancer biology is interpreted, both in the discovery of novel network alterations and in the effort to intervene with targeted drug development.

EXOME SEQUENCING OF HEAD AND NECK SQUAMOUS CELL CARCINOMA REVEALS INACTIVATING MUTATIONS IN *NOTCH1*

Nishant Agrawal, Mitchell J Frederick, Curtis R Pickering, et al.

Head and neck squamous cell carcinoma (HNSCC) is the sixth most common cancer worldwide. To explore the genetic origins of this cancer, we used whole exome sequencing and gene copy number analyses to study 32 primary tumors. Tumors from patients with a history of tobacco use had more mutations than did tumors from patients who did not use tobacco, and tumors that were negative for human papilloma virus (HPV) had more mutations than did HPV-positive tumors. Six of the genes that were mutated in multiple tumors were assessed in up to 88 additional HNSCCs. In addition to previously described mutations in TP53, CDKN2A, PIK3CA and HRAS, we identified mutations in FBXW7 and NOTCH1. Interestingly, nearly 40% of the 28 mutations identified in NOTCH1 were predicted to truncate the gene product, suggesting that NOTCH1 may function as a tumor suppressor gene rather than an oncogene in this tumor type.

Agarwal N, Frederick MJ, Pickering CR, et al. *Exome sequencing of head and neck squamous cell carcinoma reveals inactivating mutations in NOTCH1. Science. 2012;333:1154-1157.*

Commentary by: *Thomas E Carey*

The advent of high throughput genomic sequencing has enabled the rapid assessment of the complete exome sequences of multiple tumors. In the August 26, 2011, issue of Science, two landmark papers were published: "Exome sequencing of head and neck squamous cell carcinomas reveals inactivating mutations in *NOTCH1*" by Agarwal et al. and "The mutational landscape of head and neck squamous cell carcinoma" by Stransky et al. In these studies, 32 (Agarwal et al.) and 74 (Stransky, et al.) tumor normal pairs from head and neck cancer patients were sequenced to determine the mutational spectrum of this highly lethal cancer type.

As expected, the exome sequencing identified the commonly recognized genes that are mutated in head and neck cancer, including *TP53, CDKN2a, PTEN, PIK3CA*, and *HRAS*, confirming the validity of exome sequencing as a strategy to detect genetic abnormalities that define and drive individual tumors. Of particular interest in these studies was the unexpected discovery by both teams that the *NOTCH* gene family is mutated in a subset of 11–22% of head and neck squamous cell cancers. Notch had not been implicated previously in head and neck cancer. The *NOTCH* family of genes encodes cell surface receptors that mediate cell-to-cell signaling necessary in development and cell fate determinations.

NOTCH mutations have been identified in a variety of other cancer types and include both activating and inactivating mutations. The role of Notch protein is complex due to its structure and its capacity to affect both partner cells involved in cell-to-cell signaling activity. Of particular interest was the comparison of *NOTCH* mutations in head and neck squamous cell carcinoma (HNSCC) to those typically found in hematopoietic cancers and other solid tumors, as discussed in the Agarwal et al. paper. In the hematopoietic cancers, the mutational spectrum is largely focused on the juxta transmembrane domain or the C-terminal domain and is frequently associated with activation of Notch signaling. The other solid tumors have overlap with this pattern, with clusters of mutations in both sites, but among HNSCC, the majority of tumors with *NOTCH* mutations are frequently truncating, most likely inactivating and clustered in the N terminal EGF repeat domain of the extracellular region necessary for cell-to-cell signaling and the ankyrin repeat domains in the intracellular segment necessary for transactivation.

There is evidence that *NOTCH* can function either as a transforming gene as in T-cell leukemias or as a tumor suppressor gene, which is likely in HNSCC. The incidence of *NOTCH* mutations in HNSCC, including the presence of more than one *NOTCH* mutation in several tumors, strongly implicates these as driver mutations. Furthermore, knockout of *Notch* in mice leads to the development of epithelial tumors. The Cancer Genome Atlas (TCGA) has now confirmed that among 280 HNSCC tumors, *NOTCH* family mutations occur in 15–20%. Thus, this discovery marks a clear step forward in the identification of a novel cancer driver in HNSCC.

Notch therapeutics, such as gamma secretase inhibitors, now exist. This class of agent inhibits Notch function in tumors with activating mutations. The loss of function mutations observed in HNSCC are not expected to respond, and skin tumor development has been noted in people taking the inhibitors, further reinforcing the role of Notch in maintaining normal epithelial homeostasis.

The discovery of frequent *Notch* mutations also increased the level of suspicion of mutations in other genes such as *TP63* and *IRF6* involved in epidermal development. Further inspection of recurrent mutations of other genes in HNSCC as discussed in the Stransky et al. study, extended this link to include multiple other mutated genes that regulate squamous differentiation suggesting that loss of this function blocks differentiation of epidermal cells and leads to increased cell proliferation. Furthermore, defects in the murine homologs of genes mutated in HNSCC, including *Notch1, Notch2, Irf6, Tp63, Ripk4, Cdh1, Ezh2, and Dicer1*, alter squamous epithelial differentiation *in vivo*.

The examination of other less commonly mutated genes revealed additional recurrently compromised pathways in 5–10% of tumors that provide squamous cancers with survival or growth advantages, including mutations of *Casp8* and *DDX3X* genes that mediate apoptosis, and histone methyl transferases *PRDM9* and *EZH2* that regulate expression of genes involved in development and differentiation.

From these studies it is becoming clear that deregulation of the squamous epithelial differentiation machinery is an important mechanism in malignant transformation of squamous cells. This is not surprising since proliferation of the epithelium is tightly regulated and requires interaction with the basement membrane for squamous cell replication and survival. When a normal daughter cell leaves the basal cell layer it enters an irreversible differentiation pathway with progressive pyknosis and karyorrhexis of the nucleus that is incompatible with future cell division. The basal epithelial cell is also programmed to undergo anoikis if deprived of attachment to the basement membrane. Thus, mutation of pathways regulating epithelial differentiation is a requisite for cancer development.

In the last 10–15 years, there has been a significant change in the pathogenesis of head and neck cancer. The discovery that high-risk human papillomaviruses are now an important etiologic factor in head and neck cancer, especially in those cancers arising in Waldeyer's ring surrounding the oropharynx, has changed how such cancers are treated. Fortunately, HPV-positive oropharyngeal cancers are easier to treat, and for the first time, physicians are discussing and embarking on treatment de-escalation studies. In the context of these landmark papers, it is of interest that the HPV-positive cancers were shown to have a very different mutational spectrum than HNSCC associated with tobacco carcinogens. Nevertheless, the pathways affected in the HPV-driven cancers are still altered, but in this case, the changes are largely secondary to the effects of the viral oncogenes, E6 and E7. HPV-associated cancers are typically poorly differentiated and have a basaloid appearance. In the tumor sets examined in these papers, roughly 20% contained HPV16, but this is not necessarily representative of the actual incidence of HPV-positive oropharynx cancers, which at some centers reaches 90% of all oropharynx cancers. Additionally, HPV-positive oropharynx cancer is making up an increasing proportion of all head and neck cancers as smoking incidence declines. There is a strong inverse relationship between HPV and *TP53* and *CDKN2A* mutations that are very common in smoking-related HNSCC. However, as the HPV E7 and E6 oncoproteins inactivate the Rb and *p53* pathways, respectively, there is near universal disruption of these pathways in HNSCC, regardless of the etiologic mechanism.

These papers have ushered in a new era of genetic discovery in head and neck cancer and are a harbinger of the type of team science that has begun to permeate large-scale genomic investigation. Scientists working together can accomplish remarkable things that cannot be done as well working alone. These papers and TCGA demonstrate this synergy and provide huge amounts of research material for investigation and the development new strategies to counter the driver mutations affecting individual cancers. As many of the mutations that affect HNSCC are loss of function mutations, this provides a significant challenge for new therapeutics, since typical pathway inhibitors will not work. Thus, we have important research targets to move to the next level of intervention in HNSCC therapy.

Chapter 3

Staging

INCLUSION OF COMORBIDITY IN A STAGING SYSTEM FOR HEAD AND NECK CANCER

Jay F Piccirillo

The widespread use of the TNM staging system has helped standardize the classification of cancers. Despite its excellence in describing a tumor's size and extent of anatomic spread, the TNM system does not account for the clinical biology of the cancer. Clinical factors, such as symptom severity, performance status, and comorbidity, which are important for classification, prognostication, and evaluation of treatment effectiveness, remain excluded from this system. In several studies of cancer prognosis, the presence of severe comorbidity was found to dramatically influence survival statistics and the evaluation of treatment effectiveness. A statistical technique known as conjunctive consolidation was used to incorporate comorbidity into the TNM staging system and maintain the four category system. Utilizing this technique, comorbidity was added to the TNM system for laryngeal cancer to create a composite staging system. Quantitative evaluation of the new system showed that the addition of comorbidity provides improved prognostic precision over TNM stage alone.

Piccirillo JF. Inclusion of comorbidity in a staging system for head and neck cancer. Oncology. 1995;9: 831-836

Commentary by: *William M Lydiatt*

"Inclusion of Comorbidity in a Staging System for Head and Neck Cancer" was published in *Oncology* in 1995. It stands as a significant contribution to the advancement of accurate and meaningful staging. The idea of including comorbidity in head and neck staging was based on the general knowledge that anatomic prediction was not always the best predictor of outcome and that it is the patient with the disease that must be understood. Even today, the goal of achieving the described outcome of measuring comorbidity and including it as a staging criterion has not come to fruition.

Staging of cancer in general and head and neck specifically has been an attempt to define the natural history of the disease, promote comparisons of data across geographic and temporal landscapes, and to approximate prognosis for the physician and patient. The American Joint Committee on Cancer (AJCC) manual, 7th Edition, states the most important use of staging is to "provide those with cancer and their physicians the critical benchmark for defining prognosis and the likelihood of overcoming the cancer and for determining the best treatment approach fort their case".

Historically, staging was based on the size, location, and degree of invasiveness of the primary tumor, presence or absence and size, location and extent of nodal metastasis, and presence or absence of distant metastasis. These morphological criteria were developed in the 1940s by Pierre Denoix and served as a simple but powerful tool for the disease-specific prediction of outcome. Larger tumors, those with regional nodal disease, and especially those with distant disease have all been shown in work done over decades to have a negative impact on survival. The utility of this system has been born out over time.

It has been long recognized, however, that anatomic staging, while an excellent first approximation, suffers an intrinsic inexactitude for many patients. Over the years, multiple authors have suggested revisions to the staging system, from minor cosmetic reshuffling of the stage groupings to a marked revamping of the entire system. The AJCC and the Union for International Cancer Control (UICC) have conscientiously and carefully weighed the benefits of change to a more exact but demanding system against the need for simplicity and consistency over time. One of the biggest strengths of the current staging system is its longevity. This allows for reasonably uniform comparisons of treatments over time. Additional strengths of the current system are user friendliness and its ability to be easily and inexpensively used globally.

The major area for improvement cited by authors suggesting modifications to the staging system is a lack of consistency in prognostication. Throughout, several key attributes of a staging system must be balanced. The system must create groups that are internally similar but sufficiently different from the group above and below. For example, all members of stage I should have similar characteristics and prognosis, and these attributes should be measurably different than those in stage II. These two concepts are known as hazard consistency and hazard discrimination, respectively. The groups should also have generally similar numbers within each subcategory to make the process worthwhile. If 90% of patients are in one stage, the utility of staging to differentiate has been lost. Thus, each group should have roughly equal numbers within. This is known as balance. Finally, the system must have predictive power. As cited above, the AJCC manual on staging believes this is the key factor for a staging system. It is this attribute that has engendered the most debate and innovation.

Non-anatomic factors have been introduced in the staging of cancers for many years; these include age in thyroid cancer, B symptoms in Hodgkin's lymphoma, and Gleason score in prostate cancer. Biological staging was proposed by Drs Helmuth Goepfert and Stimson Schantz as a way of including emerging data into the staging system to make it more descriptive of the biological process. Schantz et al. further developed this idea in a subsequent work that allowed for a more comprehensive description of the entire process, including the incorporation of emerging biomarkers and comorbidity. The concept was to define the biology of the disease with respect to its intrinsic genetic and epigenetic characteristics but also to accommodate for the host's response to the disease. It is this aspect that the Piccirillo's work addresses.

The fundamental insight in recognizing performance status came from Karnofsky and others. They defined a rough assessment of how patients would fair with treatment based on a general assessment of their health. These scales have helped to direct clinical care and patient management decisions. They recognized that patients with other significant health problems were unable to receive or tolerate antineoplastic therapies, whether surgical, medical or radiation based. In addition, life expectancy from other disease may be more self-limiting than the cancer itself, termed prognostic comorbidity. Scales have been developed in these areas as well. They have not been readily incorporated into the staging system, however.

Using laryngeal cancer patients as the cohort and a statistical technique called conjunctive consolidation, Piccirillo demonstrated a 5-year survival rate in stage I patients without severe comorbidity of 83% compared to a 17% survival rate in those with prognostic comorbidity. This dramatic difference suggests a major problem with hazard consistency if comorbidity is not acknowledged.

The 7th edition of the staging manual instituted chart abstractions to record and measure the influence of comorbidities on patient outcomes in various head and neck sites. This important innovation was largely due to the work of Piccirillo and will potentially yield benefits on which to base future significant changes to the system. This paper stands as a testament to innovative thinking in response to basic clinical observations.

A COMPARISON OF PUBLISHED HEAD AND NECK STAGE GROUPINGS IN CARCINOMAS OF THE ORAL CAVITY

Patti A Groome, Karleen Schulze, Morten Boysen, et al.

Background: The combination of T, N, and M, classifications into stage groupings is meant to facilitate a number of activities, including the estimation of prognosis and the comparison of therapeutic interventions among similar groups of cases. We tested the UICC/AJCC 5th edition stage grouping and seven other TNM-based groupings proposed for head and neck cancer for their ability to meet these expectations in a specific site: carcinomas of the oral cavity.

Methods: We defined four criteria to assess each grouping scheme: (1) the subgroups defined by T, N, and M that make up a given group within a grouping scheme have similar survival rates (hazard consistency); (2) the survival rates differ among the groups (hazard discrimination); (3) the prediction of cure is high (outcome prediction); and (4) the distribution of patients among the groups is balanced. We identified or derived a measure for each criterion, and the findings were summarized by use of a scoring system. The range of scores was from 0 (best) to 7 (worst). The data are population based from a prospectively gathered series in Southern Norway, with 556 patients diagnosed from 1983 through 1995. Clinical stage assignment was used, and the outcome of interest was cause-specific survival.

Results: Summary scores across the eight schemes ranged from 1.66 for TANIS-3 to 6.50 for UICC/AJCC-5. The TANIS-7 staging scheme performed best on the hazard consistency criterion. The kiricuta scheme performed best on the hazard discrimination criterion. Synderman predicted outcome best overall and Berg produced the most balanced distribution of cases among its groups.

Conclusions: UICC/AJCC stage groupings were defined without empirical investigation. When tested, this scheme did not perform as well as any of seven empirically derived schemes we evaluated. Our results suggest that the usefulness of the TNM system could be enhanced by optimizing the design of stage groupings through empirical investigation.

Groome PA, Schulze K, Boysen M, et al. A comparison of published head and neck stage groupings in carcinomas of the oral cavity. Head Neck. 2001;23:613-624.

Commentary by: *Carol R Bradford*

This article by Groome et al. evaluates the utility of the UICC/AJCC stage groupings in head and neck cancer in defining subsets of patients with similar disease severity. The authors demonstrate that, at least for carcinomas of the oral cavity, the UICC/AJCC stage groupings do not accurately define subsets of patients with similar disease severity/outcome. In fact, when the UICC/AJCC stage groupings were tested against seven distinct empirically derived schemes, the empirically derived schemes outperformed the UICC/AJCC staging system. The authors chose to utilize overall survival rather that disease control in testing these various staging schemes (empiric vs UICC/AJCC).

This paper, published over a decade ago, encouraged the staging organizations (UICC/AJCC) to optimize the design of stage groupings through empirical investigation. The authors selected a dataset of 556 cases of squamous cell carcinoma of the oral cavity from Southern Norway diagnosed from 1983 through 1995 and followed for a median of 37 months. This dataset was used to validate the accuracy of the various stage grouping schemes (i.e. what T, N, and M stage comprise the various stages I–IV of head and neck cancer). While the UICC/AJCC is the schema most widely adopted to date, the authors present compelling data that alternative stage grouping schemes would be much more accurate in predicting uniform outcome than UICC/AJCC schema. The two schemes most often tested against UICC/AJCC are TANIS and Hart. Overall, the TANIS-3 grouping scheme ranked first in summary scores whereas the UICC/AJCC performed the worst.

One of the many challenges of changing the widely accepted UICC/AJCC stage grouping schemes is that it would make comparison of future outcomes to past experience very difficult. Another challenge is the simple challenge of training the world community to learn a new staging system. Finally, the AJCC and UICC organizations have continued to refine the definitions of T, N, and M since this article was published to better achieve the goal of defining subsets of patients with similar disease severity. A review of the literature reveals that Groome et al. published additional papers in 2002 asserting the same deficiencies of the UICC/AJCC stage grouping schemes in tonsillar and laryngeal cancer patients and urging the cancer community to enhance the usefulness of the TNM system by optimizing the design of stage groupings through empirical investigation.

The authors discuss four important aspects of a staging system that determine its effectiveness: hazard consistency, hazard discrimination, predictive power, and balance. Hazard consistency refers to homogeneity within the group of similarly staged patients. In other words, patients with stage I tumors of the oral cavity should have similar survival rates. Hazard discrimination refers to heterogeneity between stage groups. For example, the survival of stage II patients should be significantly different from that of stage I patients. Predictive power refers to the ability of any staging system to predict outcome of populations with a reasonable degree of accuracy. Balance refers to equivalent size of the stage groups.

While Groome et al. raised important points about the weakness of the present stage grouping schema with the UICC/AJCC systems, these stage groupings have held up in the intervening decade. The reason for this is that the present system enjoys familiarity and ease of use. More complex systems are less likely to be used consistently or accurately by clinicians. The AJCC Head and Neck Task Force has continued to advocate for ongoing significant revisions to the staging system for head and neck cancer in order to improve the system's ability to compare similarly staged patients treated with various modalities and predict outcome.

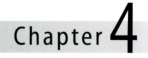

Chapter 4

Scalp and Skin

CHEMOSURGICAL TREATMENT OF CANCER OF THE SKIN
A Microscopically Controlled Method of Excision

Frederic E Mohs

The term "chemosurgery" was coined to designate a newly developed method for the treatment of cancer. The most important feature of the method is the technic by which thorough microscopic control of excision may be attained. This microscopic control makes possible, in effect, the selective destruction of cancer with the resultant dual advantages of unprecedented reliability and conservatism. The use of the method is limited to accessible regions of the body because the procedure is carried out in stages.

The development of the method, both in the laboratory and in the clinic, has been described as has been the application of the method in the treatment of cancer of the lip, nose, ear, eyelid, face, extremities and trunk. The present article concerns the chemosurgical treatment of cancer of the skin except for the orificial cancers affecting the lips, vulva, penis and anus. The therapeutic results in a consecutive series of 814 cases in which the patients were observed for a period of three years or more are presented.

Mohs FE. Chemosurgical treatment of cancer of the skin: a microscopically controlled method of excision. JAMA. 1948;564-569.

Commentary by: *Philip L Bailin, Allison T Vidimos*

Mohs surgery has had a major worldwide impact on the way challenging cutaneous malignancies are treated. Originally known as chemosurgery, it is now referred to as Mohs micrographic surgery (MMS), Mohs surgery, or less often as fresh tissue chemosurgery. The values of this technique are the combination of unmatched reliability of tumor removal coupled with a high degree of conservatism (i.e. tissue sparing). The key components are the excision of a layer of tissue; the drawing of a detailed anatomic map of the area of excision; the division of the specimen into segments with color-coded margins, and the corresponding recording of those coded segments onto the map; the cutting and staining of unique tangentially oriented frozen sections of each segment; and the microscopic analysis by the Mohs surgeon of the entire deep and lateral margins of the specimen. This process is repeated sequentially wherever any marginal tumor is identified until all margins are clear.

Frederic E Mohs MD, was a Brittingham Research Assistant to Professor Michael F Guyer, Chairman of the Department of Zoology at the University of Wisconsin in the 1930s. While studying the potential curative effects of injecting various chemicals into different neoplasms, they discovered that zinc chloride solution caused non-selective tissue necrosis but preserved microscopic features necessary for analysis. Mohs realized that his quest for a chemical cancer cure had led to a means of fixing tissue *in situ,* allowing for precise controlled excisions of cancer. Prior to this landmark 1948 publication, Mohs had published several papers, starting in 1941, which described the development of the chemosurgical paste and its use in treating cancer in rats, as well as successful use of chemosurgery in the treatment of human skin cancers on the lip, nose, ear, eyelid, face, extremities, and trunk. This seminal article detailed the method of the fixed tissue technique for skin cancer removal, which allowed optimal removal of the skin cancer cells while sparing non-involved tissue. The zinc chloride fixative paste was compounded by a local pharmacist in Madison, Wisconsin, utilizing stibnite (a granular antimony ore) and Sanguinaria Canadensis (bloodroot) powder as the vehicle. Mohs patented the paste and then generously sold the rights to the Wisconsin Alumni Association for $1 in 1944.

Mohs described the chemosurgical technique with the following steps: (1) chemical fixation *in situ* of the tissue suspected of being cancerous by applying a paste containing zinc chloride after prepping the skin with dichloroacetic acid to improve penetration of the fixative; (2) excision of a layer of the fixed tissue with precise color-coded mapping of each tissue segment; (3) slide preparation that utilized unique tangentially cut frozen sections that allowed *complete microscopic examination* of *all deep and peripheral margins* and precise location of the cancerous tissue by systematic microscopic examination of the tissue by the surgeon; (4) further chemical treatment of the areas demonstrated to be involved with tumor; and (5) repetition of the process until a tumor-free margin was obtained. An example of a large basal cell carcinoma of the temple involving periosteum of the orbital rim that necessitated four stages of chemosurgery was illustrated.

This 1948 publication in *JAMA* summarized the outcomes of the fixed tissue technique on 814 consecutively treated cutaneous basal cell carcinomas and squamous cell carcinomas, over one third of which had recurred after surgical, radiation, or caustic treatment. He reported 555 cases of basal cell carcinoma, 458 of which were determinate with a 97.4% cure rate at 3 years or longer, and 96.2% cure rate in 291 cases observed for 5 years or more. Adverse prognostic factors included large tumor size > 3 cm, recurrent lesions, infiltrative growth pattern, and location on the ear, eyelids, or nose. The cure rate was 85.6% for 222 squamous cell carcinomas observed for 3 years and 84.4% for 136 cases observed for 5 years or more. Adverse prognostic factors included large tumor size > 2 cm, recurrent tumors, higher histologic grade, location on the ear and hands, and presence of metastases. Advantages of chemosurgery using the zinc chloride paste included optimal cure rates, low operative mortality, lack of interference with second intention healing, lack of systemic toxicity, and conservation of normal tissue. The disadvantages included treatment that frequently extended over several days, as each layer took one day to complete due to the time required for the paste to fix the tissue before excision; pain, fever and lymphadenopathy associated with the fixative application; and delay in reconstruction due to postoperative sloughing of the fixed tissue, which took up to 7 days to complete. Mohs popularized using second-intention wound healing extensively, and noted superior cosmetic outcomes over first-intention surgical repairs, especially in concave areas such as the temple and medial canthus. His published cure rates using chemosurgery for cutaneous carcinomas were superior to reported outcomes of treatment of cutaneous carcinomas with wide excision, radiation, or other destructive treatments at the time.

The fresh tissue technique evolved over the next 20 years, initially when Mohs excised tumors over cartilage on the ear or nasal alas without pretreatment with the zinc chloride paste in order to spare the cartilage. Subsequently, he employed the fresh tissue technique to treat eyelid tumors and wrote about the technique in the textbook *Skin Surgery* in 1956. He presented the fresh tissue technique employed to treat nonmelanoma skin cancers in 70 patients in 1969 at the American College of Chemo-surgery and published the series of eyelid tumors in 1970 in the Bulletin of the American College of Chemosurgery. Samuel Stegman and Theodore Tromovitch subsequently published a series of patients treated with the fresh tissue technique in 1974 in the *Archives of Dermatology* after which time the technique became widely accepted for skin cancers in all anatomic locations. Mohs later published a series of 3,466 nonmelanoma skin cancer patients treated using the fresh tissue technique with a 99.8% cure rate in 1976 in the *Archives of Dermatology*. The advantages of the fresh tissue technique included the ability to remove several stages in 1 day and complete wound reconstruction on the same day without the need to allow separation of the eschar caused by the zinc chloride paste. There was no chemically induced pain or inflammation. Although the fresh tissue technique became the more widely employed, Mohs continued to use the fixed tissue technique to treat tumors invading bone, invasive melanoma, penile carcinoma, as well as osteomyelitis and gangrene. It became recognized that the key factor in the reliability of the "Mohs" technique was the uniquely precise margin control it afforded through mapping and tangential frozen section analysis rather than any destructive effect of the chemical paste on cancer cells. Another benefit of the fresh tissue technique was that it was even more tissue sparing because no additional tumor-free tissue was chemically destroyed.

The applications of MMS have extended to optimizing treatment of many other tumors including dermatofibrosarcoma protuberans, atypical fibroxanthoma, microcystic adnexal carcinoma, sebaceous carcinoma, extramammary Paget's disease, Merkel cell carcinoma, and leiomyosarcoma, among others. Tumors that do not grow in continuity or that are not easily identified on frozen sections may not be as effectively managed with MMS. The "slow Mohs" technique may be employed to excise tumors that are difficult to interpret on frozen sections and involves performing paraffin sections on the excised and color-coded tissue segments. This method may take days to complete and therefore delay reconstruction. Special immunohistochemical stains can also be done on frozen tissue in the Mohs lab to enhance the ability of the Mohs surgeon to interpret the tumor margins in such tumors as malignant melanoma, DFSP, and poorly differentiated squamous cell carcinoma. Rapid immunostains for frozen tissue are being developed to minimize the delay involved.

The multidisciplinary management of complex cutaneous tumors has optimized the management of head and neck tumors, and publications describing a team approach with the head and neck surgeon, facial plastics, or plastic surgeon excising the tumor under general anesthesia and the Mohs surgeon performing the tissue mapping and pathologic interpretation have illustrated the excellent cure rates and reconstructive outcomes with this approach. The extended operating times required by such an approach have proven justified by much improved cure rates and the avoidance of the need to operate multiple times to achieve clear margins. This approach is also highly conservative of normal tissue in critical anatomic areas so that function and cosmesis may be optimal. It also allows the surgeon to perform reconstruction with a much greater likelihood that the reconstructed area will not have to be damaged later by incomplete resection and tumor recurrence.

Formal fellowships to teach the MMS technique began in the early 1980s, and are now under the auspices of the ACGME. There are currently over 1,000 fellowship-trained Mohs surgeons in the United States. Mohs micrographic surgery is practiced worldwide and continues to provide unmatched cure rates and optimal functional and cosmetic outcomes for high-risk cutaneous tumors.

PERINEURAL INVASION IN SQUAMOUS CELL SKIN CARCINOMA OF THE HEAD AND NECK

Helmuth Goepfert, William J Dichtel, Jesus E Medina, et al.

The perineural space has been recognized as a route of spread for various types of cancer. In the past, the space was believed to be part of the lymphatic vessel network, and Ernst thought of it as the connecting channel between the central nervous system and the subarachnoid space on one end and the peripheral lymph nodes on the other. Later studies dispelled this myth. The extension of this virtual space and communication with the subarachnoid lining has been demonstrated experimentally by injection of local anesthetic and through the identification of cancer cell growth. The dissemination of tumor along this pathway assumes both a centrifugal and centripetal direction. Several reports have remarked on the propensity of squamous cell carcinoma and salivary gland carcinomas of the head and neck to disseminate preferentially in a perineural pattern, and most reports have noted this to be associated with more aggressive tumor behavior. Occasionally, basal cell carcinomas will take this route of spread. This neurotropic invasion may be the exclusive form of tumor progression, or it may be one of several manifestations of the cancer's annihilating ability.

We present our experience with patients who had squamous cell carcinomas of the skin of the head and neck with perineural invasion who were treated during a 10-year period at The University of Texas M.D. Anderson Hospital and Tumor Institute at Houston. Several parameters were investigated in these patients and were compared with those of patients admitted during that same period of time for treatment of squamous cell carcinoma of the skin without perineural invasion.

Goepfert H, Dichtel WJ, Medina JE, et al. Perineural invasion in squamous cell skin carcinoma of the head and Neck. Am J Surg. 1984;148:542-547.

Commentary by: *Richard J Wong*

Perineural invasion (PNI) has been defined by the pathologist Dr John Batsakis as the extension of tumor cells in, around, or along nerves. PNI is now widely recognized as a highly adverse pathologic factor for a variety of malignancies, and has been associated with increased local recurrence and diminished survival as an independent variable in many retrospective studies. This ominous clinical and pathologic event is particularly prevalent in cancers originating from the pancreas, prostate, head and neck, salivary glands (e.g., adenoid cystic cancer), and colon, among others.

One of the earliest and most influential reports to recognize the clinical significance of PNI appeared in 1984, when Dr Helmuth Goepfert and his colleagues reported on outcomes of PNI in head and neck skin cancer in *The American Journal of Surgery (148:542–547, 1984)*. This retrospective study is one of the largest and earliest reports to focus entirely on this specific entity. The authors reviewed a series of 520 patients with skin cancers of the head and neck treated between 1970 and 1979 at the MD Anderson Hospital. Clinical outcomes were compared between 72 patients who were found to have PNI documented in one or more "major nerve trunks" and 448 patients lacking this specific definition of PNI.

In this study, Dr Goepfert made many seminal findings of lasting importance. PNI was statistically linked to: (1) identification of regional nodal metastases, (2) identification of distant metastases, and (3) diminished survival. The sheer magnitude of the survival difference presented in this study is particularly striking, with 10-year survival rates of just under 90% for patients lacking PNI, as compared to approximately 25% for those with PNI of "major nerve trunks". The study very nicely presents the distribution of the involved cranial nerves (mostly trigeminal and facial nerves) and of the presenting symptoms (asymptomatic, followed by pain, anesthesia, and facial paralysis), along with a series of eight case reports that illustrate the spectrum of the course of this disease. Readers may note, however, that some data are lacking in this report, including descriptions of: (1) tumor differentiation, size, stage, and location, (2) patient demographics and length of follow-up, (3) pathologic criteria for PNI, (4) treatment regimens, and (5) patterns of recurrence. Nonetheless, this study clearly establishes a clear take-home point that was far ahead of its time: PNI is a distinct clinical and pathologic event that heralds poor clinical outcome.

Nearly 30 years after the publication of this work, Dr Goepfert's findings still remain highly relevant, and the scope of this study still dwarfs most clinical reports of PNI that are currently being published. Recent scientific research has now provided a glimpse into the intricate mechanisms underlying the phenomenon of PNI. There is strong evidence that nerve microenvironment is a key facilitator in the process of PNI through the release of a variety of proteins that may attract cancer cells to nerves. Studies have demonstrated that cancer cells actively migrate towards and along nerves through specific ligand-receptor interactions and downstream signaling pathway activation. This process can be interrupted at a variety of different stages (nerve ligand release, cancer cell receptor function, downstream signaling) to impede the process of PNI in both *in vitro* co-culture and animal models. This recognition that the nerve is key co-conspirator in enabling the process of PNI may hopefully lead to novel therapeutic strategies aimed at disrupting these interactions rather than simply targeting cancer cell death. Future progress in further deciphering the mechanisms of PNI will be built on the strong foundation of clinical data presented in Dr Goepfert's landmark study.

PROGNOSTIC FACTORS FOR LOCAL RECURRENCE, METASTASIS, AND SURVIVAL RATES AND SQUAMOUS CELL CARCINOMA OF THE SKIN, EAR, AND LIP
Implications for Treatment Modality Selection

Dan E Rowe, Raymond J Carroll, Calvin L Day, et al.

We reviewed all studies since 1940 on the prognosis of squamous cell carcinoma (SCC) of the skin and lip. The following variables are correlated with local recurrence and metastatic rates: (1) treatment modality, (2) prior treatment, (3) location, (4) size, (5) depth, (6) histologic differentiation, (7) histologic evidence of perineural involvement, (8) precipitating factors other than ultraviolet light, and (9) host immunosuppression. Local recurrences occur less frequently when SCC is treated by Mohs micrographic surgery. This local recurrence rate differential in favor of Mohs micrographic surgery holds true for primary SCC of the skin and lip (3.1% vs 10.9%), for ear SCC (5.3% vs 18.7%), for locally recurrent (previously treated) SCC (10% vs 23.3%), for ear SCC (5.3% vs 18.7%), for locally recurrent (previously treated) SCC (10% vs 23.3%), for SCC with perineural involvement (0% vs 47%), for SCC of size greater than 2 cm (25.2% vs 41.7%), and for SCC that is poorly differentiated (32.6% vs 53.6%).

Rowe DE, Carroll RJ, Day CL, et al. Prognostic factors for local recurrence metastasis, and survival rates and squamous cell carcinoma of the skin, ear, and lip: Implications for treatment modality selection. J Am Acad Dermatol. 1992;26:976-990.

Commentary by: *Randal S Weber*

In 1992, Rowe et al. published a meta-analysis of several selected papers published on the influence of clinico-pathologic factors and the type of treatment administered for patients with cutaneous squamous cell carcinoma of the head and neck and how these factors influenced outcome. Multiple scientific papers that consistently reported demographics, tumor site, stage, presence of immunosuppression, treatment modality, duration of follow-up, histopathologic data on tumor size, depth of invasion, presence or absence of perineural invasion, and tumor differentiation were examined to determine their impact on local-regional control and survival. The authors also examined how patterns of failure were related to the length of follow-up. They defined short-term follow-up as < 5 years and long-term follow-up as ≥ 5 years. Through a broad literature search incorporating the following treatment-related variables: radiation, curettage, electrodessication, cryotherapy, or Mohs excision versus conventional surgical resection, duration of follow-up, 71 studies were identified that met the inclusion criteria from which a pooled data set was developed. Outcome measures of local, regional, and distant failure were stratified by the length of follow-up into short term or long term. In addition, the primary site was evaluated with respect to its influence on the rates of local, regional, and distant failure. Primary tumor sites were defined as general skin, ear, lip, and whether or not the tumor arose within a pre-existing scar. A subset of 43 manuscripts was included to determine the impact of immuno-suppression, histologic differentiation, size of the primary tumor, prior treatment, depth of invasion, and perineural spread.

Regardless of the treatment modality administered, curettage, electro-dessication, radiation therapy, MOHS excision, or conventional excision, local recurrence rates increased as a function of longer follow-up. The longer latency period noted for some recurrences may be a biologic characteristic of cutaneous SCC or may represent new adjacent second primaries. For patients who presented with locally recurrent tumors who were treated for cure, their local recurrence rate was 23.3% with 5 or more years of follow-up and exceeded the failure rate for those patients without prior treat-ment. Another risk factor for recurrence was tumors arising on the pinna, which had an 18% risk of local recurrence.

In this review, metastatic rates increased with longer follow-up irrespec-tive of tumor site. The metastatic rate for sun-exposed sites of the head and neck increased from 2.3% to 5.2% with longer follow-up. For patients with squamous carcinomas arising within a pre-existing scar, metastatic rates were 26% and 38% with shorter and longer intervals of follow-up, respectively. Within the entire analysis of nearly 1,000 patients, the overall regional metastatic rate was 11%. Ninety-five percent of the local recurrences or metastasis were noted within 5 years of follow-up. The majority of regional metastasis, or 91%, were detected within 2 years of initial treatment.

Numerous factors were evaluated to assess their relationship with the risk of local failure and regional metastasis. Using these data the clinician is able to identify patients at higher risk for local-regional failure who might benefit from more frequent surveillance and/or adjuvant radiation. The local recurrence rate for patients with tumors greater than 2 cm was 15.2% and the metastatic rate was 30% as opposed to a 7.4% local recurrence rate and a 9% metastatic rate for patients with smaller tumors. For thicker tumors defined as greater than or equal to 4 mm or with Clarke's level IV or V invasion, local recurrence and metastatic rates were 17% and 45%, respectively, as opposed to 5.3% and 6.7% local failure and metastatic rates among patients with thinner tumors (Clarke's Level I–III). Differentiation had a significant impact on both local recurrence and regional metastatic rates, with nearly 30% of patients with poorly differentiated tumors having local recurrence or metastasis, whereas the more well-differentiated tumors had a 13% and a 9% incidence of local failure and regional metastasis. Other factors significant for higher risk of local and regional failure included recurrence after prior treatment and perineural invasion. The latter had a nearly 50% local recurrence rate and a 50% metastatic rate.

The authors compare conventional surgical resection with MOHS excision from the perspective of local-regional control. They also examined other histopathologic factors and their influence on tumor control as a function the treatment modality administered. In every histopathologic category the authors reported better outcomes with MOHS surgery: tumors greater than 2 cm and well-differentiated histology vs poorly differentiated tumors. Interestingly, for neurotropic tumors that are associated with high local-regional failure rates, conventional surgical excision had a 47% local failure rate as opposed to 0% for MOHS. Likewise, the metastatic rate for patients treated by conventional excision was 47%, and for MOHS surgery it was 8.3%. In evaluating patients with regional metastasis the authors found that patients who had surgery followed by radiation had a cure rate of 25% versus 45% for surgery alone. The analysis also highlighted the impact of immunosuppression either from organ transplant, leukemia, or lymphoma and its influence on recurrence rates, which were 5- to 20-fold higher in the immunocompromised patient. The authors admit that a direct comparison of MOHS excision versus conventional surgery is problematic given the retrospective nature of the data, thus making sweeping generalizations difficult. The authors, however, did conclude that, overall, MOHS surgery produces better local-regional control and survival than conventional surgical excision.

The significance of this study is the examination of a large cohort of patients with cutaneous SCC, permitting an analysis of the impact of clinical, pathologic, and treatment factors that impact recurrence rates and survival. Important findings were the impact of tumor site, tumor thickness, prior treatment, length of follow-up, and the type of treatment rendered. The data allows the clinician to identify the patient at high risk for local-regional recurrence who might benefit from the addition of radiation following surgical excision to decrease the risk for recurrence. These findings have been demonstrated in prior studies and are associated with little controversy. Where the results and conclusions are less substantiated is the advocacy for MOHS surgery being more efficacious than conventional excision. First, the data with respect to the type of excision is retrospective rather than prospectively acquired. To actually compare the two modalities directly, a randomized prospective trial would be necessary, with stratification for tumor site, stage, thickness, and prior treatment. Obviously, this would be a complex undertaking and possibly not feasible given the extreme heterogeneity of the disease. Aggressive cutaneous SCC is a lethal disease that deserves respect. Inadequately treated patients will recur, and 30–40% of patients will die of their disease. The premise that MOHS surgery has a higher margin clearance rate than en bloc surgical resection is untested. It defies the biology of aggressive cutaneous SCC to consider narrow margin surgery as is performed by most MOHS surgeons as being more effective than an oncologic resection. Aggressive tumors are often associated with deep invasion, cranial nerve invasion and regional metastasis, all requiring an oncologic approach in their management. Furthermore, selection bias may exist when deciding which patients should have MOHS surgery over conventional excision. Patients with deeply invasive cutaneous SCC over the parotid gland are more likely to undergo en bloc resection and parotidectomy as opposed to MOHS excision. Finally, many confounding variables likely exist as the authors attempted to compare conventional resection with MOHS surgery.

IMPLICATIONS FOR CLINICAL STAGING OF METASTATIC CUTANEOUS SQUAMOUS CARCINOMA OF THE HEAD AND NECK BASED ON A MULTICENTER STUDY OF TREATMENT OUTCOMES

Jennifer L Andruchow, Michael J Veness, Gary J Morgan, et al.

Background: Cutaneous squamous cell carcinoma (SCC) of the head and neck is a common cancer that has the potential to metastasize to lymph nodes in the parotid gland and neck. Previous studies have highlighted limitations with the current TNM staging system for metastatic skin carcinoma. The aim of this study was to test a new staging system that may provide better discrimination between patient groups.

Methods: A retrospective multicenter study was conducted on 322 patients from three Australian and three North American institutions. All had metastatic cutaneous SCC involving the parotid gland and/or neck and all were treated for cure with a minimum follow-up time of 2 years. These patients were restaged using a newly proposed system that separated parotid disease (P stage) from neck disease (N stage) and included subgroups of P and N stage. Metastases involved the parotid in 260 patients (149 P1; 78 P2; 33 P3) and 43 of these had clinical neck disease also (22 N1: 21 N2). Neck metastases alone occurred in 62 patients (26 N1: 36 N2). Ninety percent of patients were treated surgically and 267 of 322 received radiotherapy.

Results: Neck nodes were pathologically involved in 32% of patients with parotid metastases. Disease recurred in 105 (33%) of the 322 patients, involving the parotid in 42 neck in 33 and distant sites in 30. Parotid recurrence did not vary significantly with P stage. Disease-specific survival was 74% at 5 years. Survival was significantly worse for patients with advanced P stage: 69% survival at 5 years compared with 82% for those with early P stage (P = 0.02) and for those with both parotid and neck node involvement pathologically: 61% survival compared with 79% for those with parotid disease alone (P = 0.027). Both univariate and multivariate analysis confirmed these findings. Clinical neck involvement among patients with parotid metastases did not significantly worsen survival (P = 0.01).

Conclusions: This study, which included a mixed cohort of patients from six different institutions, provides further information about the clinical behavior of metastatic cutaneous SCC of the head and neck. The hypothesis that separation of parotid and neck disease in a new staging system is supported by the results. The benefit of having subgroups of P and N stage is uncertain, but it is likely to identify patients with unfavorable characteristics that may benefit from further research.

Andruchow JL, Veness MJ, Morgan GJ, et al. Implications for clinical staging of metastatic cutaneous squamous carcinoma of the head and neck based on a multicenter study of treatment outcomes. Cancer. 2006;106:1078-1083.

Commentary by: *Fernando L Dias*

Cutaneous squamous cell carcinoma of the head and neck (CSCCHN) represents 25% of all nonmelanoma skin cancers. Because skin cancer is known to be induced by sunlight exposure, CSCCHN incidence directly relates to the proximity to the equator as well as to the predominant population, particularly Caucasians and Anglo Celtic descents. The impact of the previously mentioned characteristics is responsible for the contrast between the annual incidence of CSCCHN ranging from 16/100000 in central Europe to 300/100000 in Australia. In most patients with CSCCHN, the prognosis is good, with cure rates exceeding 95% when the primary tumor can be completely excised; the reported risk for local recurrence, regional metastases, and distant metastases is 5%, 5%, and 1%, respectively.

Given the high incidence of CSCCHN to low metastatic rate, most of these tumors are not investigated or treated for occult metastases but rather treated based on positive clinical examination. Nevertheless, the rates of metastatic disease associated with CSCCHN in patients with selected high-risk features may exceed 20%, with a significant impact on survival. Several clinicopathological factors associated with an increased risk of lymph node metastases have been identified in the literature. Certain characteristics such as increased tumor size, thickness, poor differentiation, desmoplasia, perineural and lymphovascular invasion, as well as immunosuppression have been associated with an increased risk of nodal involvement and poor outcome. This is known to be a biologically aggressive disease with a high incidence of extranodal spread, usually requiring aggressive combined treatment.

The most common sites of nodal metastases from CSCCHN are the parotid gland, in particular the parotid tail/external jugular lymph node junction, and the upper cervical nodes. There is also considerable data indicating that the location of the primary tumor predicts the site of nodal disease. Retrospective data from Australian cancer centers, analyzing a large cohort of patients with CSCCHN undergoing neck dissections, demonstrated that the parotid gland was involved in 75% and level II in approximately 40% of patients.

Previously, the TNM staging system used internationally for CSCCHN had a simple classification for regional metastatic disease with minimal clinical applicability and limited prognostic value. This has prompted a number of studies aimed at designing a staging system that could be applied incorporating the already known clinicopathological high-risk criteria for T staging as well as N staging criteria identical to those of mucosal head and neck squamous cell carcinoma (SCC).

The independent significance of lymph node metastases in the parotid gland and neck was suggested by various studies. O'Brien, in 2002, therefore proposed the P/N staging system to allow better assessment of prognostic factors and treatment outcomes in patients with CSCCHN. In this study, clinical staging was carried out prospectively in 87 patients. The extent of parotidectomy was based on the clinical extent of disease, so that patients with mobile localized tumors and normal facial nerve (FN) function had, in general, conservative parotidectomies, preserving the FN. Those patients with massive tumors or FN involvement, on the other hand, had radical excisions, sacrificing the nerve. The multivariate analysis demonstrated that increasing P stage, positive margins, and failure to have postoperative radiotherapy independently predicted for decreased control in the parotid region. Survival did not correlate with P stage, probably due to the fact that many patients staged P1 and P2 also presented with lymph node metastases. Clinical and pathologic N stage significantly influenced survival, as expected. The authors stressed that the principal aim of this study was to draw attention to the limitations of the staging system used at that time for cutaneous malignancy recommended by the AJCC (2002). They concluded that the proposed system or some other model should be tested with a much larger patient cohort to confirm whether the extent of metastatic disease in the parotid gland has prognostic significance.

Based on previous studies, which highlighted the limitations with the TNM staging system for metastatic skin carcinoma, a multicentric study was conducted by Andruchow et al. to test a new staging system that may provide better discrimination among patient groups. Clinical and pathologic information of 322 patients from three Australian and three North American institutions was retrospectively accrued. To be eligible, patients needed to be previously untreated and to have received definitive therapy with the aim of cure (with histologically proven metastatic SCC involving the parotid gland and/or lymph nodes of the neck with at least 2 years of follow-up). Patient data were de-identified and clinically restaged according to the proposed new staging system. The majority of patients (67%) had disease only in the parotid gland, and the majority of these (130 of 217) had early stage disease (P1). Neck disease alone was found in only 19% of patients, with more than half of these N2 disease. False positive rates for clinical examination of the parotid gland and neck in this retrospective study were 13% and 14%, respectively. Once again, the authors found a nonsignificant trend towards a worse survival as P stage increased, but this became statistically significant when patients staged P1 were separated from those clinically staged P2 and P3 (p = .022). Likewise, clinical N stage only had a significant influence on survival when patients clinically staged N0 were separated from those clinically staged N1 and N2 (p = .026). Survival was also worse among patients with metastatic involvement of the parotid gland and neck nodes (p = .027). When multivariate analysis was carried out, clinical parotid stage (P3), and pathologic neck stage (N1, N2) had independent influence on survival (p = .033 and p = .005, respectively). The authors analyzed their own study as an honest attempt to gather data from a number of centers to increase knowledge on the clinical behavior of CSCCHN.

The authors made it clear that the TNM staging classification used at that time had a simplistic and limited power to adequately discriminate the prognosis of these patients. The N1 staging classification at that time would apply equally to a patient with a single 2 cm parotid metastases, a patient with a larger (6 cm) parotid metastases with FN invasion, and a patient with metastases in both parotid gland and neck nodes. Although local control in the parotid bed did not vary statistically significantly with P stage, this study was able to prove its influence in survival. The authors also adequately analyzed the impact of clinical neck disease in addition to parotid disease on survival, recognizing the potential confounding effect of false-positive and false-negative neck disease rates in this study. Although the application of this staging system was an important achievement and that the discrimination between parotid (P) and neck metastases (N) underlies our current treatment philosophies, the value of subgrouping within the P and N stages remained uncertain.

Additional staging systems have been published in an attempt to simplify the O'Brien P/N system, such as the ITEM prognostic score (incorporating the Immunosuppression, Treatment, Extra-nodal spread, and Margin status [ITEM] into three risk groups for assessment of treatment outcomes) and the N1S3 system (New staging system according to the number and size of involved lymph nodes, incorporating the parotid gland as one of the regional levels), contributing to better understanding of the biological behavior of CSCCHN.

Finally, the 7th edition of the AJCC staging manual has incorporated the current information available to make substantial changes to the T and N staging criteria. The T stage incorporates size, bone invasion, as well as pathological high-risk criteria (thickness, perineural invasion, site, and differentiation). The N staging criteria became identical to those of mucosal head and neck SCC. The article entitled "Implications for Clinical Staging of Metastatic Cutaneous Squamous Carcinoma of the Head and Neck Based on a Multicenter Study of Treatment Outcomes" has provided important information about the clinical behavior of CSCCHN, confirming the importance of adding P and N stages for the prognostication of cancer-specific survival in these patients.

PATTERNS OF LYMPH NODE SPREAD OF CUTANEOUS SQUAMOUS CELL CARCINOMA OF THE HEAD AND NECK

Tom J Vauterin, Michael J Veness, Garry J Morgan, et al.

Background: Among patients with cutaneous squamous cell carcinoma (SCC) of the head and neck, recent studies have shown that those with involvement of the parotid gland also have a high incidence of neck node involvement. Treatment of the neck by either surgery or radiotherapy is therefore recommended among patients with parotid SCC, even if clinical examination is negative. The aim of this study was first to analyze patterns of metastatic spread in the parotid and cervical lymph nodes and then to correlate the pattern of involved nodes with the primary cutaneous site in order to guide the appropriate extent of surgery, should neck dissection be used to treat the neck in patients with parotid SCC.

Methods: A cohort of 209 patients with cutaneous SCC of the head and neck and clinically evident regional metastatic disease was reviewed retrospectively from 3 Australian institutions. The distribution of involved nodes was obtained from pathology reports; the anatomic sites of primary cutaneous cancers were then correlated with these findings.

Results: Among 209 patients 171 (82%) had clinical parotid involvement. Of these, 28 had clinical neck disease, whereas 143 had parotid disease alone. Thirty-eight (18%) patients had neck disease only. A total of 199 patients were treated surgically, whereas 10 received radiotherapy alone. Surgery included 172 parotidectomies and 151 neck dissections (93 of which were elective). Primary sites were cheek (21.7%), pinna (20.4%), temple (15.8%), forehead (15.8%), postauricular region (5.9%), neck (5.3%), anterior scalp (5.3%), posterior scalp (3.3%), periorbital (3.3%), nose (2.6%), and chin (0.6%). Among pathologically positive necks, level II was most frequently involved (79%). Level IV (13%) and level V (17%) were only involved in extensive lymph node disease, the exception being for isolated level V metastases from the posterior scalp.

Conclusions: Primary sites were mainly localized to the lateral aspect of the head. Among patients with cutaneous SCC involving the parotid and neck level II was the most commonly involved neck level. The distribution of involved nodes suggests that in a patient with parotid involvement and a clinically negative neck with an anterolateral primary, a supraomohyoid neck dissection, always including the external jugular lymph node(s) would be appropriate. In the case of a posterior primary, level V should be dissected as well. In patients with parotid SCC and a clinically positive neck, a comprehensive neck dissection is recommended.

Vauterin TJ, Veness MJ, Morgan GJ, et al. Patterns of lymph node spread of cutaneous squamous cell carcinoma of the head and neck. Head Neck. 2006;28:785-791.

Commentary by: *Ashok R Shaha*

Vauterin and his colleagues from Australia clearly have great experience in the management of cutaneous squamous cell carcinoma and metastatic disease to the parotid region and neck. Prognostically, even though squamous cell carcinoma and basal cell carcinoma are considered to show excellent long-term outcome, patients who present with metastatic disease to the parotid region or the neck generally have a much poorer prognosis and a high incidence of recurrence and subsequent mortality. The management of advanced cutaneous carcinoma is quite complex, not only for the wide excision of the lesion, appropriate reconstruction and follow-up, but also in relation to the metastatic disease involving the parotid region and upper neck. The resection of tumor in the parotid region was mainly based around the identification of all gross tumors and the preservation of facial nerve function. The oncologic principle of the removal of all gross tumors is extremely critical, along with understanding the patterns of metastatic disease to the upper neck when the parotid shows metastatic squamous cell carcinoma.

Chris O'Brien had a long-standing interest in head and neck cutaneous malignancies, including squamous cell carcinoma, and a special interest in melanoma. His contributions in the field of melanoma are well recognized around the world. Unfortunately, he passed away a few years back at a very young age of a brain tumor; however, his contributions are long lasting, and I am very happy to summarize his philosophy in the management of cutaneous squamous cell carcinoma. Recent studies have shown that with involvement of the parotid gland, there is also a high incidence of neck node involvement. The authors have therefore recommended either surgery or radiation therapy for patients with parotid squamous cell carcinoma even if clinical examination is negative. This manuscript describes the patterns of metastatic spread to the parotid and cervical lymph node. They reviewed an experience of 209 patients with cutaneous squamous cell carcinoma of the head and neck from three Australian institutions. Among the 209 patients studied in this manuscript, 171 (82%) had clinical evidence of parotid involvement, while only 28 had clinical evidence of neck disease. Surgery included 172 parotidectomies and 151 neck dissections, 93 of which were considered elective. The primary sites were the cheek, pinna, temple, forehead, postauricular region, scalp, periorbital area, nose, and chin. Among the pathologically positive necks, level II was most frequently involved (79%), while level IV (13%) and level V (17%) were only involved in extensive lymph node metastasis. Isolated level V metastasis was rarely seen in tumors originating primarily in the posterior scalp.

The authors concluded that in patients with cutaneous squamous cell carcinoma involving the parotid and neck, level II was the most commonly involved neck level. They recommended, based on the distribution of the involved nodes, that in patients with parotid involvement and clinically negative neck with anterolateral primary, a supraomohyoid neck dissection should be considered. While in patients with posterior primary level V should be dissected as well. In patients with parotid squamous cell carcinoma and a clinically positive neck, a comprehensive neck dissection is recommended.

Cutaneous malignancy is a common disease in Australia, with the majority of the skin cancers originating in the head and neck region. Understanding the etiology, pathophysiology, and patterns of spread with special emphasis on the parotid and neck region is extremely critical in the overall management of squamous cell carcinoma. The true incidence of lymph node metastasis from squamous cell carcinoma of the head and neck remains somewhat uncertain; however, it is well known that the parotid gland is the most common site of metastatic disease, and clearly, the management of this region revolves around an appropriate parotidectomy and the preservation of facial nerve function. The authors have previously demonstrated the high incidence of clinical (26%) as well as occult neck disease (35%) in patients with metastatic cutaneous squamous cell carcinoma involving the parotid. The patterns of nodal metastasis are very well described from many different institutions, with the highest incidence of metastatic disease to level II. The surgical procedure generally should include a supraomohyoid neck dissection, with the removal of the lymph nodes at levels I, II and III; however, if the primary originated in the posterior scalp region, level V should be included. Appropriate skeletonization of the accessory nerve is critical, and dissection and preservation of the facial nerve is also important. In the O'Brien study, the lateral aspect of the head and neck (cheek, pinna, and temple) was the most common site of origin, followed by lesions of the forehead and postauricular region.

There continues to be considerable debate about sentinel node biopsy in patients with high-risk cutaneous squamous cell carcinoma. Even though there appears to be some enthusiasm in a few institutions, the authors do not have major support for sentinel node biopsy as the incidence of nodal disease is quite high and a formal surgical procedure would be much more beneficial. However, patients with recurrent disease, larger tumors or thickness more than 4 mm may be considered for sentinel node biopsy. The authors have interestingly described the presence of external jugular lymph node, which usually lies superficial to the anterior border of the sternomastoid muscle and now a part of a specific level, but it is a common site for metastatic spread. The authors have recommended the excision of this lymph node in any lymphadenectomy for cutaneous cancer including squamous cell carcinoma and melanoma. Due attention should be paid to the superficial occipital nodes in patients presenting with primary tumor involving the posterior aspect of the head, and surgery should also incorporate the removal of occipital nerves. Kraus et al. from Sloan-Kettering have reviewed their experience with 41 patients undergoing neck dissection for regional metastatic disease from squamous cell carcinoma of the head and neck. Eighty percent of the patients received postoperative radiation therapy. The majority of the patients had tumors larger than 2 cm and a depth more than 4 mm. However, the overall 2- and 5-year survival rates were dismal–33% and 22%, respectively. The clinical staging of the neck proved to be the major prognostic factor. Their studies also reported patients with impaired immune system exhibiting high incidence of nodal metastasis.

A similar study predicting the patterns of regional metastasis was also published by Ibrahimi and O'Brien from the Sydney Cancer Center in Australia. Their recommendations regarding selective neck dissection remained the same, including levels I-III for facial primaries, level II and III for anterior scalp, and level II-V for posterior scalp and neck primaries. Furthermore, in 2010 the authors stated that the dissection of levels IV and V could safely be omitted, except in patients with posterior scalp or neck primaries. They also concluded that level I dissection is only necessary in patients with facial primaries.

Iyer and O'Brien in 2009 discussed the extent of parotidectomy and the implications of microscopic residual disease along the facial nerve. They recommended preservation of the functioning facial nerve. They definitely recommended postoperative radiation therapy in this group of patients. Every attempt should be made to preserve the functioning facial nerve; however, radical parotidectomy may be considered in patients presenting with preoperative facial nerve palsy or bulky metastatic disease either involving or encircling the facial nerve. They concluded that facial nerve preservation followed by postoperative radiation therapy is a reasonable option in patients with microscopic residual disease involving the facial nerve and normal preoperative facial nerve function. In a multi-institutional study, Andiuchow and O'Brien reported the experience from six international institutions for clinical staging of metastatic cutaneous squamous cell carcinoma. There appears to be a consensus to stage parotid metastatic disease and separate it from nodal disease in the neck. The benefit of having subgroups of parotid and neck stage is uncertain, but it is unlikely to identify patients with unfavorable characteristics that may benefit from further studies. Palme Carsten in 2003 concluded that the extent of metastatic disease in the parotid gland significantly influences the outcome and suggests that staging the parotid separately in metastatic cutaneous squamous cell carcinoma may be useful.

The conclusions made by the Sydney Cancer Center and O'Brien's group are very important and help to elucidate the patterns of nodal metastasis and prognosis and overall management of these patients with cutaneous malignancy and metastatic disease to the parotid and upper neck area. The role of radiation therapy and the long-term outcome with radiation therapy still remains somewhat unclear; however, the general consensus is to consider postoperative radiation therapy in these individuals. Whether, in N0 set up, radiation therapy alone would be of equal help remains unclear.

Chapter 5

Sinuses, Orbit and Skull Base

ORBITAL TUMORS
RESULTS FOLLOWING THE TRANSCRANIAL OPERATIVE
ATTACK *BY WALTER E DANDY*
Oskar Piest, New York, 1941. Pp. xv + 168

The publication of a monograph by Dr Dandy is always an event of considerable interest to neurological surgeons. The present work should be of even greater interest to the ophthalmologists. Based upon the study of thirty-one cases of tumors involving the orbit, it was found that 80 percent of these tumors either arose in or extended to the cranial cavity. The selection of cases excluded the small anterior orbital tumors. The more common pathological types were: meningioma with hyperostosis, Schüller-Christian's disease, and glioma.

The transcranial operative approach, used in most of the cases, is the logical method for dealing with posterior orbital and intracranio-orbital tumors. It has proved extremely safe in the author's hands. It is regrettable that certain errors escaped correction in the final proofreading.

WJ German

Dandy WE. Orbital tumors: results following the transcranial operative attack. New York, Oscar Piest, 1941

Commentary by: *Steven A Newman*

In 1941, in a short 168-page monograph, Walter Dandy, one of the early acolytes of Harvey Cushing and the Johns Hopkins Hospital and at the time the director of the "brain team" at Johns Hopkins, described his experience in approaching tumors of the orbit. His series consisted of 24 operative cases (and an additional 7 cases were observed) of patients with orbital tumors treated between 1921 and 1940. Analyzing the results of these cases, Walter Dandy concluded that the transcranial operative approach was the ideal way of dealing with orbital tumors.

Dandy's transcranial approach was certainly not the first attempt at operating on the orbit. Prior to the advent of general anesthesia, orbital surgery was limited to crude exenteration and enucleations, as illustrated by Bartish in 1583. Even after the advent of anesthesia in the mid-19th century, surgical approaches were uncommonly employed, consisting mainly of anterior transcutaneous or transconjunctival approaches when the orbital lesion could be palpated. It was not until 1886 that Krönlein described removing the lateral rim of the orbit up to the inferior orbital fissure as a means of approaching lesions within the orbital cavity. In spite of his description, orbital surgery remained extremely uncommon, as indicated by Henry Stallard in his 1973 presidential address on the history of orbital surgery (with essentially no cases done either in the US or England in the first third of the 20th century). This was largely due to the inability to preoperatively diagnose orbital lesions. Even after the advent of radiography in 1895, plain films rarely truly outlined pathology within the orbit, unless the bony walls were involved.

What Dandy had fortuitously found in the early 1920s was that removal of the orbital roof presented a panoramic view of the superior anatomy of the orbit. His technique used gravity to displace the frontal lobes from the orbital roof, and he was able to further decompress the brain by draining cerebrospinal fluid from the chiasmatic cistern. Alan Woods, who was Chairman of the Department of Ophthalmology and successor to William Holland Wilmer at Hopkins, strongly supported Dandy's efforts, forming an early example of a team approach to lesions involving the areas of the skull base.

In Dandy's series, not surprisingly, meningiomas made up almost one-third of the patients, followed by patients diagnosed with Schüller-Christian disease. It is likely, in retrospect, that many of those cases would today be recognized as variants of idiopathic orbital inflammatory disease (and perhaps would not be candidates for surgery). It also is likely that some of the bony tumors described actually represented fibrous dysplasia or ossifying fibromas.

The publication of Dandy's monograph and his suggestion that all orbital tumors be approached transcranially produced a not surprising backlash from orbital surgeons, particularly Henry Stallard in England and Algernon Reese in the United States. They questioned Dandy's suggestion that most orbital pathology extended outside the orbit and suggested, not inappropriately, that there was a significant referral bias in the patients that Dandy treated. This, combined with the limited series of pathology involving the orbit, clearly demonstrated the propensity for individuals to see things based on their own limited experience.

Although the last three decades have produced substantial improvements in the transcranial approach, including the removal of the orbital rim as described by John Jane and colleagues and more extensive bony openings as with the orbito-zygomatic approach, many of the techniques employed by Dandy, including the cutaneous incision, advancement of the galeal flap, avoiding the frontal sinuses and making a bone flap, are not dissimilar to current practice. Although his approach at the time included opening the frontal dura to access the perichiasmatic cistern for decompression, he recognized the importance of avoiding cerebrospinal fluid leak by staying out of the ethmoid sinuses. His knowledge of orbital anatomy seemed to be somewhat limited, since although he identified the rectus muscles and moved them with silk sutures, there is no comment in the monograph on the levator. Dandy recognized the theoretical potential of producing pulsatile exophthalmos when removing the orbital roof, since in his surgery, the roof was not reconstructed. He, however, did point out that this was never a clinical problem; something that we recognize today (preferentially not reconstructing the roof). He further pointed out the importance of intraosseous involvement of meningiomas, the indication for extensive bone resection, and an early observation about the technical difficulty of removing the meningioma from the carotid artery (the cause of his one mortality). True appreciation for meningioma invasion of the carotid artery would take another 50 years for recognition.

The importance of Dandy's approach was recognized even by Harvey Cushing, who mentioned Dandy's earlier work in his 1938 monograph on meningiomas. It was also recognized by Horax, another one of Cushing's students. Other neurosurgeons had described approaches through the orbital roof, including Naffzinger, who in 1931 described this technique for the decompression of thyroid orbitopathy.

The controversy set off by Dandy on one side (supported by subsequent neurosurgery series including those of the Mayo Clinic) and Reese and Stallard on the other over which was the "best approach" to orbital pathology lasted 30 years, until the advent of CT scanning in 1973, which demonstrated that there was no one "best approach" but rather surgery should be determined by the location within the orbit, particularly with respect to the optic nerve, the expected pathology, and the goal of surgical intervention. Extensive series of orbital pathology, such as those published by Rootman, including more than 4,000 orbital cases pointed out that greater than 60% of orbital lesions were inflammatory and did not require surgery (other than possible decompression). The common lesions of Dandy (meningiomas) and the ophthalmologists (hemangiomas) made up barely 2% or less each of the orbital series. Even with these common tumors, more recent studies have suggested that many hemangiomas do not need surgery, as they often do not grow, and meningiomas are not often "cured" by surgery.

Although preceding the pioneering work in orbital decompression by approaching the orbit through the floor and medial wall as published by Walsh and Ogura in 1957 and combined sinus and orbital approaches such as those pioneered by Connelly in 1962, Dandy's monograph clearly increased our options of approaches to lesions involving the anterior skull base and set an example for the application of team approaches to the skull base.

Clearly, this monograph was a milestone for those of us who practice orbital surgery and is one of the pioneering works in the development of an approach to anterior skull base pathology. Further refinements including the direct transorbital approach to intracranial contents through an eyelid key hole and endoscopic approaches will continue to represent evolutionary changes in what was started by Dandy and his "brain team" more than 70 years ago.

A COMBINED INTRACRANIAL FACIAL APPROACH TO THE PARANASAL SINUSES

Alfred S Ketcham, Robert H Wilkins, John M Van Buren, et al.

Neoplasms arising in the paranasal sinuses have usually extended beyond the site of origin when symptoms suggest this diagnosis. As a result of the delay in diagnosis, most sinus cancers are associated with bone invasion and extension to adjacent regions. When caner arises from or extends into the frontal or ethmoid sinuses, complete excision has often been considered to be impossible due to its proximity to the inner table of the cranial bones. While there has been a trend toward more radical excision of nasal and paranasal neoplasms, the intracranial extent of disease cannot be accurately evaluated prior to attempts at excision. Neither can the resection be directed through adjacent uninvolved tissues and, therefore, encompass a true en bloc resection.

The combined intracranial facial approach to the paranasal sinus areas, which was reported by Smith, Williams and Klopp in 1954, allows a more accurate determination of the true extent of disease and also allows en bloc resection of certain of the paranasal sinuses in continuity with the cribriform plate area of the anterior cranial fossa and the medial wall of the orbit. The present report will discuss the results of this type of operation in nineteen patients treated at the Surgery Branch of the National Cancer Institute.

Ketcham AS, Wilkins RH, Van Buren JM, et al. A combined intracranial facial approach to the paranasal sinuses. Am J Surg. 1963;106:698-703.

Commentary by: *Jatin P Shah*

Ketcham and his colleagues reported on a consecutive series of 19 patients who underwent an intracranial facial approach for en bloc resection of malignant tumors of the paranasal sinuses. Thirteen of these 19 patients were previously treated and had either persistent or recurrent disease. Although Ketcham and his colleagues were not the first to report such resection for malignant tumors, their series was the first to report on outcomes from this ground breaking surgical approach. Smith, Klopp and Williams had reported earlier, in 1954, a combined cranial facial approach for the excision of malignant tumors of the frontal sinuses; however, Ketcham and his colleagues are to be complimented for their detailed description of the surgical technique of accomplishing a mono-bloc resection and reporting oncologic outcomes.

Ketcham's work is particularly important since this work was done in the days when radiological evaluation of tumors involving the skull base was limited to anterior, lateral and Water's views of the skull and conventional coronal tomograms to assess intracranial extension. No wonder, by modern day standards, to do an exploratory craniotomy to assess the intracranial extent of tumor would be considered archaic at best. In spite of this handicap, they were successful in achieving complete resection of tumor in

10 of their 19 patients. The remaining patients had microscopically positive margins and required further adjuvant treatment.

In the introduction to the manuscript, Ketcham and his colleagues rightfully noted that extension of tumors of the nasal cavity and paranasal sinuses thru the roof of the orbit or the cribriform plate and into the frontal sinus made a conventional facial approach unsuitable for complete excision of the tumor. However, the inability to assess intracranial extent of the tumor prior to surgery using the facial approach would lead to failure of facial approaches employed for resection of tumors approaching or involving the skull base. The fundamental reason for craniotomy proposed by Ketcham et al. was to assess the presence and/or extent of intracranial invasion by tumor and allow the feasibility of a mono-bloc resection.

Ketcham's series included patients with squamous cell carcinomas, other epithelial malignancies including poorly differentiated carcinomas and minor salivary gland tumors as well as sarcomas. They had a single operative mortality secondary to meningitis in this series, while other complications were relatively minor.

By modern day standards, the use of an split thickness skin graft would hardly be considered optimal in the repair of skull base defects. In spite of this, they achieved satisfactory healing in the majority of their patients who were ready to be treated further with adjuvant postoperative radiotherapy. Three of 6 patients with epidermoid carcinoma, 5/7 patients with sarcoma, and 3/5 patients with other carcinomas were alive and free of disease at the time of last follow-up. This is a remarkable achievement reported nearly 50 years ago, and we have made little progress in improving survival outcomes for patients with locally advanced malignant tumors involving the anterior skull base since then. Ketcham and his colleagues were correct in pointing out that 6/7 patients who were not cured had positive surgical margins and they pointed out that local recurrence was a major factor in treatment failure. This observation has been seen in numerous subsequent studies on larger series of patients, indicating that surgical margins remain a significant obstacle in achieving an oncologically complete resection, leading to local failure and thus lack of improvement in long-term survivorship.

This early report by Ketcham and his colleagues from the National Cancer Institute in the United States paved the way for encouraging numerous head and neck surgeons around the world to embark upon such a radical surgical approach to achieve enblock resection of advanced tumors of the paranasal sinuses approaching or involving the skull base. Clearly, his report opened the doors for modern day craniofacial surgery and stimulated dozens of young surgeons in the 1970s and 80s to improvise upon his techniques to reduce morbidity and improve curability. Ketcham's work will remain as pioneering work in the field of craniofacial surgery for malignant tumors involving the anterior skull base and is an important milestone in the archives of head and neck cancer surgery.

COMBINED SURGERY, RADIOTHERAPY, AND REGIONAL CHEMOTHERAPY IN CARCINOMA OF THE PARANASAL SINUSES

Yasuo Sato, Mamoru Morita, Hiro-omi Takahashi, et al.

Since 1964, we have been using the simultaneous combined therapy of surgery, radiotherapy, and regional chemotherapy in treating malignant tumors of the paranasal sinuses. Total number of cases treated was 68. In 57 cases of carcinomas 38 showed disappearance of tumor by this therapy and among these, 22 required no further treatment. In 19 cases of still existing tumor at the end of the therapy, partial resection of the maxilla or intracavitary irradiation was effective in eradication the residue of the tumor. Thus, no total resection of the maxilla has been required even in advanced cases since May 1965. This therapy reduced the rate of local recurrences and consequently has been improving survival rate. The curtailment of surgery increased the number of patients who rehabilitated successfully and able to return to their occupations soon after the treatment.

Sato Y, Morita M, Takahashi H, et al. Combined surgery, radiotherapy, and regional chemotherapy in carcinoma of the paranasal sinuses. Cancer. 1970;25:571-579.

Commentary by: *Paul P Knegt*

As a young resident in ENT halfway through the 70s of the last century, I was instructed to prepare a lecture on paranasal sinus carcinoma. At that time, I was very much impressed by a patient who had had a total maxillectomy and postoperative radiotherapy for a carcinoma of the maxillary sinus. The old lady with her deformed face, difficult speech, unpleasant odor, and continuous pain apparently was in a deplorable condition. Soon I would find out that most of the patients treated for cancer of the paranasal sinuses in those years had the same problems, and moreover, that many of them died within a year after treatment of uncontrolled tumor growth.

A comparison of the treatment results of paranasal sinus cancer in the literature of the 50s, 60s, and early 70s was hindered by the absence of a generally accepted TNM classification for carcinoma of the paranasal sinuses. But it was clear that the survival rates that could be achieved in those years (5-year survival rate of 25%) were very disappointing. The main cause of these poor results was an extremely high rate of local recurrences.

However, one of the publications we studied reported better results and less mutilation.

This was the article of Yasuo Sato et al. published in the journal *Cancer* in March 1970 (*Combined surgery, radiotherapy, and regional chemotherapy in carcinoma of the paranasal sinuses*). Sato (1921–2010) was dissatisfied with the results of total maxillectomy and high doses of radiotherapy for carcinoma of the paranasal sinuses. Therefore, beginning in 1965, he combined radiotherapy (50–70 Gy), intra-arterial chemotherapy (20 × 250 mg 5-FU), and daily cleaning of the maxillary sinus by removal of necrotic tumor. With this treatment he not only reduced the local recurrence rate to 27% (< 1965 ± 80 %) and improved the 2-year survival to 75% (< 1965 ± 29%), but he also could avoid total maxillectomy in all cases. In his article, Sato stressed the importance of the combination of all three components: radio-therapy, chemotherapy, and antral cleaning. If one of the three components was left out, the results were disappointing. In 1978, the authors published the 5-year survival rate of the 77 patients treated according to the described method from 1965–1968; the rate was 55%.

In those years, the results as described by Sato were very favorable. We could hardly believe that such good results could be achieved: "*probably the tumors in Japan are different from tumors in Western Europe and the United States*"; "*manipulation of the tumor will without any doubt cause a lot of metastases in the neck*"; "*this man is an impostor*". To disprove these negative comments, we decided to study Sato's treatment method in more detail, and in 1974, I was sent to Tokyo with hundreds of critical questions. Professor Sato started very early in the morning and worked till late in the evening. His staff and residents would do the same. Sato instructed one of his senior staff members (Professor Takeo Kobayashi) to translate our 200 questions from English into Japanese and his answers back from Japanese into English, a task that required angelic patience. Thus, we were able to achieve a good insight into his unconventional treatment. He allowed me to choose randomly histological coupes of his patients. Back home the diagnosis of high grade malignant carcinoma could be confirmed in all cases.

During my visit in 1974, it became evident that the method as described in *Cancer* in 1970 was no longer used. Due to the observation that during infusion of 5-FU and BUdR the tumor started to disappear clinically and histologically with a low dose of radiotherapy, Sato adapted his treatment scheme and lowered the dose of radiotherapy (10–15 Gy).

He also had noticed that in patients in whom intra-arterial chemotherapy for some reason failed, the tumor still started to disappear. Consequently, he replaced intra-arterial 5-FU by local application of 5-FU. Sato felt that, according to the at-that-time prevailing opinion about tumor immunology, on one hand the number of tumor cells should be reduced but on the other hand the immunological defense of the patient should be spared by keeping the dose of radiotherapy and of chemotherapy as low as possible. So the method as described in this article evolved from high dose radiotherapy and intra-arterial chemotherapy in 1964 to low dose radiotherapy and topical chemotherapy in 1974. But the essential part of the treatment in all those years was the surgical removal of necrotic material by daily antral cleaning. The results with low dose radiotherapy, low dose topical chemo-therapy, and daily removal of necrotic material remained very favorable, and with his method, he was able to achieve the highest survival percentages

(5-year survival rate of 75%), with the lowest discomfort for the patients. The fear that manipulation of the tumor by daily antral cleaning might increase the number of neck nodes and distant metastases was not confirmed; these percentages (15% and 12%, respectively) remained the same for treatment without and with manipulation of the tumor.

Sato was able to use his observations to effectuate changes in treatment. He was not impressed by the repeated remarks in those years (and sometimes even in more recent years) that *"more radical surgery, higher dose radiotherapy and more aggressive chemotherapy might improve survival"*, and he showed that with less aggressive treatment, better results could be achieved, while the maxilla could be spared. His treatment is one of the earliest forms of organ preservation surgery in the history of head and neck cancer

We adopted his treatment for paranasal sinus carcinoma. At first we used it only for patients with a local recurrence, knowing that we had very little to offer with conventional treatment. Within one year, it became clear that the results for this group were extremely good.

So we started a prospective study to verify the hypothesis that the treatment according to Sato results in improved survival compared with the treatment previously used. Our results, published in 1985 in *Cancer* and in 2001 in the *Archives of Otolaryngology*, were similarly good and comparable to the results of Sato (5-year survival rate of 65%). The results were even better for adenocarcinoma of the ethmoidal sinus complex (5-year survival rate of 87%). In 2008, Almeyda and Capper (Berks and Wycombe, UK) with this treatment achieved a 5-year survival rate of 86% in woodworkers with adenocarcinoma.

In animal experiments, it has been demonstrated that local chemotherapy not only causes necrosis of tumor cells but also initiates a strong potentiation of the immune system. This is one possible explanation for the apparent success of this form of treatment.

It remains unclear to us why in the past decades this form of treatment has not been more widely accepted for its simplicity, but more importantly for its higher success rates, when compared with other forms of conventional therapy.

TEMPORAL BONE RESECTION
Review of 100 Cases

John S Lewis

One hundred cases of temporal bone resection for cancer of the ear were reviewed retrospectively, allowing for a survival five-year follow-up period in all cases. Operative technique previously described varied from case to case but essentially involved subtotal resection of the mastoid, petrous pyramid and squamosa of the temporal bone, temporomandibular joint, base of zygoma, and attached adjacent soft tissues. The procedure sacrifices the facial nerve and hearing in the involved ear. Preoperative radiation or a sandwich technique of preoperative and postoperative radiation was used. Many complications were encountered, but with hypotensive agents, high-speed air drills, and adequate coverage of the defect, the death rate was reduced from 10% in 1954 to 5% in recent years. The overall five-year cure rate was 27%, with a 25% cure rate for squamous carcinoma.

Lewis JS. Temporal bone resection: review of 100 cases. Arch Otolaryngol. 1975;101:23-25.

Commentary by: *Michael Gleeson*

In the modern era, not one surgeon has treated more cancers of the external auditory canal than John S Lewis. Few surgeons have the experience of more than 25 patients with the disease in their professional lifetime. Multi-institutional studies struggle to find more than 75 patients, and only a meta-analysis of all published cases in the literature has been based on more than 100 cases. These data alone suggest that an analysis of 100 patients who have undergone a temporal bone resection for cancer of the ear, performed by one surgeon, is likely to be a seminal text. Better still, 80 of Lewis's patients had tumors that arose from the external ear canal, middle ear, or mastoid. Only 20 patients had tumors that had developed from the pinna and infiltrated the temporal bone, a completely different disease. Furthermore, all had at least 5 years of clinical follow-up. This publication was the culmination of 20 years of experience and a professional lifetime devoted to the management of a lethal disease.

Squamous cell carcinoma of the temporal bone is a rare and invariably aggressive tumor, with an estimated incidence of 1 per million per year. Even today, management of this disease remains a challenge in the hands of skilled skull base surgeons and radiation oncologists. The prognosis for patients has remained poor despite the development and employment of different surgical and radiation techniques throughout the years. At the outset of Lewis's study, one in every 10 patients never left the hospital, as his operative mortality was 10%. Within 20 years, Lewis had reduced the operative mortality rate to 5%. By any standards and in any era, a surgical procedure that halves the operative mortality must be considered revolutionary.

Lewis identified the pitfalls of delayed diagnosis: the chronically infected external ear canal that failed to respond to antibiotics or local medications.

He decried the reluctance of clinicians to biopsy early and estimated that most patients experienced a diagnostic delay of at least 6 months from the onset of symptoms to the clinical diagnosis. It was too late by the time blood-tinged otorrhoea or severe pain had developed from bone erosion. So what has changed? Sadly, nothing! Preoperative assessment relied heavily on plain X-rays of the mastoid and temporal bone tomograms to assess bone erosion. Retrograde jugular venography was introduced to detect possible invasion of the lateral sinus or jugular bulb. Lewis stopped short of defining clinical indications that might mitigate against anything other than palliative care. Perhaps this was rarely a consideration.

The operation that Lewis described involved a subtotal petrosectomy that at the outset must have been a formidable procedure. It was a combined intracranial and extracranial approach using a temporal craniotomy. An en bloc technique was attempted in all cases but, just as today, this was not always possible, and the deeper aspects of the resection were piecemeal. If necessary, the root of the zygoma was removed together with the temporomandibular joint. Lewis had to wait until the latter part of his career before high-speed air drills became available and anesthetic techniques could provide him with a better operative field by the use of controlled hypotension.

Reduction of cerebrospinal fluid (CSF) pressure was achieved by the withdrawal of 50–100 mLs of CSF by lumbar puncture with malleable needles or the use of diuretics. Presumably, the intraspinal needles would not have been left in place during the postoperative period. Lewis would not have had the benefit of continuous lumbar drainage devices, as they were not available. Resections often included dura, and the resultant dural defects were repaired with temporalis fascia grafts. Water-tight closure of the dura must have been difficult but absolutely essential. CSF leaks were not uncommon, and those that did not seal spontaneously within 10 days required secondary closure, and that could not have been easy. Meningitis and brain abscess—unusual complications today—were constant hazards and must have been responsible for much of the mortality.

It is quite remarkable that Lewis managed to restrict his average blood loss to 1.5 L. While hemorrhage was usually confined to venous loss from the external jugular and the superior petrosal sinus, there were frequent occasions when the lateral sinus was damaged and had to be controlled with vascular silk and oxidised cellulose. Lewis also encountered intra-operative lacerations of the internal carotid artery that required repair. Those that he was able to stop bleeding had a high incidence of delayed thrombosis and, as a consequence, hemiplegia.

Many of Lewis's patients had already been given a full course of radiotherapy prior to their referral. Most would have received 35–50 Gy some time earlier. This must have had a negative impact on healing. He had to rely on scalp flaps to repair the operative defect. Today, these flaps would be the ultimate refuge for the despairing head and neck surgeon and for good reason. They always seem to be the final insult following a mutilating operation. However, at a time when antibiotic prophylaxis consisted of a combination of Ampicillin and Coly-Mycin M, at least they gave some robustness to local skin closure, though most likely under some tension. Gram negative septicaemia with wound breakdown and cerebral herniation was a fearsome complication. Lewis reported frequent partial loss of skin cover as one could imagine. Areas of local breakdown were managed by regular acetic acid dressings. When clean, further local flaps and probably split skin grafts were used to gain coverage. Whenever possible, Lewis gave postoperative radiotherapy, recognizing the importance of combined treatment.

We now know that survival is related to the stage of the tumor at presentation but is independent of histological grade of the tumor. Patients that have positive nodal disease or recur inevitably succumb to their tumor, and often very quickly. Treatment failure usually declares itself in the first 2 years. Another 20 years passed before the staging system we use today and which guides our treatment management was published. There was no staging system when Lewis undertook his study and probably most of the tumors he treated were advanced. He achieved a 25% 5-year cure rate.

Cure rates for squamous cell carcinoma of the external auditory canal have improved since Lewis reported his monumental series. But, are today's series directly comparable? Almost certainly not! A number of series are so small, that no meaningful inferences about treatment efficacy can be drawn. Small T1 tumors, those restricted to the external canal without bone erosion, that are rarely found but skew overall statistics, are cured in greater than 95% of patients. T2 tumours, those restricted to the external canal with evidence of bone erosion, that are adequately resected and given post-operative radiotherapy, should be cured in greater than 50% of cases. These early tumors are often picked up by the ubiquitous CT scan and often more by luck than judgment. More extensive tumors, T3, require subtotal petro-sectomy and postoperative radiotherapy. Cure rates for these patients are a little unpredictable. When the dura is involved or brain infiltrated, T4, the patient is rarely cured, though some claim surgery can achieve worthwhile palliation, albeit with significant morbidity. Patients with nodal metastases in the neck all die. Overall survival rates of 50–60% are usually quoted, but all single-institution and surgeon series have the disadvantage of being very small. Skilled palliative care is also an option for our patients today that many choose or have chosen for them. They never appear in the statistics of modern day series and so never dilute the survival statistics. While the extent of Lewis's surgery is rarely repeated today, his management philo-sophy remains the cornerstone of treatment, and his series lives on as the historical standard against which all others are compared.

What of the man himself? John Lewis was presented with a lifetime award at the North American Skull Base Society Annual Meeting in February 2004, which was held in New Orleans. I had the privilege of meeting him there and having supper in his company. I wasted no time in making his acquaintance. John Lewis was a quiet, gentle, and thoughtful man who was not shy to share his clinical experiences with someone probably 40 years his junior. It was difficult to imagine him as the bold surgeon going where no surgeon had gone before. Lewis recounted those days of heroic surgery with modesty and intrinsic honesty. He gave me his time for which I will be eternally grateful.

NONOCULAR CANCER IN RETINOBLASTOMA SURVIVORS

David H Abramson, Robert M Ellsworth, Lorenz E Zimmerman

The occurrence of a second malignant nonocular tumor in patients who have been successfully treated for retinoblastoma has been recognized since the first report of the treatment of bilateral retinoblastoma with radiation and surgery. (For the purpose of this study, a second tumor is defined as an extraocular tumor in any part of the body representing either a new primary neoplasm or a lesion indistinguishable from a late [greater than five years] metastasis of retinoblastoma). In that report, Reese et al. recorded one case of fatal rhalxlomyosarcoma and one fatal maxillary sinus sarcoma following the treatment of 55 cases of bilateral retinoblastoma with combined surgery and radiation. The association of radiation therapy and the second malignancies has been emphasized by Forrest and others. In almost all of these cases, the tumors appeared following high doses of radiation, long latent period, and in the area of radiation beam, and have therefore, previously been classified as "radiation induced".

Recently, however, we have been seen patients who developed second tumors in the field of radiation with low doses (3,500 to 4,500 rads). In addition, a significant number of patients have appeared with second tumors clearly distant from the radiation site, for example, the femur. Finally, three patients have been seen who developed second tumors despite the fact that they and never received any radiation for their retinoblastoma.

It was the purpose of this study to review all cases of second malignancies in survivors of retinoblastoma therapy seen at the Columbia-Presbyterian Medical Center (CPMC) Eye Tumor Clinic between 1922 and 1972 and those cases on file at the Armed Forces Institute of Pathology (AFIP) through 1972. Over 2,300 cases were reviewed, and the results indicate that retinoblastoma patients have a definite predilection for the development of fatal second malignancies despite adequate control of their original eye tumor and, perhaps, unrelated to radiation treatment.

Abramson DH, Ellsworth RM, Zimmerman LE. Nonocular cancer in retinoblastoma survivors. Trans Sect Ophthalmol Am Acad Ophthalmol Otolaryngol. 1976;81:454-457.

Commentary by: *Brian P Marr*

Dr David H Abramson's pivotal article "Nonocular cancers and retinoblastoma survivors" was published in May 1976. At the time of this publication, the first author was working with co-author Robert M Ellsworth MD, a leader in the retinoblastoma field, and collaborated with Lorenz E Zimmerman, MD, at the Walter Reed Army Medical Center, in the Armed Forces Institute of Pathology (AFIP). The study was proposed to seek the incidence of second cancers in the retinoblastoma population from the extensive data collected by the AFIP and Columbia-Presbyterian Medical Center (CPMC). Two thousand three hundred two patients were reviewed, and the incidence of second tumors was recorded. The observation that second tumors occurred in the field of radiation was not unexpected, and many previous publications of radiation-induced tumors were cited in the paper. The interesting observation and important discovery was that the vast majority of patients who developed second malignancies had bilateral retinoblastoma disease. Also interesting was that all bilateral retinoblastoma survivors who developed second tumors did not develop them in the field of radiation, and some patients did not have radiation at all. The majority of tumors were sarcomas, but other non-sarcoma tumors also appeared in the same time period. This suggested that radiation was not the sole cause of the tumors, but there existed a predisposition for second tumors in children who had the germline form of retinoblastoma. This paper was the first step in realizing that the retinoblastoma gene was a tumor suppressor gene and the reason for these second malignancies. At the same time, in 1976, papers by Alfred G Knudson, Jr. elucidated the genetic impact of genes on childhood cancers using retinoblastoma as a model, Uta Francke identified the location of the mutation for retinoblastoma to chromosome 13, and later Ted Dryja found its location on that chromosome. Years later, the genes role as a tumor suppressor was discovered.

The standard treatment of intraocular retinoblastoma in 1976 was enucleation and radiation. External beam radiotherapy was used successfully to salvage the eyes of patients with bilateral disease to preserve vision. However, advanced cases still developed metastatic retinoblastoma; this occurred early, and usually patients succumbed to their disease. It was thought that some patients developed "late metastasis" of retinoblastoma. These tumors were diagnosed differently depending on their site of origin and the pathologist reading the slides; some were called sarcoma others metastatic retinoblastoma. We know today that most of these tumors were in fact secondary tumors and not metastatic disease. The fact that a genetic predisposition existed for second tumors in patients with the germline form of retinoblastoma was not known until this paper.

No longer is radiation primary treatment for retinoblastoma. The awareness that not only treatment doses of radiation but low doses of radiation puts patients with bilateral retinoblastoma at risk for second cancers has steered the innovation of new treatments and surveillance protocols for patients with retinoblastoma. The need to avoid radiation has driven the field to develop chemotherapy treatment strategies that not only cure intraocular retinoblastoma but also save eyes, with useful vision. Surveillance for second malignancies has been tailored to avoid radiation and monitor different areas when they are at their greatest risk. Today, it is well known that retinoblastoma is caused by a mutation of the retinoblastoma gene on chromosome 13. This gene codes for a tumor suppressor protein that has been implicated in many other types of cancer in addition to retinoblastoma. The genetics of retinoblastoma are understood, and families can be tested to identify if they have or carry a mutation. It is Dr David H Abramson's paper in conjunction with concurrent research, which became the bases for our current knowledge of radiation's effect on patients with retinoblastoma. This discovery changed the way we view this disease and spurred advancements in treatment and patient care.

THE INFRATEMPORAL FOSSA APPROACH FOR THE LATERAL SKULL BASE

Ugo Fisch, Paul Fagan, Anton Valavanis

Until recently lesions of the lateral skull base have been relatively inaccessible to the surgeon. Control of the carotid artery in the temporal bone has been inadequate, the great venous sinuses have been a source of uncontrollable hemorrhage, and the facial nerve lies across the middle of the operative field.

Large glomus tumors, clivus chordomas, petrous apex cholesteatomas, and extensive juvenile angiofibromas of the nasopharynx are life threatening disease that are best treated by surgical ablation. To reach such lesions, many surgical approaches to the skull base have been developed. The facial nerve, to a greater of lesser degree, has prevented adequate access in the approaches of Conley, Mullen et al. House and Hitselberger, and Gardner et al. The central, inferior approaches of Biller and of Guiot et al. are hampered by the long working distance and the necessity for traversing a potentially septic field.

Further, the combined superior and lateral approaches of Hilding and Greenberg and Kempe et al. are hampered by the retained facial nerve and by wide dural incisions, which can lead to cerebrospinal fluid leaks and serious complications.

The infratemporal fossa approach to the skull base provides for direct surgical access to the entire length of the intratemporal carotid artery and for control of the great venous sinuses. The facial nerve is dealt with according to the site of the lesion, which also determines which of the three infratemporal fossa approaches will be employed. These infratemporal fossa approaches provide access as follows:

1. *Type A. Access to the temporal bone in its infralabyrinthine and apical compartments and its inferior surface.*
2. *Type B. Access to the clivus.*
3. *Type C. Access to the parasellar region and nasopharynx.*

The type A approach is most commonly used and is described in the greatest detail. For each approach the indications, results, and complications are described.

Fisch U, Fagan P, Valavanis A. The infratemporal fossa approach for the lateral skull base. Otolaryngol Clin North Am. 1984;17:513-552.

Commentary by: *Chandranath Sen, Donato Pacione*

The area of the skull base has been an anatomical border zone for neuro-surgeons and head and neck surgeons and neuro-otologists. Tumors involving the temporal bone, clivus, and the infratemporal fossa were, and even now remain, a difficult problem. Barriers to access result from being in a deep location at the center of the head surrounded by critical structures such as the facial nerve, otic capsule, the jugular foramen, the internal carotid artery, and the cavernous sinuses. Although the nasopharynx, the nasal and oral cavities provided a direct access to the clivus, the problem of adequate visualization, contamination, cerebrospinal fluid fistula formation, and usually resulting infection was a feared complication. Tumors in this region were generally considered incurable. Diagnosing and accurately defining the anatomical extent of the tumor was limited to computed tomographic scans at best. Added to these factors was also the problem of uncontrolled hemorrhage from many of the tumors that occur here that tend to be very vascular. Managing the internal carotid artery, which was often involved by these tumors was not well defined.

With the advent and refinement of the CT scan in the 70s, images were able to provide unprecedented clarity of the skull base. Embolization of the tumors by interventional neuro-radiologists and assessment of the cerebrovascular reserve by balloon test occlusion of the internal carotid artery substantially improved the evaluation and treatment of patients with such tumors. Surgeons were emboldened to take on these formidable tumors.

At the time of the publication of "The Infratemporal Fossa Approach for the Lateral Skull Base", Ugo Fisch was the only surgeon to have previously published work related to the infratemporal fossa approach. The concept of skull base surgery as a distinct specialization did not exist. Although others had discussed combined superior and lateral approaches, Fisch's approach addressed many of the difficulties previously encountered regarding the constraints of the facial nerve, petrous carotid, and venous sinuses. As a true skull base approach, it also avoided the necessity for large dural exposure/incisions and potential for cerebrospinal fluid leak—common in the combined transcranial approaches. Fisch demonstrated the ability to control and mobilize key structures, such as the petrous carotid artery, facial nerve and sigmoid sinus, in order to facilitate visualization and resection of difficult skull base tumors.

The landmark article by Ugo Fisch has been cited 124 times since its publication in 1984. In the first 10 years after its publication it was referenced 44 times. Of the articles that cite this paper, 16 of the top 20 most cited works were written in the first 10 years after its publication. The number of citations decreased in the years following the initial skull base boom. However, from 2007–2012, this article was cited another 29 times. The recent resurgence in citations of Fisch's article appears to be related to the development of expanded endonasal approaches to the infratemporal fossa.

Prior to its publication, there were only three articles published regarding skull base approaches to the infratemporal fossa, all of which were written by Fisch. In searching the terms skull base and surgery, only 27 citations are found in the literature from 1900–1984. Comparatively, from August 1984 to January of 2013 there are 4,398 citations regarding this topic. Overall, there are only three articles, two of which are written by Fisch, regarding skull base and the infratemporal fossa, which have been cited more times than this article.

From a literature impact, the importance of this article is obvious, especially during the first 10 years after its initial publication, as it was instrumental in ushering in the development of modern skull base surgery. Beyond what is evident in the literature, Fisch demonstrated a brave pioneering mentality and pushed the limits of what was known to be possible at the time. When taken in the context of the low-resolution CT imaging available at the time, Fisch's endeavors could be likened to that of the early explorers attempting to navigate safely to the new world. After the publication of his success with the infratemporal fossa approach, other skull base surgeons adopted and expanded on these techniques. He trained a whole generation of surgeons, many of whom became prominent in their own right. In the present skull base world, surgeons are continuing to expand the limits through the use of extended endoscopic approaches to the central skull base through the nasal passages. This has avoided many of the accepted morbidities associated with the open lateral approach. Ironically, one of Fisch's major concerns of morbidity that was driving the lateral approach was avoiding entry into the sinuses and nasal cavity. Although Van Buren and Ketcham introduced the concept of interdisciplinary collaboration between neurosurgeons and head and neck surgeons in the arena of the anterior skull base surgery, this concept was now carried into the lateral skull base. The skull base techniques that were introduced with this article have withstood the test of time and are even used now for many pathological processes. Approaches to the central skull base have been largely supplanted by endoscopic endonasal operations.

With the publication of the infratemporal fossa approach, Ugo Fisch did more than provide the skull base community with a new surgical technique. He forged into the unknown and fostered the development of modern day multidisciplinary skull base surgery.

PRESERVATION OF THE EYE IN PARANASAL SINUS CANCER SURGERY

Christopher Perry, Paul A Levine, Brian R Williamson, et al.

Forty-one patients undergoing surgery between 1977 and 1985 for malignant tumors of the paranasal sinuses abutting or eroding the orbital walls were studied for the need to remove the orbital contents. All patients had preliminary computed tomographic scans to delineate the extent of orbital invasion. All were treated with preoperative readiotherapy. If the tumor mass could be peeled from the periorbita, the eye was saved. Preservation of eyes in the patients without periosteal invasion did not after survival. Frozen-section control may be used to determine periorbital involvement. If the periorbita was minimally involved, it was locally resected. If invasion of the periorbita was extensive, an orbital exenteration was done. Only five of 41 patients required exenteration. Local recurrence of disease in the orbit has not occurred in these patients.

Perry C, Levine PA, Williamson BR, et al. Preservation of the eye in paranasal sinus cancer surgery. Arch Otolaryngol Head Neck Surg. 1988;114:632-634.

Commentary by: *Peter E Andersen*

The paper entitled "Preservation of the Eye in Paranasal Sinus Cancer Surgery" by Perry, Levine, Williamson, and Cantrell describes the results of surgery without orbital exenteration in a select group of patients with cancers of the nasal cavity and paranasal sinuses. The authors present evidence to dispute the belief, which was common prior to this publication, that any bony transgression of the orbital wall required orbital exenteration for oncologic control. As such, it resulted in a change of thought regarding the management of said tumors.

The paper presents a retrospective consecutive sample of 41 patients with cancers of the nasal cavity and paranasal sinuses treated between 1977 and 1985. All patients had preoperative computed tomography scans and adequate follow-up, although the actual length of follow-up is not specified in the manuscript. Fifteen patients who met the initial criteria were excluded due to inadequate follow-up data, death due to intercurrent disease or the fact that the tumors represented recurrent disease. The average age of the patients was 51 years (range, 18–77). It is not stated in the manuscript exactly where the tumors were located, i.e., maxillary sinus vs nasal cavity. The predominant histologic type was esthesioneuroblastoma in 19 patients; squamous carcinoma, adenocarcinoma, adenoid cystic carcinoma, melanoma, small cell carcinoma, undifferentiated carcinoma, and malignant mixed tumor were present in 8, 6, 3, 2, 1, 1, and 1 patient, respectively. All patients were treated with preoperative radiation therapy, although there is no mention of the dosages received.

The endpoints studied were local recurrence and survival. The authors broke out the results based upon the integrity of the orbital wall observed at surgery. Fifteen patients had intact orbital walls both radiographically and grossly at the time of surgery. In 5 patients, the bone was thinned by the tumor but still intact. In an additional 14 patients, the bone was transgressed by the tumor but the periorbita was intact; and in 7 patients, the periosteum of the orbit was invaded. In the 15 patients with intact orbital walls, 9 patients were alive and free of disease with follow-up periods ranging from 26–120 months (mean, 71 months). Two patients in this group had adenoid cystic carcinoma and developed pulmonary metastases without local recurrence but were still alive, while two additional patients died of distant metastasis without local recurrence. The remaining 2 patients developed a local recurrence; however, it was not within the orbit. Thus, in this group with intact orbital walls, the local recurrence rate was 2 of 15 patients, with no recurrences occurring within the orbit itself.

In the group with thinned but still intact orbital walls, 4 of 5 were alive and free of disease. The other patient died of recurrent disease in the neck and skin of the face. Thus, in this group, the local recurrence rate was 1 of 5 patients, and none of the recurrences were in the preserved orbit.

In the group in which the bony orbital wall was transgressed but the periosteum was not invaded, 10 of 14 patients were alive and disease free at last follow up. One patient was alive with distant metastasis present. One patient died with a local recurrence outside of the orbit, and 2 patients recurred within the orbit and died. Thus, in this group, the local recurrence rate was 3 of 14 patients, and the orbital recurrence rate was 2 of 14.

In the group with gross invasion of the periorbita, 5 of 7 patients required orbital exenteration. Of the other 2, in one patient with minimal invasion the eye was preserved but the patient succumbed to distant metastases, and the other patient had the surgery aborted due to unresectable disease being found. Of the 5 patients who had exenterations, 2 were alive and free of disease, 2 died of distant metastases, and 1 died of recurrence within the orbital cavity.

This series lends support to the concept that the decision to perform an orbital exenteration should be based upon the individual nature of the tumor and that there is not a one-size-fits-all approach. The authors demonstrated that it is certainly possible in selected cases to preserve the eye with acceptable oncologic results. This would indicate that in the absence of gross invasion of the eye it is reasonable to surgically explore the area to determine orbital involvement prior to orbital exenteration and that bony invasion of the orbital wall alone does not necessarily mean that exenteration is required. However, it should be recognized that the presence of an eye does not necessarily imply that the eye is functional or even useful. When presented with the option of an attempt to preserve the eye, many patients will express a desire to do so; however, it may not be clear to the patient at the time of such a decision just how miserable it is to have a painful, exposed eye that really gives no functional vision and is cosmetically unappealing. Attention should be given to the state of the surrounding supporting structures of the eye, including the eyelids, lacrimal system and the extent of orbital wall remaining after the tumor is removed. If the supporting structures will not be present to allow the eye to function, then perhaps the eye should not be saved, even if it is oncologically sound to do so. While some would argue that the presence of the eye has cosmetic value, I believe this argument fails if the eye that remains is crippled by dystopia, exposure, ectropion, or blindness. Of course there are varying degrees of these problems, and the surgeon must use their judgment and experience as to how severe the problem may be and consider the patient's wishes when making the decision to preserve or exenterate the orbit.

There are some peculiarities of this study that bear comment. One is the fact that all these patients had undergone preoperative radiation therapy. While this may be the preferred treatment at the author's institution, it is not so everywhere. It may be that the results would be different when applied to a group of patients who have not been previously irradiated. In addition, the patient population described has an excess of esthesioneuroblastomas. This is likely due to the fact that these patients are more likely to have disease confined to the nose, and thus orbital preservation can be considered. It is possible that a sample with higher numbers of squamous carcinomas or melanomas would give different results.

ORBITAL PRESERVATION IN MAXILLECTOMY

Scott J Stern, Helmuth Goepfert, Gary Clayman, et al.

Twenty-eight previously untreated patients with squamous carcinoma of the maxillary sinus underwent maxillectomy with preservation of the orbital contents at the MD. Anderson Cancer Center between 1971 and 1986. Eighteen patients had part or all of the orbital floor resected; nine patients were treated with radiotherapy, and nine had surgery only. Only 3 of 18 patients in this group (17%) retained significant function in the ipsilateral eye. Furthermore, local recurrence in this group was common (44%), regardless of whether postoperative radiotherapy was used. Ten patients retained the bony orbital floor; it the radiation fields did not include the eye, problems were minimal. Strong consideration should be given to orbital exenteration at the time of surgery, when the orbital floor is resected—especially if postoperative radiation fields will include the eye.

Stern SJ, Goepfert H, Clayman G, et al. Orbital preservation in maxillectomy, Otolaryngol Head Neck Surg.1993;109:111-115.

Commentary by: *Dennis H Kraus*

The article from Stern et al. from the University of Arkansas and MD Anderson Cancer Center represents a sentinel work in describing the outcome of patients undergoing maxillectomy with or without postoperative radiation, with the endpoint focusing on orbital function and local recurrence. The authors are applauded for their decision to utilize a homogenous group of patients, namely those with squamous carcinoma of the maxillary sinus undergoing either partial or total maxillectomy.

A review of the data reveals a total of 9 patients who underwent orbital floor resection with postoperative radiation. Nine patients had orbital floor resection with no postoperative radiation. There were 10 patients who had orbital floor preservation, 4 of whom received postoperative radiation, and 6 of whom did not. Within the 9 patients who underwent orbital floor resection with postoperative radiation, 5 of 9 had local failure, and only 1 of 9 had a functional eye. Within the 9 patients who had orbital floor resection with no radiation, 3 of 9 had a local failure, and 6 of 9 had a functional orbit. Lastly, within the group of patients who had orbital floor preservation, 7 of 10 had local failure, but 8 of 10 had a normal or functional eye after completion of treatment. In discussing their results, the authors noted that a previous experience from MD Anderson revealed that when the patients had a small lens block compared to a complete eye shielding, there was an increased incidence of orbital complications. If the ipsilateral orbit was irradiated, 79% of patients lost ocular function. Contralateral blindness occurred in 5% of patients within their series. They noted that complications have reportedly decreased since the advent of a three-field technique. Certainly, in the modern era (not included in this series), the use of intensity modulated radiation therapy (IMRT) has decreased the incidence of orbital complications.

The authors cited the work of Bridger et al. indicating that the patients undergoing orbital exenteration had worse survival and local regional control in comparison to patients in whom the eye was preserved. They suggested that the patients undergoing orbital exenteration are a proxy for more advanced disease stage, and this accounts for the worse outcome.

For the orbital floor resection group, local recurrence developed in 43%. Thirty-three percent were alive without disease, and 83% had significant orbital dysfunction. In the patients with orbital floor preservation, all patients initially had good eye function. Survival was reported at 33%, and local recurrence was noted in 70%. The authors stated that no difference in local control or survival existed between the patients undergoing orbital exenteration versus preservation. They did note a potential selection bias, with the patients undergoing orbital exenteration having more advanced cancer. In summarizing, the authors noted that within this experience, orbital floor resection with or without postoperative radiation resulted in poor ocular function.

In their conclusion, the authors stated that there were new techniques for orbital floor reconstruction in development. They questioned the wisdom of the conventional use of skin grafting for reconstruction of the orbital floor. They noted there is a group of patients who may undergo orbital preservation who develop recurrence, and thus suffer worse outcomes. Most importantly, the authors noted that when the orbital floor is resected and radiation includes the eye, exenteration should be performed due to the chance for good ocular function being extremely low and ocular complaints may significantly diminish quality of life.

The tremendous value of this work is to identify in essence what represents a two-hit model for visual impairment in patients with squamous carcinoma of the maxillary sinus. The combination of orbital floor resection with radiation of the globe is associated with poor orbital function. It is this observation that led to parallel developments addressing each of these issues. Many surgeons identified the inadequacy of skin grafting for providing orbital support. This led to complex reconstruction, often including bone grafting for recreation of the orbital floor, followed by soft tissue obliteration of the maxillary defect. An experience reported by Cordeiro et al. examined the Memorial Hospital experience for orbital floor reconstruction. Markedly improved outcomes were reported in terms of orbital function, speech, swallowing, and cosmesis.

The second advancement is the development of more directed radiation delivery utilizing IMRT for the purpose of preserving normal structures. As this relates to the maxillary sinus, it obviates the need for complete irradiation of the globe. An experience by Hoppe from Memorial Hospital showed a marked decrease in orbital complications as a consequence of the early application of directed radiation therapy in this patient population. It should be noted that many of the patients included in this experience also had the aforementioned orbital floor reconstruction addressed in the Cordeiro paper.

In summary, the landmark work by Stern et al. identifies a high-risk group of patients undergoing maxillectomy including the orbital floor and irradiation of the orbit. These patients were at high risk for ocular dysfunction as well as local recurrence. Utilizing a combination of more aggressive surgical resection, immediate complex reconstruction, and intensity-modulated radiation therapy, there are data that suggest we have improved both local control and functional outcome for this challenging patient population.

The true value of the Stern article is to identify factors that must be addressed to improve outcome for this patient population. Fortunately, we see continued progress in the field by which we have been able to improve survival and functional outcome for this compelling patient population.

CRANIOFACIAL SURGERY FOR MALIGNANT SKULL BASE TUMORS
Report of an International Collaborative Study

Snehal G Patel, Bhuvanesh Singh, Ashok Polluri, et al.

Background: Malignant tumors of the skull base are rare. Therefore, no single center treats enough patients to accumulate significant numbers for meaningful analysis of outcomes after craniofacial surgery (CFS). The current report was based on a larger cohort that was analyzed retrospectively by an International Collaborative Study Group.

Methods: One thousand three hundred seven patients who underwent CFS in 17 institutions were analyzable for outcome. The median age was 54 years (range, 1–98 years). Definitive treatment prior to CFS had been administered in 59% of patients (12%), and surgery in 523 patients (40%). The majority of tumors (87%) involved the anterior cranial fossa. Squamous cell carcinoma (29%) and adenocarcinoma (16%) were the most common histologic types. The margins of surgical resection were reported close/positive in 412 patients (32%). Adjuvant postoperative radiotherapy was received by 510 patients (39%), and chemotherapy was received by 57 patients (4%).

Results: Postoperative complications were reported in 433 patients (33%), with local wound complications the most common (18%). The postoperative mortality rate was 4%. With a median follow-up of 25 months, the 5-year overall, disease specific, and recurrence-free survival rates were 54%, 60%, and 53%, respectively. The histology of the primary tumor, its intracranial extent, and the status of surgical margins were independent predictors of overall, disease-specific, and recurrence-free survival on multivariate analysis.

Conclusions: CFS is a safe and effective treatment option for patients with malignant tumors of the skull base. The histology of the primary tumor, its intracranial extent, and the status of surgical margins are independent determinants of outcome.

Patel SG, Singh B, Polluri A, et al. Craniofacial surgery for malignant skull base tumors: report of an international collaborative study. Cancer. 2003;98:1179-1187.

Commentary by: *Dan M Fliss, Ziv Gil*

Surgical treatment of anterior skull base tumors dates back to 1963 when the first series of patients undergoing combined craniofacial resection (CFR) was reported by Ketcham and colleagues. Since then, the craniofacial approach and its modifications became the standard of care for treatment of malignant tumors involving the anterior skull base. During the last four decades, we have witnessed outstanding improvements in preoperative imaging, techniques of tumor resection, reconstruction methods, effectiveness of radiotherapy, case selection, cooperation of multidisciplinary clinical teams, and quality of life assessments. Recent data from Memorial Sloan-Kettering Cancer Center and Tel Aviv Medical Center showed that these developments contributed to a significant improvement in the overall and disease-specific survival rates of these patients. Such improvements may also be attributed to a cumulative 5-fold increase in the number of surgeries per year.

Studies reporting the outcome of CFRs were traditionally based on single-institution experiences with small numbers of patients. The main achievement of these earlier publications was to provide evidence that CFR is a valid method for the removal of anterior skull base tumors. However, due to the large variability in underlying histologies, patient characteristics, adjuvant treatment modalities and surgeon's experience, there were contradictions in the rates of mortality and complications and in outcome data. Because of the relative rarity of these tumors, there were simply not enough patients to accumulate significant numbers for meaningful outcome analyses. To overcome this difficulty, an international collaborative study group was launched in 1999. This endeavor was set up to report the collective experience of 17 institutions in performing craniofacial surgery, with the objective of assessing the safety and efficacy of the procedure. An important related aspect of this study was the standardization of data management from one country to another, thus affording greater compatibility in the expertise, quality control, and research capabilities across the globe.

The data on a total of 1,541 patients were available for analysis, representing a range of 13–205 patients per investigator. Of these, 234 patients (~15%) had to be excluded, leaving 1,307 patients upon whom this report was based.

The first important contribution of this paper was the characterization of the population of patients with anterior skull base tumors. Most of them had squamous cell carcinoma, one-half had orbital involvement, one-third had bone invasion, and one-third had intracranial invasion. The results of the study revealed that surgery achieved disease-free margins in only one-half of the patients. Inspection of the data also showed that stage grouping was available in only two-thirds of the patients and a considerable variability in the adjuvant treatment provided to the patients.

Another valuable contribution of this work was the establishment of CFR as a safe procedure, with acceptable mortality and complication rates (4% and 30%, respectively). In addition, this report set a standard for patient outcome, with a reported 5-year overall survival rate of 53%. The study defined the most important factors influencing survival as being histological grade, intracranial extension, and status of surgical margins. For example, esthesioneuroblastoma was shown to be associated with a relatively good outcome (5-year overall survival rate of 80%) in contrast to mucosal melanoma, which was associated with a dismal prognosis and a relative risk that was 8-fold higher than that for esthesioneuroblastoma.

Overall, this collaborative effort has led to the publication of six manuscripts, which have received over 300 citations in a short period of time. Patel and colleagues provided well-researched and objective data that replaced the earlier hypotheses and assumptions that had been derived from small case series. This project is an example of successful international research collaboration that conferred clear benefits to the scientific progress of the field of skull base surgery. It advanced the knowledge and strengthened the research capacity of a relatively small medical specialty.

It should be noted that this collaborative effort took advantage of the large variability in environmental conditions across continents; this is of utmost importance when working on treatment guidelines to ensure the standard of care in countries with such a variety in the quality of healthcare facilities. The great success of this project should motivate collaborative research not only in head and neck cancer but in the study of all rare diseases. Collaborative research such as this will not progress spontaneously. Specific professional societies and research agencies should encourage and guide teams of investigators to pursue similar endeavors, especially when dealing with uncommon neoplasms. Cross-border multicenter studies such as this one are invaluable for identifying different risk factors for cancer development and for establishing standards for treatment and health policies worldwide.

ENDOSCOPIC RESECTION OF SINONASAL CANCERS WITH AND WITHOUT CRANIOTOMY
Oncologic Results

Ehab Hanna, Franco DeMonte, Samer Ibrahim, et al.

Objective: To evaluate the oncologic outcomes of patients with sinonasal caner treated with endoscopic resection.

Design: Retrospective review.

Setting: Tertiary care academic cancer center.

Patients: All patients with biopsy-proved malignant neoplasm of the sinonasal region who were treated with endoscopic resection between 1992 and 2007 were included in the study, and their charts were reviewed for demographics, histopathologic findings, treatment details and outcome.

Main Outcome Measures: Oncologic outcomes, including disease recurrence and survival.

Results: Of a total of 120 patients, 93 (77.5%) underwent an exclusively endoscopic approach (EEA) and 27 (22.5%) underwent a cranioendoscopic approach (CEA) in which the surgical resection involved the addition of a frontal or subfrontal craniotomy to the transnasal endoscopic approach. Of the 120 patients, 41% presented with previously untreated disease, 46% presented with persistent disease that had been partially resected, and 13% presented with recurrent disease after prior treatment. The most common site of tumor origin was the nasal cavity (52%), followed by the ethmoid sinuses (28%). Approximately 10% of the tumors had an intracranial epicenter, most commonly around the olfactory groove. Tumors extended to or invaded the skull base in 20% and 11% of the patients, respectively. An intracranial epicenter (P < .001) and extension to (P = .001) or invasion of (P < .001) the skull base were significantly more common in patients treated with CEA than in those treated with EEA. The primary T stage was evenly distributed across all patients as follows: T1, 25%; T2, 25%; T3, 22%; and T4, 28%. However, the T-stage distribution was significantly different between the EEA group and the CEA group. Approximately two-thirds (63%) of the patients treated with EEA had a lower (T1-2) disease stage, while 95% of patients treated with CEA had a higher (T3-4) disease stage (P < .001). The most common tumor types were esthesioneuroblastoma (17%), sarcoma (15%), adenocarcinoma (14%), melanoma (14%), and squamous cell carcinoma (13%). Other, less common tumors included adenoid cystic carcinoma (7%), neuroendocrine carcinoma (4%), and sinonasal undifferentiated carcinoma (2%). Microscopically positive margins were reported in 15% of patients. Of the 120 patients, 50% were treated with surgery alone, 37% received postoperative radiation therapy, and 13% were treated with surgery, radiation therapy, and chemotherapy. The overall surgical complication rate was 11% for the whole group. Postoperative cerebrospinal fluid leakage occurred in 4 of 120 patients (3%) and was not significantly different between the CEA group (1 of 27 patients) and the EEA group (3 of 93 patients) (P > .99). The cerebrospinal fluid leak resolved spontaneously in 3 patients, and the fourth patient underwent successful endoscopic repair. With a mean follow-up of 37 months, 18 patients (15%) experienced local recurrence, with a local disease control of 85%. Regional and distant failure occurred as the first sign of disease, recurrence in 6% and 5% of patients, respectively. The 5- and 10-year disease-specific survival rates were 87% and 80%, respectively. Disease recurrence and survival did not differ significantly between the EEA group and the CEA group.

Conclusions: To the best of our knowledge, this is the largest US series to date of patients with malignant tumors of the sinonasal tract treated with endoscopic resection. Our results suggest that, in well-selected patients and with appropriate use of adjuvant therapy, endoscopic resection of sinonasal cancer results in acceptable oncologic outcomes.

Hanna E, DeMonte F, Ibrahim S, et al. Endoscopic resection of sinonasal cancers with and without craniotomy: oncologic results. Arch Otolaryngol Head Neck Surg. 2009;135:1219-1224.

Commentary by: *Carl H Snyderman*

Oncologic head and neck surgery is in a transition period with the introduction of new technologies and challenges to existing dogma. In the mid-1980s, Kennedy and others introduced endoscopic sinus surgery in the United States. The benefits of endoscopic techniques for inflammatory sinus disease were readily apparent, and the indications for endoscopic surgery gradually expanded as surgeons gained experience. Endoscopic excision of benign neoplasms of the nasal cavity and paranasal sinuses was a natural extension, and early reports demonstrated efficacy. For example, endoscopic excision of inverting papillomas is the new standard of surgical care, and open approaches (Caldwell Luc procedure, lateral rhinotomy) are rarely used. The treatment of sinonasal malignancy with endoscopic techniques has met with greater resistance, however, and remains controversial as surgeons continue to debate the relative advantages of endoscopic and open approaches. Contributing factors to the debate are the involvement of rhinologists without a background in head and neck oncology and a lack of clinical outcomes data.

Most surgical advances occur in a relative vacuum of clinical outcomes data due to the difficulty of performing randomized surgical trials and the rapid evolution of surgical techniques. Review of the medical literature demonstrates the usual deficiencies—small case series with short follow up. Early reports from Casiano and others have focused on esthesion-euroblastoma, an ideal candidate for endoscopic cranial base surgery due to its location and biological behavior. The results of endonasal surgery for other types of sinonasal cancer are not widely described and are limited by diverse histologies with small numbers, inadequate surgery, and limited follow up.

The study by Hanna et al. attempts to answer the question: "What are the oncologic outcomes of patients with sinonasal cancer treated with endoscopic resection?" This publication is significant on multiple levels. First of all, it represents the largest US series of patients with malignant tumors of the sinonasal tract treated with endoscopic resection. There is a fairly even distribution of patients across pathologic types, with inclusion of early and advanced stage tumors. Although the series covers 15 years, all of the patients were treated in the modern era of endoscopic surgery, increasing the relevance of the conclusions.

Another strength of this study is that it was performed at a single institution by an experienced cranial base team. The team includes surgeons from surgical specialties (otolaryngology, neurosurgery) as well as radiation and medical oncologists. The surgeons have a strong background in head and neck oncology and apply these principles to their endoscopic techniques. As such, the results reported here represent the best outcomes that can be expected. In conjunction with the other large endoscopic series reported by Nicolai and Castelnuovo, these results are the benchmark for all future studies of endoscopic surgery for sinonasal malignancy. Treatment outcomes are dependent on multiple factors. One of the strongest prognostic factors is the presence of positive margins. As demonstrated in this study, careful case selection and flexibility in surgical approaches minimizes the risk of a positive margin. Although not randomized, Hanna et al. provide important information regarding the selection of cases for an exclusively endoscopic approach versus a cranioendoscopic approach. They adopted a justifiably conservative approach and thus were able to demonstrate the benefits of endoscopic techniques in a way that advances surgical innovation without compromising patient care. Endoscopic surgeons who do not adhere to oncological principles risk positive margins and tumor recurrence. If endoscopic surgery is associated with poor outcomes due to inadequate surgery, the medical community may conclude prematurely that endoscopic techniques should be abandoned. Hanna et al. adopt a rational and responsible approach that is incremental and allows us to make valid conclusions regarding the role of endoscopy.

The difficulty of performing a long-term study like this cannot be overemphasized. Prior attempts to establish a similar benchmark for open cranial base surgery were complicated by incomplete retrospective data collection, multiple institutions with small volumes, diverse pathology, inconsistent treatment philosophies, and unknown quality of diagnosis and treatment. Although important historical data was obtained, it is of limited value and leaves many questions unanswered. The study by Hanna et al. is much more rigorous and provides a strong foundation for comparison. It is a model for future studies and will help direct subsequent clinical trials and surgical innovation for many years to come.

Chapter 6

Oral Cavity

"FIELD CANCERIZATION" IN ORAL STRATIFIED SQUAMOUS EPITHELIUM
Clinical Implications of Multicentric Origin

Danely P Slaughter, Harry W Southwick, Walter Smejkal

Squamous-cell or epidermoid carcinoma is the most common cancer affecting the human body. This tumor prototype may originate in more anatomical sites than any other form of carcinoma, since it is the usual cancer of the skin, lip, oral cavity, pharynx, larynx, bronchi, esophagus, anus, vulva, vegina, cervix, urethra, penis, and even bladder and renal pelvis. Rarely, it may occur primarily or as a metaplastic variant in other organs. Since the behavior patterns of this morphological entity would seem to have many similar characteristics in its differing locations and microscopic variations, detailed knowledge of the natural history of this disease is of some importance.

As our most readily available source of squamous-cell carcinoma, oral cancers were studied from the standpoint of their origins and manner of spread. Tumors of the lip, oral cavity, and pharynx in 783 patients have been reviewed, with findings that reinforce the concept of multifocal growth of these tumors. The multicentric origin of epidermoid carcinoma is not widely accepted, although such occurrence in the skin is generally recognized and studies of in situ carcinoma of the cervix uteri are indicative of this origin.

Slaughter DP, Southwick HW, Smejkal W. "Field cancerization" in oral stratified squamous epithelium: clinical implications of multicentric origin. Cancer. 1953;6:963-968.

Commentary by: *Diane Carlson, Isaäc van der Waal*

■ FOLLOWING COMMENTARY BY: DIANE CARLSON

In the 60 years since Drs Slaughter, Southwick, and Smejkal wrote their landmark paper regarding "Field Cancerization in the Oral Cavity", much has changed, while much has remained the same. Their original work was presented at the Sixth Annual Cancer Symposium of the James Ewing Society on March 7, 1953.

As stated by these gentlemen, and enduring as fact, squamous cell carcinoma (SCC) is the usual cancer of the oral cavity. Following their evaluation of 783 patients with oral cancers, the authors reported observations, including that a squamous mucosa that grossly appeared normal beyond the boundaries of a malignant tumor was histologically abnormal. Separate foci of *in situ* carcinoma and isolated islands of invasion were identified in resection specimens. They therefore concluded that microscopically related foci of neoplasia grow independently. They went on to hypothesize that, "epidermoid carcinoma of the oral stratified squamous epithelium originates by a process of "*field cancerization*", in which an area of epithelium has been preconditioned by an as-yet-unknown carcinogenic agent" (p. 967). These physicians were able to appreciate the influence of offensive agents deemed *carcinogens*, although science had not yet identified those of which we are presently aware.

Slaughter et al. demonstrated a straightforward application of reason and logic, providing evidence for support of the concept of microscopic multicentric origin for squamous cell carcinoma. The repeated exposure of the entire oral cavity to tobacco, alcohol and viruses increases the risk for the development of multiple independent synchronous or metachronous premalignant or malignant neoplasms. Synchronous lesions are characterized by skip lesions. Their astute observation that, "This pattern of distribution is of interest because it suggests a regional carcinogenic activity of some kind, in which a preconditioned epithelium has been activated over an area in which multiple cell groups undergo a process of irreversible change toward cancer" (p. 967) remains accurate and has defined the concept of "premalignant".

Over time, and with the characterization of distinct molecular mechanisms, research has been able to link specific substances to carcinogenesis. The identification of genetic pathways involved in cellular alterations and mutagenesis continues to be better elucidated. What has changed significantly since the 1953 publication of Slaughter et al. particularly over the past 20 years, is the growing number of patients with human papillomavirus (HPV)-associated oropharyngeal squamous carcinomas, who are without exposure to the classical common causal agents and are a younger cohort. Here, one is less likely to see the consequence of *field cancerization*, with a different underlying mechanism of disease evolution and progression.

The observations and suppositions of Slaughter et al. have also directly impacted the clinical approach to oral cavity dysplasia. Through their research efforts at the University of Illinois College of Medicine and the Presbyterian Hospital of Chicago, not only did this paper create defining terminology, establish a foundation and basis for a concept, which explains disease progression, it further substantially contributed by establishing a foundation for standards of treatment and care. Furthermore, *field cancerization* and the notion of preneoplasia can be applied to explain the high risk for local failure postoperatively, which remains the greatest challenge to the practicing clinician, and simultaneously for the decrease in local failure secondary to treatment with postoperative radiation therapy.

It is in these ways that Dr Slaughter and his colleagues have contributed to the advancement of the field of head and neck cancer, and he would surely be in awe of the Head and Neck Program at Memorial Sloan-Kettering Cancer center as it celebrates a centennial anniversary.

■ FOLLOWING COMMENTARY BY: ISAÄC VAN DER WAAL

The authors acknowledged that the oral cavity is an easily accessible part of the body for the study of the origin of squamous cell carcinomas (SCCs) and their manner of spread. In their study of 783 patients with oral cancer, they made the interesting observation that the majority of SCCs had wider horizontal spread than infiltration in depth, being suggestive of growth by a process of what they called lateral cancerization. Furthermore, they drew attention to the fact that on histopathologic examination of grossly normal-looking surgical margins of the mucosa a wide range of abnormalities could be observed. These abnormalities varied from stromal changes to, particularly, intraepithelial ones such as atypia and carcinoma *in situ*. Even in SCCs less than 1 cm, separate foci of *in situ* cancer cells or isolated islands of invasive SCC were encountered. These observations led the authors to hypothesize that such microscopic related foci grow independently and eventually coalesce to produce the clinical picture of a single ulcerative tumor.

In their series of 783 patients, 88 patients (11.2%) were found to have two or more independent SCCs involving the mucosa of the upper alimentary and respiratory tract. In half of these cases, two separate tumors occurred in the same anatomical area of the oral cavity, probably being the result of a regional carcinogenic activity of some kind—obviously, the etiologic role of tobacco and alcohol was not identified at that time, let alone the possible etiologic role of some of the human papillomaviruses—in which a precon-ditioned epithelium has been activated over an area in which multiple cells undergo a process of changes toward cancer. For this phenomenon the authors introduced the term "field cancerization". They explicitly concluded that oral SCCs arise from multifocal areas of precancerous changes and not from one cell that suddenly becomes malignant. The lateral cancerization could thus be explained by the progressive change to cancer of peripheral cells rather than by the expansion and destruction from pre-existing cells. This concept would explain in part the high local recurrence rate in oral cancer, both after surgery and radiotherapy.

The paper by Slaughter et al. is probably the most cited one in the literature related to the biologic behavior of oral cancer and precancer. The concept of field cancerization in the oral cavity and actually also in the upper aerodigestive tract has been, and still remains, the subject of num-erous studies related to the cause of local recurrences and second primary SCCs. Through developments in the field of molecular biology, information has become available beyond the microscopic level, confirming the presence of genetic damage in clinically normal-looking mucosa well away from an SCC. However, because of anatomical limitations, this finding does not easily allow us to extend the limits of surgical excision or radiotherapy, as was also mentioned already by Slaughter et al.

In contrast to Slaughter et al.'s hypothesis of independent growth of multicentric foci of cancerous cells, the present view, based on immunohistochemical studies and genetic profiling, points to a monoclonal origin of SCC. In the latter concept, the cancerous or precancerous cells spread laterally in the surface epithelium, either being clinically invisible for an unknown period of time or detectable as leukoplakia or erythroplakia. Although the present explanation of field cancerization differs from that suggested by Slaughter et al. the clinical implications remain the same.

The concept of field cancerization has strongly influenced the surgical and radiotherapeutical protocols; it also has stimulated the search for medical treatment strategies. Apart from conventional chemotherapeutic agents, the focus has become more and more on targeted treatment with tumor- and patient-specific biologicals. Photodynamic therapy is another example of a treatment modality that may overcome the challenges posed by field cancerization. This may also be true for manipulated adenoviruses, for instance incorporated into a mouthwash, which specifically may destroy cells with a defective *p53* pathway.

In summary, the paper by Slaughter et al. has had and still has a major impact on both treatment strategies and research in the field of oral cancer.

RADICAL SURGERY IN CANCER OF THE HEAD AND NECK
The Changing Trends in Treatment

Hayes E Martin

Up until the late 1930s, the development of radical surgery for cancer of the head and neck lagged far behind that of cancer surgery in other areas of the body. Operations within the mouth, pharynx and larynx were associated not only with a fairly high operative mortality, but with almost inevitable failure of primary union and a prolonged morbidity. Since primary union rarely could be achieved, endothermy and the actual cautery were commonly used for growths within the mouth, deliberately leaving the wounds open to heal by granulation.

Martin HE. Radical surgery in cancer of the head and heck: the changing trends in treatment. Surg Clin N Am. 1953;33:1-22.

Commentary by: *Elliot W Strong*

The article "Radical Surgery in Cancer of the Head and Neck: The Changing Trends in Treatment" by Hayes Martin was published in 1953. The report was directed to the surgical community at large. Doctor Martin described recent advances in anesthesia, blood transfusions, prevention/control of infection, surgical equipment, and techniques that enabled surgeons to provide more effective and safer radical surgical procedures in the treatment of head and neck cancer.

Prior to this era, the surgical management of head and neck cancer had been limited and done by few practitioners with results significantly compromised by life-threatening complications, especially infection, in the postoperative period, accompanied by significant morbidity and mortality. Doctor Martin and his colleagues on the Head and Neck Service at Memorial Hospital had developed a philosophy of aggressive surgical treatment of head and neck cancer. Doctor Martin was committed to meticulous record keeping and publishing the complete results of the Service's experience. Employing the extensive support services and personnel of Memorial Hospital, the Head and Neck Service acquired a considerable experience in the management of all varieties of head and neck neoplasia and liberally shared that experience with the surgical community. This article, authored by Dr Martin himself, is an excellent example of that work. For perhaps the first time, a detailed report of the decision-making, pre-, intra- and postoperative management of patients with all stages of head and neck cancer, together with the rationale for the decisions made and the treatment rendered, was available. The article clearly and concisely outlines the management of the patient, including patient education with discussion of operative risk and consent, the absolute importance of biopsy, detailed description of preoperative evaluation and preparation, intra- and postoperative management and potential complications, and ancillary procedures. The value of this surgical experience and the admittedly aggressive philosophy of the author are obvious. Much of the information reported in this article was subsequently incorporated into Doctor Martin's very successful book "Surgery of the Head and Neck Tumors", published in 1957, as perhaps the first "modern" resource extensively covering this subject.

For the first time, this article provided a detailed and logical How-I-Do-It discussion appropriately based upon vast and well-studied experience. The impact upon the surgical community was considerable. Young surgeons were stimulated to seek further training, knowledge, and experience in the management of head and neck cancer. The challenge of a complex and varied disease occurring in a vital and critical region of the body was met with increased interest, clinical research, and knowledge. Centers of excellence were established, thus further adding interest, knowledge, and experience to the surgical management of head and neck cancer. This all led to the increased understanding of the complexities of the disease and its treatment, with the resultant improved management of the patient and his/her disease, better results of treatment, and improved reconstruction, rehabilitation, survival, and quality of life.

ROUTES OF ENTRY OF SQUAMOUS CELL CARCINOMA TO THE MANDIBLE

Alan D McGregor, D Gordon MacDonald

A recent preliminary report of a study to determine the patterns of invasion of squamous cell carcinoma to the nonirradiated edentulous mandible indicated that tumor entered mainly through the residual alveolar occlusal ridge. This study has now been extended and includes both nonirradiated and irradiated mandibles. Of a total of 46 nonirradiated mandibles (10 partially dentate and 36 edentulous) invaded by tumor, 41 were invaded through the occlusal surface. This confirms the findings of the preliminary report. These findings indicate that there is a rational basis on pathologic grounds for adopting a conservative approach to the nonirradiated mandible. In 16 irradiated mandibles, the routes of tumor entry were found to be much more variable than in the nonirradiated mandible, and multiple foci of tumor invasion of the bone were often present wherever tumor in adjacent soft tissues approached the bone. This variability of tumor entry means that a conservative approach to mandibular excision cannot be pursued in the previously irradiated mandible and full-thickness segmental resection is necessary if bone involvement appears likely.

McGregor AD, MacDonald DG. Routes of entry of squamous cell carcinoma to the mandible. Head Neck Surg. 1988;10:294-301.

Commentary by: *Guillermo Raspall*

Squamous cell carcinoma is the most common primary malignant tumor of the oral cavity. The optimal treatment for all squamous cell carcinomas of the oral cavity should fulfil the following principles:

1. Complete eradication of carcinoma, with vast safety margins
2. Preserving or restoring functions of the oral cavity (mastication, speech)
3. Conservation or restoration of orofacial aesthetics
4. Minimization of those sequelae secondary to treatment
5. Prevention of recurrences.

To try to achieve these principles, three treatment modalities have been widely established:

1. Surgery
2. Radiotherapy
3. Chemotherapy.

Current strategies in the initial treatment of squamous cell carcinoma of the oral cavity differ, depending on the TNM staging: in early stages of oral cavity squamous cell carcinomas, surgical resection highlights as the appropriated treatment, while more advanced tumor stages require the combination of two or even three therapeutic modalities.

The choice of surgical approach for squamous cell carcinoma of the oral cavity depends on:

1. Tumor location
2. Tumor size

3. Depth of tumor invasion
4. Proximity to maxilla/mandibular bone
5. Superficial maxilla/mandibular bone infiltration
6. Deep maxilla/mandibular bone infiltration.

At this point, the role of the mandibular bone in the context of squamous cell carcinomas of the oral cavity should be focused on, as the adopted surgical approach has evolved over the years. Until the publication of this article in 1988, there was little knowledge about the mechanism(s) by which the mandibular bone could be affected by squamous cell carcinoma, so segmental mandibular bone surgical resection was carried out, with the consequent functional and esthetic sequelae.

The segmental mandibulectomy was performed routinely, not only to obvious mandibular invasion by squamous cell carcinoma, but also to healthy bone near the tumor. The need for vast surgical resection margins, along with the fear of possible recurrences, were other reasons leading to segmental mandibular resection.

To clarify the mechanisms by which squamous cell carcinomas invade the mandibular bone (nonirradiated and dentated, nonirradiated and edentulous, irradiated), the article by McGregor et al. should be considered revolutionary, because it changed the surgical approach adopted on mandibular bone, introducing the concept of marginal mandibulectomy or mandibular bone resection with preservation of the basal cortical

McGregor found that squamous cell carcinomas of the oral cavity are usually spread over the mucosal surface and submucosal soft tissues to reach the gingiva at its lingual, buccal, or oral side. At this point, the tumor does not extend directly to the periosteum and mandibular bone, but it is directed towards the alveolus and, from there, it reaches the trabecular mandibular portion.

These results significantly changed the surgical approach to the mandibular bone: mandibular bone is completely resected when the trabecular portion is invaded by the tumor, but in those cases in which the trabecular portion is unharmed, the marginal mandibulectomy should be considered as a valid alternative to segmental mandibulectomy.

The importance of this article is based on the following:

1. It provides knowledge about the mechanisms by which a squamous cell carcinoma of the oral cavity invades a dentated nonirradiated mandibular bone
2. It provides knowledge about the mechanisms by which a squamous cell carcinoma of the oral cavity invades an edentulous nonirradiated mandibular bone
3. It provides knowledge about the mechanisms by which a squamous cell carcinoma of the oral cavity invades a previously irradiated mandible

4. It introduces the concept of marginal mandibulectomy
5. It introduces the concept of unnecessary segmental mandibulectomy
6. It changes the surgical approach, defining the mandibular trabecular bone invasion as the delimiting factor in mandibular surgical resection
7. It defines the surgical indications of marginal mandibulectomy
8. It redefines the surgical indications of segmental mandibulectomy
9. It reduces the number of unnecessary segmental mandibulectomies
10. It allows many patients to maintain masticatory function
11. It allows many patients to maintain speech
12. It allows many patients to preserve their orofacial esthetics.

Since the publication of this article in 1988, our surgical approach has changed: in some cases, squamous cell carcinoma of the oral cavity that involves or abuts the mandible can be eradicated without sacrificing all of the mandibular bone; surely, our oncological patients are thankful for this new surgical approach reported by McGregor et al.

Chapter 7

Nasopharynx

STAGE CLASSIFICATION OF NASOPHARYNGEAL CARCINOMA: A REVIEW

John HC Ho

The extent of a cancer in a patient is best described by the extent of its primary tumor, the extent of involvement of the regional lymph nodes and the clinically demonstrated presence or absence of metastases. Although the spread of cancer is a continuous process, there is a practical need to classify cancer cases into groups according to certain stages, for the following purposes:
1. *To guide treatment planning*
2. *To give some indication of prognosis*
3. *To help in the evaluation and comparison of treatment results, especially those from different centers*
4. *To facilitate cancer research*

In order to achieve the latter two goals, general agreement on the stage classification to be adopted is essential. At present, a number of stage classifications of nasopharyngeal carcinomas (NPC) are used, but none has yet received general acceptance.

Ho JHC. Stage classification of nasopharyngeal carcinoma: a review. IARC Sci Publ. 1978;(20):99-113.

Commentary by: *Bhadrasain Vikram**

John Ho, the author of this seminal article, was born and raised in Hong Kong and became interested in nasopharyngeal carcinoma (NPC) as a medical student there. During WWII he spent almost 5 years in the Chinese army, which brought him into contact with villagers in Southern China. Insights into the way those villagers lived and raised their children proved quite valuable in his later discoveries.

From the 1950s to the 70s, as an oncologist in Hong Kong, Ho treated and gathered data on a large number of patients with NPC and conducted systematic and painstaking analyses that culminated in this landmark paper in 1978. It clarified the natural history of NPC and assisted physicians worldwide (such as myself who had just become an attending radiation oncologist at MSKCC) in treating and analyzing our own NPC patients.

In addition to his clinical staging system, Ho also described an association between the stage of NPC and the EB virus titer. In the mid-1960s,

---

*This commentary was written by Dr Vikram in his personal capacity; the views expressed herein do not necessarily reflect the positions of the NIH or the DHHS.

the legendary Lloyd Old of Sloan-Kettering Institute was researching the association between the EB virus and Burkitt's lymphoma in Africa. He used blood from NPC patients as controls and ended up serendipitously discovering that NPC was also associated with the EB virus. Ho and his colleagues in 1974 showed that the viral antigens were produced by viral genetic material integrated within the tumor cells. Subsequently, they used EB virus serology for screening first-degree relatives of NPC patients who constituted a very high-risk population. A genetic predisposition for NPC is now well established although not yet completely understood. Genome wide association studies will, we hope, soon change that.

The then prevailing wisdom as well as common sense suggested that any environmental cause of NPC would likely be an inhalant. From studies in Singapore, it was found that Indians there had, as in the case of Chinese, a high incidence of EBV infection in childhood, but they had a very low incidence of NPC. Consequently, either they had some unknown protective factors against a possible carcinogenic action of the virus or, more likely, Ho thought, there were other co-factors involved in the carcino-genesis in Chinese but not in Indians. To narrow down the enormous number of possible co-factors for study, he first proceeded to find out whether they were inhalants or ingestants. The fact that Indians and Chinese living in the same general environment in Singapore had a marked difference in the incidence of NPC, and second-generation Chinese in the U.S. still had a high incidence of the cancer, although lower than that of the first-generation immigrants, made him suspect ingestants rather than inhalants to be the more likely culprit. As he was pondering the matter one day, a junk manned by fisherfolks was serenely sailing past his office at Queen Mary Hospital. An idea immediately flashed through his mind. The fisherfolks in Hong Kong traditionally lived in and worked from their boats or junks, and cooked in the open. They should have a lower incidence of the cancer if household carcinogenic inhalants were the culprit. He therefore studied and compared the incidence of NPC in the boat-dwelling fisherfolks and the land-dwelling population. To his big surprise, the fisherfolks had an incidence double that of the land-dwellers, the majority of whom lived in congested dwellings with poor ventilation.

The end result of these and many more painstaking studies was that Cantonese salted fish, given to children in rice porridge (congee) as early as during the weaning period, was identified as the likely culprit, and it was subsequently designated a Group 1 human carcinogen by the International Agency for Research on Cancer. In Ho's own words "We inherit from our forbearers not only their genes, but frequently also their peculiar food culture".

The combination of EB virus infection, a genetic predisposition and dietary carcinogens is now believed to be the triad culminating in NPC. The extraordinary economic development in Hong Kong during the last 30 years has been associated with a plummeting by 50% of the age-standardized incidence rate of NPC. Decreased consumption of salted fish and tobacco, increased consumption of fresh vegetables, and intermarriage of the genetically high-risk population with persons at lower genetic risk probably all played a role.

Until the advent of megavoltage radiation therapy, NPC used to be a death sentence. Pioneers such as Ho showed us the possibility of curing some patients without metastatic disease by radiotherapy. His staging system provided physicians like me with a framework for radiotherapy dose escalation to 70 Gy and more, which by the mid-1980s resulted in 5-year survival rates in excess of 70% and local control rates in excess of 90% at MSKCC, even without any chemotherapy. Those results were made possible by not only the availability of megavoltage radiotherapy but of megavoltage portal imaging, computed tomography, magnetic resonance imaging, and brachytherapy. Megavoltage portal imaging allowed adequate coverage of the primary tumor without injuring the spinal cord, optic chiasm, or brainstem. Brachytherapy proved particularly useful for reducing the toxicity of external beam radiation to the salivary glands and temporal lobes. The roles of intensity modulated radiation therapy and particles such as protons and carbon ions are now being investigated. Another very important factor contributing to improvements in tumor control was improved supportive care and the recognition that interruptions during radiation therapy could have devastating consequences for tumor control.

By the mid-1980s distant metastases were becoming the predominant cause of death, especially among patients with bulky nodal metastases. The intergroup 0099 study established concurrent and adjuvant chemotherapy as a standard of care, although the value of adjuvant therapy still remains in doubt, and the optimal sequencing of systemic and radiation therapy remains an active area of investigation. Although the intergroup study showed a modest reduction in the rate of distant metastases, the prevention and treatment of distant metastases still remains the most problematic area in the treatment of NPC. Targets such as VEGF and EGFR are being studied along with many others for improving the dismal prognosis of patients with M1 disease, which hasn't changed very much since Ho's landmark paper.

The association between EB virus and NPC was suspected about the same time as the association between HPV and cancer of the uterine cervix. Unfortunately, the success in preventing cervical cancer by vaccination against HPV has yet to be replicated in the case of NPC. Ho's work, however, raised hopes that NPC was a preventable disease; in part, that hope has already been realized, and we can hope that in the not too distant future most, if not all cases can be prevented.

RETROSPECTIVE ANALYSIS OF 5037 PATIENTS WITH NASOPHARYNGEAL CARCINOMA TREATED DURING 1976–1985: OVERALL SURVIVAL AND PATTERNS OF FAILURE

Anne W Lee, Poon YF, William Foo, et al.

This is a retrospective analysis of 5037 patients with squamous cell carcinoma of the nasopharynx treated during the years 1976–1985. The stage distribution according to Ho's classification was 9% Stage I, 13% II, 50% III, 22% IV, and 6% Stage V. Only 4488 (89%) patients had full course of megavoltage radiation therapy. The median equivalent dose to the nasopharyngeal region was 65 Gy and cervical region in node-positive patients 53 Gy. Seventy percent (906/1290) of the node-negative patients had no prophylactic neck irradiation. The overall actuarial 10-year survival rate was 43%, and the corresponding failure-free survival 34%. Altogether, 4157 (83%) patients achieved complete remission lasting more than 6 months, but 53% (2205/4157) of them relapsed after a median interval of 1.4 years. The 10-year actuarial local, regional, and distant failure-free rates were 61%, 64%, and 59%, respectively. Thirty-eight percent (338/891) of all patients with local recurrence achieved second local remission. The local complete remission rate with aggressive re-irradiation alone was 47% (333/706). But 37% (124/338) of the responders recurred the second time. The incidence of distant failure correlated significantly with both the N-stage and the T-stage, with the highest (57%) occurring in patients with N3 disease. The incidence of nodal relapse in node-negative patients was 11% (44/384) among those given prophylactic neck irradiation, but 40% (362/906) among those without. Therapeutic irradiation achieved a complete regional remission rate of 90% (306/339). However, despite successful salvage, these patients had a significantly higher distant failure rate than those without nodal relapse, even if they remained local-failure-free (21% vs 6%). Patients treated during 1981–1985 achieved significantly better treatment results than those treated during 1976–1980, especially in terms of the overall survival (57% vs 47% at 5-year), the overall failure-free survival (42% vs 35% at 5-year), and the local failure-free rate (70% vs 63% at 5-year). The possible contributing factors are discussed.

Lee AW, Poon YF, Foo W, et al. Retrospective analysis of 5037 patients with nasopharyngeal carcinoma treated during 1976–1985: overall survival and patterns of failure. *Int J Radiat Oncol Biol Phys. 1992;23:261-270.*

Commentary by: *Ivan Tham, Shie-Lee Cheah, Yoke-Lim Soong, Joseph Wee*

Nasopharyngeal carcinoma (NPC) is a fairly rare malignancy worldwide, but ranks among the top 10 cancers in endemic regions, including East and Southeast Asia. While it is likely to make up only a minor component of the practice of an average head and neck oncologist in North America or Europe, it may constitute the bulk of the work of his/her colleague in China, Hong Kong, Taiwan, or Singapore. The senior radiation oncologist in these parts would have experienced large and rapid changes in the imaging and treatment for this disease over the past 20 years. While advances have been made internationally, one can look to the "Hong Kong School" for many of the key developments in this field.

Treating NPC is somewhat analogous to *kung fu,* with its different "schools" and techniques. While *kung fu* has its Shaolin, Wudang and Ermei schools, the Hong Kong School has dominated the NPC scene in East Asia and possibly the world in the last half century. Started in the 1950s by the original Great Grand Master—the late Professor John Ho—its influence is evident by the adoption of the term "Cantonese Cancer" as being synonymous to NPC. This paper by Professor Anne Lee, current Grand Mistress of the HK School, is an excellent example of why the HK School has managed to influence NPC treatment for such a long period of time.

Key Lessons from the "Hong Kong School".

1. *Meticulous records of past efforts*

   By the accumulation of this very large case series across the different centers in Hong Kong, this and other publications have set the baseline for treatment outcomes in the two-dimensional radiation therapy era.

2. *Standardization of staging and treatment*

   The uniform application of Ho's staging, itself a product of the HK School, allowed detailed analysis stratified by the main prognostic factor and was an important influence in the evolution of an international UICC/AJCC staging system. Results of the standardized megavoltage radiation therapy technique (commonly termed "Ho's technique") also set the benchmark for future comparisons with more conformal techniques.

3. *Relapse patterns of NPC*

   Besides overall treatment results, Lee's paper also highlighted other key points, including the high rate of nodal relapse in the absence of prophylactic nodal irradiation and the relatively low rate of durable response for re-irradiation in local recurrences. These findings resulted in the adoption of prophylactic nodal irradiation as standard of care and spurred efforts to improve local control in the first treatment episode.

4. *Continued innovation*

   The paper noted a survival improvement of 10% over a decade. The reasons are likely multi-fold, but innovation and rapid adoption of new imaging and treatment techniques are likely to be significant factors. This motivation to improve continues to be seen in the HK School, with multiple subsequent studies exploring the role of magnetic resonance imaging, intensity modulated radiation therapy, and systemic therapy in NPC.

CHEMORADIOTHERAPY VERSUS RADIOTHERAPY IN PATIENTS WITH ADVANCED NASOPHARYNGEAL CANCER: PHASE III RANDOMIZED INTERGROUP STUDY 0099

Muhyi Al-Sarraf, Michael LeBlanc, Shanker Giri PG, et al.

Purpose: The Southwest Oncology Group (SWOG) coordinated an Intergroup study with the participation of Radiation Therapy Oncology Group (RTOG), and Eastern Cooperative Oncology Group (ECOG). This randomized phase III trial compared chemoradiotherapy versus radiotherapy alone in patients with nasopharyngeal cancers.

Materials and Methods: Radiotherapy was administered in both arms: 1.8- to 2.0-Gy/d fractions Monday to Friday for 35 to 39 fractions for a total dose of 70 Gy. The investigational arm received chemotherapy with cisplatin 100 mg/m^2 on days 1, 22, and 43 during radiotherapy; postradiotherapy, chemotherapy with cisplatin 80 mg/m^2 on day 1 and fluorouracil 1,000 mg/m^2/d on days 1 to 4 was administered every 4 weeks for three courses. Patients were stratified by tumor stage, nodal stage, performance status, and histology.

Results: Of 193 patients registered, 147 (69 radiotherapy and 78 chemoradiotherapy) were eligible for primary analysis for survival and toxicity. The median progression-free survival (PFS) time was 15 months for eligible patients on the radiotherapy arm and was not reached for the chemoradiotherapy group. The 3-year PFS rate was 24% versus 69%, respectively (P < .001). The median survival time was 34 months for the radiotherapy group and not reached for the chemoradiotherapy group, and the 3-year survival rate was 47% versus 78%, respectively (P = .005). One hundred eighty five patients were included in a secondary analysis for survival. The 3-year survival rate for patients randomized to radiotherapy was 46%, and for the chemoradiotherapy group was 76% (P < .001).

Conclusion: We conclude that chemoradiotherapy is superior to radiotherapy alone for patients with advanced nasopharyngeal cancers with respect to PFS and overall survival.

Al-Sarraf M, LeBlanc M, Giri PG, et al. Chemoradiotherapy versus radiotherapy in patients with advanced nasopharyngeal cancer: phase III randomized Intergroup study 0099. J Clin Oncol. 1998; 16:1310-1317.

Commentary by: *Anne WM Lee*

Hidden at the center of the head, surrounded by critical structures, nasopharyngeal cancer (NPC) was invariably lethal a century ago. The advent of megavoltage radiotherapy (RT) brought the first chance of cure. With improving knowledge about the natural behavior of this cancer, advancing technology and optimization of dose fractionation, the average 5-year survival rates increased steadily to 30% in the 1960–70s, 50% in the 1980s, and 70% in the 1990s.

Excellent control can be achieved for patients with early disease by RT alone, but further improvements are still needed for the majority of patients presenting with advanced locoregional diseases. One unique feature of NPC is the notorious predilection for distant metastases; incorporation of effective systemic treatment is indicated.

The chemo-sensitive nature of NPC was first reported in the mid 1970s; cisplatin-containing regimens were developed in the 1980s. However, early randomized trials using RT plus induction and/or adjuvant chemotherapy failed to achieve a significant survival benefit. It was not until the late 1990s that we had the first major breakthrough by the Intergroup-0099 Study from America. This landmark trial, led by Dr Al-Sarraf, used cisplatin in concurrence with RT followed by adjuvant chemotherapy with combination of cisplatin plus fluorouracil. The first report published in the *Journal of Clinical Oncology* in 1998 was based on 147 patients eligible for primary analyses, and the median follow-up was only 2.7 years. The magnitude of benefit was astoundingly impressive: the 3-year progression-free survival (PFS) by concurrent-adjuvant chemoradiotherapy (CRT) was 35% higher than RT alone (69% vs 34%), and the corresponding overall survival (OS) was 31% higher (78% vs 47%). The Intergroup-0099 regimen immediately became advocated for patients with locoregionally advanced NPC.

However, when this was first published, there were serious concerns, particularly from Asian centers, where NPC is most prevalent. Firstly, the true magnitude of benefit might be smaller, as the result of the RT arm in the Intergroup-0099 Study was substantially poorer than contemporary results (most centers could achieve a 3-year OS $\geq$ 70% by RT alone for patients with similar stages). Secondly, the ultimate impact on therapeutic ratio is unknown, as there were no data on late toxicities. Thirdly, the proportions of patients who could complete the scheduled concurrent and adjuvant chemotherapy in the Intergroup-0099 Study were only 63% and 55%, respectively; the tolerance in Asian patients is worrisome. Hence, this trial sparked off four confirmatory trials from Singapore, Hong Kong, and Mainland China.

The Intergroup-0099 Study has stood the test of external validation and the test of time. Subsequent trials consistently concurred that concurrent-adjuvant CRT could significantly improve tumor control. The absolute increase in 5-year PFS ranged from 29% in the Intergroup-0099 Study to 13% in the trial by Wee et al., and 9% in the NPC-9901 Trial by the Hong Kong NPC Study Group, due to marked variation in results by RT alone, but the improvements were all statistically significant. The corresponding increase in 5-year OS varied more widely from 40% to 18% and 4%, respectively. Our trial, the only trial that showed statistically insignificant improvement in OS, raised concerns that the potency of the current regimen might not be adequate for distant control in patients with N2–3 disease, and a worrisome increase in non-cancer deaths was observed even though the overall late toxicity rate was not statistically excessive.

One major question regarding the design of the Intergroup-0099 regimen is the contribution of the adjuvant phase, because available randomized trials and meta-analyses showed that adjuvant chemotherapy per se had no significant impact for all endpoints. A review of randomized trials using concurrent-alone CRT showed less consistent conclusions. Two trials (Kwong et al. and Chan et al.) only showed borderline improvement in OS ($P \geq 0.06$) and no statistically significant improvement in failure-free rates ($P \geq 0.14$). Two trials reported a statistically significant benefit in both event-free survival and OS, but subsequent reanalysis of the trial by Lin et al. showed that the benefit was insignificant for high-risk patients, and the trial by Zhang et al. only had preliminary 2-year results.

Preliminary results from a randomized trial by Chen et al. comparing concurrent-adjuvant CRT versus concurrent-alone CRT showed no significant difference in 2-year failure free survival ($P = 0.13$). However, the results must be interpreted cautiously because 18% of the patients allocated to concurrent-adjuvant CRT were actually treated by concurrent-alone CRT and another 20% discontinued after starting adjuvant chemotherapy. Despite such deviations and suboptimal dose intensity, the concurrent-adjuvant group achieved a favorable trend, with a hazard ratio of 0.74 (95% CI, 0.49–1.10) on multivariate analyses.

Our exploratory analyses of patients accrued into the NPC-9901 and NPC9902 trials showed that the actual treatment given was important: the number of concurrent cycles affected locoregional control, while adjuvant cycles significantly affected distant control. Hence, further external validation and long-term results are needed to address this controversy; a meta-analysis based on updated patient data of all trials has been launched, and hopefully this will provide more information to guide clinical practice. In the current Clinical Practice Guidelines in Oncology by the National Comprehensive Cancer Network (NCCN), the Intergroup-0099 regimen remains the standard recommendation (Category 1 evidence).

Building on the undoubted success of concurrent chemotherapy, one strategy for further improvement is to change the sequence to induction-concurrent CRT. Meta-analyses showed that induction chemotherapy per se could statistically significantly reduce both locoregional and distant failures, Induction chemotherapy is much more tolerable; the upfront use of a potent combination of cytotoxic drugs at optimal dose intensity would theoretically be more effective for the eradication of micrometastases. Furthermore, shrinkage of tumor bulk would give wider margins for subsequent RT, an advantage that is particularly needed for patients with extensive locoregional infiltration infiltrating/abutting critical neurological structures. Since the first report by Rischin et al. in 2002, 16 single-arm phase II studies have reported very encouraging results. The current NCCN Guideline has included induction-concurrent CRT as an option for patients with locoregionally advanced NPC (Category 3 evidence). But the two available randomized studies (Hui et al. and Fountzilas et al.) showed conflicting results, and five more randomized trials are currently ongoing. Our NPC-0501 Trial comparing induction-concurrent CRT versus the Intergroup-0099 regimen has just completed accrual; the results are keenly awaited to see if we can really achieve further improvement.

To celebrate the century of progress in the fight against head and neck cancers, I would like to pay my tribute and deepest respect to Dr Al-Sarraf for his exemplary contribution to the treatment of NPC. It is extremely difficult to conduct a randomized trial on NPC in America, because this cancer is rare in the Western world; yet, Dr Al-Sarraf successfully conducted the Intergroup-0099 Study—the most important landmark trial that changed our clinical practice for the past 14 years. Should we be able to achieve further improvement in the future, it is because we are standing on the shoulders of our giant forefathers.

QUANTIFICATION OF PLASMA EPSTEIN–BARR VIRUS DNA IN PATIENTS WITH ADVANCED NASOPHARYNGEAL CARCINOMA

Jin-Ching Lin, Wen-Yi Wang, Kuang Y Chen, et al.

Background: We investigated the clinical significance of plasma concentrations of Epstein–Barr virus (EBV) DNA in patients with advanced nasopharyngeal carcinoma.

Methods: Ninety-nine patients with biopsy-proven stage III or IV nasopharyngeal carcinoma and no evidence of metastasis (M0) received 10 weekly chemotherapy treatments followed by radiotherapy. Plasma samples from the patients were subjected to a real-time quantitative polymerase-chain-reaction assay. EBV genotypes of paired samples from plasma and primary tumor were compared.

Results: Plasma EBV DNA was detectable before treatment in 94 of the 99 patients, but not in 40 healthy controls or 20 cured patients. The median concentrations of plasma EBV DNA were 681 copies per milliliter among 25 patients with stage III disease, 1703 copies per milliliter among 74 patients with stage IV disease, and 291, 940 copies per milliliter among 19 control patients with distant metastasis $(P < 0.001)$. Patients with relapse had a significantly higher plasma EBV DNA concentration before treatment than those who did not have a relapse (median, 3035 vs 1202 copies per milliliter; $P = 0.02$). The consistent genotyping of EBV DNA between paired samples of plasma and primary tumor suggested that the circulating cell-free EBV DNA may originate from the primary tumor.

Unlike the rebound of plasma EBV DNA concentrations in the patients who had a relapse, the plasma EBV DNA concentration was persistently low or undetectable in patients with a complete clinical remission. Overall survival $(P < 0.001)$ and relapse-free survival $(P = 0.02)$ were significantly lower among patients with pretreatment plasma EBV DNA concentrations of at least 1500 copies per milliliter than among those with concentrations of less than 1500 copies per milliliter. Patients with persistently detectable plasma EBV DNA had significantly worse overall survival $(P < 0.001)$ and relapse-free survival $(P < 0.001)$ than patients with undetectable EBV DNA one week after the completion of radiotherapy.

Conclusions: Quantification of plasma EBV DNA is useful for monitoring patients with nasopharyngeal carcinoma and predicting the outcome of treatment.

Lin JC, Wang WY, Chen KY, et al. Quantification of plasma Epstein-Barr virus DNA in patients with advanced nasopharyngeal carcinoma. N Engl J Med. 2004;350:2461-2470.

Commentary by: *Nancy Y Lee*

The current standard treatment for loco-regionally advanced nasopharyngeal carcinoma (NPC) is concurrent high-dose CDDP (100 mg/m² every 3 weeks for 3 cycles) and RT, preferably with intensity-modulated radiation therapy followed by adjuvant CDDP (80 mg/m²) and 5-FU (1000 mg/m² over 4 days every 28 days for 3 cycles) based on the US Intergroup 0099 trial. The benefit of chemotherapy has been seen in several studies, including those from our Asian colleagues. The use of IMRT has been directly compared with conventional radiotherapy techniques for this disease site and has shown superior loco-regional control as well as improved patient quality of life. The RTOG cooperative group also showed benefit of IMRT in two trials for this disease site. The predominant failure pattern in patients treated with IMRT consists of mainly distant failures, and patient selection is the key to determine which NPC patients need further treatment or a different chemotherapy regimen than the current standard.

Nasopharyngeal carcinoma, in particular undifferentiated and poorly differentiated subtypes, is unique among head and neck cancer in its association with the Epstein-Barr virus (EBV). Real-time polymerase chain reaction (PCR) technology can quantitatively detect circulating EBV DNA in the plasma in > 95% of NPC patients. Tumor cells are hypothesized to release EBV DNA directly into the circulation such that the EBV DNA level reflects tumor burden and microscopic residual disease after RT. Multiple studies have demonstrated an association between the level of circulating EBV DNA and disease stage, tumor recurrence, and patient survival after chemoradiation. Therefore, plasma EBV DNA analysis is a valuable tool in monitoring response to therapy for NPC.

Pre-treatment EBV DNA in plasma has been proven to correlate with cancer stage, clinical outcome, and prognosis in patients with endemic NPC. Post-treatment plasma EBV DNA has an even better correlation with prognosis and has been used to monitor recurrence after definitive therapy. The work by Lin et al. from Taiwan has shown early detection of tumor recurrence based on EBV DNA plasma level, which predates imaging studies. Undetectable levels of plasma EBV DNA are observed in patients who remained in remission.

In another large (n = 170) NPC study in which most patients were treated uniformly with definitive RT, the levels of post-treatment plasma EBV DNA strongly predicted for progression-free ($p < 0.001$) and overall survival ($p < 0.001$), and it dominated the effect of pre-treatment EBV DNA. The 1-year PFS was 93% among patients with post-treatment EBV DNA ≤ 500 copies/mL and 48% for those with > 500 copies/mL. EBV DNA levels were detected several months prior to the documentation of tumor recurrence. In another NPC radiotherapy study in which all patients also received neoadjuvant chemotherapy followed by radiotherapy, the investigators also showed that NPC patients with persistently detectable plasma EBV DNA had significantly worse overall survival ($p < 0.001$) and relapse-free survival (RFS, $p < 0.001$) than patients with undetectable EBV DNA 1 week after the completion of RT (Figs 1A and B). Lin et al. confirmed their initial report that post-treatment EBV DNA was the strongest prognostic factor in this patient group. The 2-year RFS was approximately 90% for patients with undetectable level versus 28% for those with detectable level.

The difference is striking when using plasma EBV DNA to predict which patients have a higher chance of relapse. This information is key for all future studies, and currently the RTOG is developing the next phase II-III multi-center study to address several questions, one being how to further improve upon the current results. Until then, despite the excellent and meticulous work by Lin et al. the information obtained from EBV DNA is only prognostic.

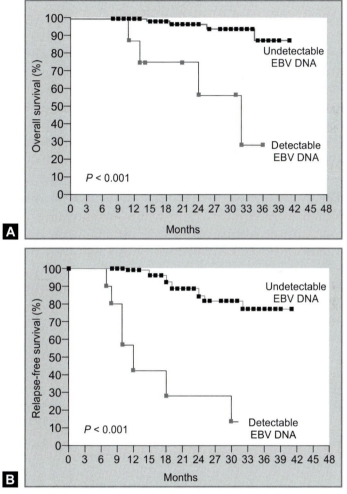

Figs 1A and B: Overall survival and relapse-free survival in 99 LA-NPC patients by post-treatment plasma EBV DNA

RANDOMIZED TRIAL OF RADIOTHERAPY VERSUS CONCURRENT CHEMORADIOTHERAPY FOLLOWED BY ADJUVANT CHEMOTHERAPY IN PATIENTS WITH AMERICAN JOINT COMMITTEE ON CANCER/INTERNATIONAL UNION AGAINST CANCER STAGE III AND IV NASOPHARYNGEAL CANCER OF THE ENDEMIC VARIETY

Joseph Wee, Eng Huat Tan, Bee Choo Tai, et al.

Purpose: The Intergroup 00-99 Trial for nasopharyngeal cancer (NPC) showed a benefit of adding chemotherapy to radiotherapy. However, there were controversies regarding the applicability of the results to patients in endemic regions. This study aims to confirm the findings of the 00-99. Trial and its applicability to patients with endemic NPC.

Patients and Methods: Between September 1997 and May 2003, 221 patients were randomly assigned to receive radiotherapy (RT) alone (n = 110) or chemoradiotherapy (CRT; n = 111). Patients in both arms received 70 Gy in 7 weeks using standard RT portals and techniques. Patients on CRT received concurrent cisplatin (25 mg/m^2 on days 1 to 4) on weeks 1, 4, and 7 of RT and adjuvant cisplatin (20 mg/m^2 on days 1 to 4) and fluorouracil (1,000 mg/m^2 on days 1 to 4) every 4 weeks (weeks 11, 15, and 19) for three cycles after completion of RT. All patients were analyzed by intent-to-treat analysis. The median follow-up time was 3.2 years.

Results: Distant metastasis occurred in 38 patients on RT alone and 18 patients on CRT. The difference in 2-year cumulative incidence was 17% (95% CI, 14% to 20%; P = .0029). The hazard ratio (HR) for disease-free survival was 0.57 (95% CI, 0.38 to 0.87; P = .0093). The 2- and 3-year overall survival (OS) rates were 78% and 85% and 65% and 80% for RT alone and CRT, respectively. The HR for OS was 0.51 (95% CI, 0.31 to 0.81; P = .0061).

Conclusion: This report confirms the findings of the Intergroup 00-99 Trial and demonstrates its applicability to endemic NPC. This study also confirms that chemotherapy improves the distant metastasis control rate in NPC.

Wee J, Tan EH, Tai BC, et al. Randomized trial of radiotherapy versus concurrent chemoradiotherapy followed by adjuvant chemotherapy in patients with AJCC/UICC stage III–IV nasopharyngeal cancer of the endemic variety. J Clin Oncol. 2005;23:6730-6738.

Commentary by: *Vincent Gregoire*

Nasopharyngeal carcinoma (NPC) is an endemic disease in Southeast Asia, where the rates vary from 30 to 50 per 100,000 people, in Inuits in Greenland, and in some countries around the Mediterranean Sea (e.g. Turkey). It is also observed quite frequently in Northern America immigrants of Asian origin. On the other hand, it is quite rare in Caucasian populations.

In Asia, undifferentiated WHO type III carcinoma constitutes more than 90% of the NPCs diagnosed, whereas in North America, up to 25% of NPC patients have keratinizing WHO type I tumors.

Radiotherapy has always been the main treatment modality for NPC, with cure rates in the order of 50–60% in Asian countries. The management of NPC is challenging for several reasons. It typically affects young patients in the middle of their professional life, and social reinsertion is a key issue; the diagnosis is often made when tumor stage is quite advanced; the rate of distant metastases is not insignificant, especially for patients with lower neck nodal disease; and treatment morbidity can be significant, especially when no Intensity Modulated Radiation Therapy (IMRT) is used, which was typically the case before the 2000s.

In this framework, Joseph Wee and colleagues from Singapore designed in the late 1990s a randomized phase III trial for stage III and IV NPC to compare radiotherapy to concomitant chemoradiotherapy followed by adjuvant chemotherapy (Wee 2005). The primary objective of the trial was to demonstrate an increase in 2-year overall survival (OS) from 55% with radiotherapy alone to 80% with combined modality. For radiotherapy, conventional two-dimensional radiation techniques (parallel opposed lateral fields and anterior field, 6-MV photons and electrons) were used up to a total dose of 60 Gy for prophylactic neck nodes and up to 70 Gy for the primary tumor and the therapeutic neck. Three cycles of 3 weekly cisplatin (25 mg/m^2 daily for 4 days) were delivered during radiotherapy, and 3 additional courses of cisplatin (20 mg/m^2 daily for 4 days) + 5Fu (1,000 mg/m^2 daily for 4 days) were delivered as adjuvant treatment.

From 1997 to 2003, 221 patients were included in the study, all but one with stage III or IV disease, the majority presenting with large T and N stage. The study showed a modest improvement in 2-year OS from 78% in the control group to 85% in the experimental arm, and a much larger improvement at 3 years from 65% to 80%, respectively. It also showed a significant reduction of distant metastasis at 2 years from 30% in the control arm to 13% in the experimental arm. Lastly, it showed that the experimental arm was associated with a significant increase in early toxicity, including mucositis/pharyngitis, anorexia, and emesis. Hematologic toxicities were also observed both during the concomitant and the adjuvant chemotherapy in the experimental arm. No late toxicity was reported.

This study was the first to demonstrate the benefit of adding chemotherapy to radiotherapy for the treatment of undifferentiated nasopharyngeal carcinoma (WHO type III) in Asia, thus confirming what has been previously demonstrated in the US Intergroup 0099, but which included 25% of keratinizing type (WHO type I) NPCs (Al-Sarraf 1998). Strangely, in the study from Wee et al., the benefit mainly occurred after 2 years of follow-up, indicating that the benefit may primarily come from the reduction of the rate of distant metastases rather than from a decrease in loco-regional recurrence. A similar study was conducted in Hong Kong from 1999 to 2005 and also concluded on the benefit of concomitant chemoradiotherapy followed by adjuvant chemotherapy over radiotherapy alone for the treatment of locally advanced NPC (Lee 2011). In that study, although disease-specific survival was significantly increased, OS was identical in the two arms due to increased deaths from toxicity or incidental causes in the experimental arm.

Unfortunately, these two studies do not answer the question as to whether the observed benefit comes from the concomitant use of chemotherapy, the adjuvant use of chemotherapy, or both. Recent randomized studies have demonstrated the dismal benefit of induction or adjuvant chemotherapy in patients with NPC (Chen 2012, Fountzilas 2012). For stage II disease, it has also been demonstrated that concomitant chemoradiotherapy without adjuvant chemotherapy significantly improved OS, emphasizing again the importance of loco-regional control on survival (Chen 2011). But in that study, only stage II patients were included, i.e. patients with a lower risk of distant metastases.

As observed for other head and neck tumors, the use of concomitant chemoradiotherapy significantly increased acute radiation toxicity, emphasizing the importance of adequate supportive care during treatment in order to avoid any interruption in the radiotherapy delivery (Wendt 1998). According to the authors, the use of fractionated delivery of cisplatin (25 mg/m^2 daily for 4 days) explained why almost three quarters of the patients received the three courses of concomitant chemotherapy, which indeed is higher than what has been reported with a higher dose of cisplatin (i.e. 100 mg/m^2 3-weekly) for head and neck tumors (Bernier 2004, Cooper 2004). In the paper of Wee et al., there was unfortunately no mention of late radiation toxicity, which is typically high in patients treated for NPC, at least in the pre-IMRT era (Lee 2012).

Another issue of this study is that radiation delivery did not include any IMRT, which might have impacted on both the loco-regional control probability and the late side effects. A prospective randomized study demonstrated a significant increase in OS (from 67.1% to 79.6%) in patients treated with IMRT compared to patients treated with conventional radiotherapy (Peng 2012). In that study, significantly less toxicity was observed in the IMRT group. Retrospective studies have also shown local control above 90% when IMRT was used, although the majority of these patients presented with locally advanced NPC (Lee 2002, Kam 2004, Wolden 2006). The use of IMRT also decreases the rate of late toxicity as demonstrated in two randomized studies showing a significant decrease in xerostomia after IMRT compared to conformal or 2-dimention radiotherapy (Pow 2006, Kam 2007).

In conclusion, there is much evidence demonstrating that concomitant chemoradiotherapy is the standard treatment for locally advanced nasopharyngeal carcinoma in 2014. Although more studies involving WHO type III nasopharyngeal carcinoma have been conducted, this conclusion can be extended to keratinizing type (WHO type I) tumors. The benefit of induction or adjuvant chemotherapy is more controversial, and on the basis of the more recent studies, it seems appropriate to only use it in the framework of randomized trials. Lastly, regarding the radiation technique, there is evidence demonstrating that all patients with NPC should get IMRT, irrespective of tumor stage.

SURGICAL SALVAGE OF PERSISTENT OR RECURRENT NASOPHARYNGEAL CARCINOMA WITH MAXILLARY SWING APPROACH—CRITICAL APPRAISAL AFTER 2 DECADES

William I Wei, Jimmy Yu Wai Chan, Raymond Wai-Man Ng, et al.

Background: The purpose of this study was to report on our experience on salvage nasopharyngectomy using the maxillary swing approach for persistent or recurrent nasopharyngeal carcinoma after primary treatment.

Methods: Over the past 2 decades, we have performed salvage nasopharyngectomies for 246 patients. Thirty-seven patients (15%) had persistent disease and 209 (85%) had recurrent tumors.

Results: All patients survived the operation with minimal morbidity. Negative resection margins were achieved in 191 patients (78%), and 55 patients (22%) had microscopic residual disease. The median follow-up was 38 months. The 5-year actuarial control of disease in the nasopharynx was 74%. The 5-year disease-free survival was 56%. Cox regression model identified the negative resection margin and the size of the tumor as 2 independent factors that affected local control of disease and survival.

Conclusion: Maxillary swing nasopharyngectomy is an effective salvage procedure for a small, persistent, or recurrent tumor in the nasopharynx after primary therapy.

Wei WI, Chan JYW, Ng RW, Ho WK. Surgical salvage of persistent or recurrent nasopharyngeal carcinoma with maxillary swing approach—critical appraisal after 2 decades. Head Neck. 2011;33: 969-975.

Commentary by: *Willard E Fee, Jr*

In 1988 or 1989, I gave a lecture at the University of Hong Kong on the first nine transpalatal, transcervical, and transmaxillary nasopharyngectomy procedures I performed at Stanford. Little did I realize that William Wei, then a senior registrar in Otolaryngology, would take my recommendation seriously—that is, to resect these local recurrences rather than place transpalatal gold seeds into them as they were doing at that time. And off he ran to stellar heights initially under the guidance of one of Hong Kong's great general surgeons, KH Lam, and later to become Chief of Otolaryngology.

This paper, published in July 2011, represents the largest open nasopharyngectomy experience in the world by a master surgeon, which probably will never be duplicated, nor should be. The majority of cases presented in this paper no longer need an open approach but can be done by an intranasal approach with scopes by surgeons experienced in functional endoscopic sinus surgery, with probably much less morbidity, shorter hospital stay, and equal oncologic results.

However, the approach discussed in this paper has the serious deficiency of not being able to control tumor very well when it extends laterally into the paranasopharyngeal space (stage T2b lesions). In my experience, almost all of these T2b tumors come to lie in very close proximity to, or right up against, the internal carotid artery. Therefore, I prefer to identify the internal carotid artery in the neck up to its entrance into the carotid canal, dissect and protect the glossopharyngeal nerve if possible, and place a pledget on the medial and anterior surface of the internal carotid artery prior to resecting the primary tumor transpalatally and/or transmaxillary.

Dr. Wei and colleagues must have very sensitive fingers indeed in that they claim on page 970 to be able to "frequently" identify the vessel by palpation of its pulsation; in approaching the vessel through the neck, I lose the ability to palpate a pulsation about 1.5–2 cm beyond the carotid bifurcation—it is most unusual in my experience to be able to feel a pulsation of the artery in the paranasopharyngeal space in either Asian or Caucasian patients. The transnasal, endoscopic approach will also have this liability for any patient stage T2b and above. In my opinion, when tumor extends laterally, a transcervical approach to protect the artery should be combined with a transnasal approach or any other approach. That may have avoided the three episodes of internal carotid injury that occurred in this paper.

Most importantly, the management of these recurrences can also be successfully dealt with by a second course of radiation therapy. Deciding which treatment will be most efficacious depends upon the local expertise of the local physicians and which complications the patients (and physicians) are willing to accept/endure. There is no doubt that both therapies are efficacious. How wonderful for patients that they have this opportunity to choose between two excellent oncologic therapies. What is needed is a randomized, prospective study comparing the two techniques with long-term (5–10 years) follow-up, so we can see the side effects of a second course of radiation therapy and quality of life data for both techniques.

The authors are to be congratulated for such a large experience with such excellent results. Fortunately for patients, intranasal techniques have replaced the open approach in most of our cases at Stanford with seemingly excellent oncologic results and definitely less morbidity.

Chapter 8

Oropharynx

RANDOMIZED TRIAL OF RADIATION THERAPY VERSUS CONCOMITANT CHEMOTHERAPY AND RADIATION THERAPY FOR ADVANCED-STAGE OROPHARYNX CARCINOMA

Gilles Calais, Mare Alfonsi, Etienne Bardet, et al.

Background: We designed a randomized clinical trial to test whether the addition of three cycles of chemotherapy during standard radiation therapy would improve disease-free survival in patients with stages III and IV (i.e. advanced oropharynx carcinoma).

Methods: A total of 226 patients have been entered in a phase III multicenter, randomized trial comparing radiotherapy alone (arm A) with radiotherapy with concomitant chemotherapy (arm B). Radiotherapy was identical in the two arms, delivering, with conventional fractionation, 70 Gy in 35 fractions. In arm B, patients received during the period of radiotherapy three cycles of a 4-day regimen containing carboplatin (70 mg/m² per day) and 5-fluorouracil (600 mg/m² per day) by continuous infusion. The two arms were equally balanced with regard to age, sex, stage, performance status, histology, and primary tumor site.

Results: Radiotherapy compliance was similar in the two arms with respect to total dose, treatment duration, and treatment interruption. The rate of grades 3 and 4 mucositis was statistically significantly higher in arm B [71%; 95% confidence interval (CI) = 54%–85%] than in arm A (39%; 95% CI = 29%–56%). Skin toxicity was not different between the two arms. Hematologic toxicity was higher in arm B as measured by neutrophil count and hemoglobin level. Three-year overall actuarial survival and disease-free survival rates were, respectively, 51% (95% CI = 39%–68%) versus 31% (95% CI = 18%–49%) and 42% (95% CI = 30%–57%) versus 20% (95% CI = 10%–33%) for patients treated with combined modality versus radiation therapy alone (P = .02 and .04, respectively). The locoregional control rate was improved in arm B (66%; 95% CI = 51%–78%) versus arm A (42%; 95% CI = 31%–56%).

Conclusion: The statistically significant improvement in overall survival that was obtained supports the use of concomitant chemotherapy as an adjunct to radiotherapy in the management of carcinoma of the oropharynx.

Calais G, Alfonsi M, Bardet E, et al. Randomized trial of radiation therapy versus concomitant chemotherapy and radiation therapy for advanced-stage oropharynx carcinoma. J Natl Cancer Inst. 1999;91: 2081-2086.

Commentary by: *Jonas T Johnson*

Earlier reports from the American literature had suggested that organ preservation, specifically avoidance of laryngectomy, could be achieved in a majority of patients with laryngeal cancer if irradiation therapy was combined with chemotherapy. This effort to avoid surgical intervention in patients with advanced cancer was the basis for the French "Groupe d'Oncologie Radiothérapie Tête et Cou" (GORTEC) trial that was initiated in 1994. In this trial, patients with oropharyngeal cancer, stage III or IV, without evidence of distant metastasis were randomly assigned to receive either radiation alone or concurrent chemoradiation. The chemotherapy chosen was 5-fluorouracil (5-FU) plus carboplatin. Chemotherapy administration was done in 3 cycles on days 1, 22, and 43 of the irradiation treatment. A total of 226 patients were enrolled, of whom 4 were eventually found to be ineligible.

Overall, compliance with treatment was excellent. No difference in the frequency of treatment breaks was observed. However, when a treatment break was required because of toxicity, the duration of radiation interruption in the combined treatment arm exceeded that of the radiation-alone arm (8.9 days vs 6.2 days, respectively). A total of 71 patients (65%) in the combined treatment group received 3 cycles of chemotherapy as planned. Thirty-eight patients (35%) did not receive a third cycle.

One patient died of treatment toxicity. The incidence of grades III–IV mucositis was higher in the combined treatment than in the radiation therapy arm (71% vs 39%, respectively). Consequently, a greater proportion of patients in the combined treatment group lost more than 10% of body mass and required temporary enteral feeding.

During follow-up (mean, 35 months), 69 patients in the radiation-only group had died, while 47 patients in the combined treatment group had died. Median survival was 15.4 months in the radiation-only group and 29.2 months in the combined therapy group. The 3-year overall survival was 51% for combined therapy versus 31% for radiation alone. The 3-year disease-free survival was 42% versus 20% and local-regional control of disease was 66% versus 42%, respectively. The overall severe late toxicity incidence was 9% in the radiation therapy arm and 14% in the combined treatment arm.

The era of "organ preservation" was introduced by the Department of Veterans Affairs Laryngeal Cancer Study Group. Organ preservation was defined as avoidance of laryngectomy. The concept, however, was quickly embraced in this and other multi-institutional studies that equate avoidance of surgery to "organ preservation". Today we recognize that functional limitations attributable to chemoradiation (CRT) treatment toxicity may result in problems such as dependence upon a feeding tube, tracheotomy, or even laryngectomy. These observed treatment-related toxicities have refocused the entire discussion to one of "functional organization preservation".

The community of head and neck oncologists has quickly embraced the availability of level 1 evidence as a new standard for which we should aspire. However, this trial failed to consider surgical intervention, which for many head and neck sites was, and still is, the legitimate standard of care. The community of head and neck surgeons especially must understand the need for level 1 evidence to influence changing therapeutic paradigms.

The recognition of HPV as a causal agent in oropharyngeal cancers, the opportunity for robotic and other minimally invasive approaches to enhance functional recovery, and the suggestion that surgery might allow for de-intensification of CRT are all factors which may allow opportunities for improved outcome in the future.

EVIDENCE FOR A CAUSAL ASSOCIATION BETWEEN HUMAN PAPILLOMAVIRUS AND A SUBSET OF HEAD AND NECK CANCERS

Maura L Gillison, Wayne M Koch, Randolph B Capone, et al.

Background: High-risk human papillomaviruses (HPVs) are etiologic agents for anogenital tract cancers and have been detected in head and neck squamous cell carcinoma (HNSCCs). We investigated, retrospectively, an etiologic role for HPVs in a large series of patients with HNSCC.

Methods: Tumor tissues from 253 patients with newly diagnosed or recurrent HNSCC were tested for the presence of HPV genome by use of polymerase chain reaction (PCR)-based assays, Southern blot hybridization, and in situ hybridization. The viral E6 coding region was sequenced to confirm the presence of tumor-specific viral isolates. Exons 5-9 of the TP53 gene were sequenced from 166 specimens. The hazard of death from HNSCC in patients with and without HPV-positive tumors was determined by proportional hazards regression analysis.

Results: HPV was detected in 62 (25%) of 253 cases [95% confidence interval (CI) = 19%–30%]. High-risk, tumorigenic type HPV16 was identified in 90% of the HPV-positive tumors. HPV16 was localized specifically by in situ hybridization within the nuclei of cancer cells in preinvasive, invasive, and lymph node disease. Southern blot hybridization patterns were consistent with viral integration. Poor tumor grade [odds ratio (OR) = 2.4; 95% CI = 1.2–4.9] and oropharyngeal site (OR = 6.2; 95% CI = 3.1–12.1) independently increased the probability of HPV presence. As compared with HPV-negative oropharyngeal cancers, HPV-positive oropharyngeal cancers were less likely to occur among moderate to heavy drinkers (OR = 0.17; 95% CI = 0.05–0.61) and smokers (OR = 0.16; 95% CI = 0.02–1.4), had a characteristic basaloid morphology (OR = 18.7; 95% CI = 2.1–167), were less likely to have TP53 mutations (OR = 0.06; 95% CI = 0.01–0.36), and had improved disease-specific survival [hazard ratio (HR) = 0.26; 95% CI = 0.07–0.98]. After adjustment for the presence of lymph node disease (HR = 2.3; 95% CI = 1.4–3.8), heavy alcohol consumption (HR = 2.6; 95% CI = 1.4–4.7), and age greater than 60 years old (HR = 1.4; 95% CI = 0.8–2.3), all patients with HPV-positive tumors had a 59% reduction in risk of death from cancer when compared with HPV-negative HNSCC patients (HR = 0.41; 95% CI = 0.20–0.88).

Conclusions: These data extend recent molecular and epidemiologic studies and strongly suggest that HPV-positive oropharyngeal cancers comprise a distinct molecular clinical, and pathologic disease entity that is likely causally associated with HPV infection and that has a markedly improved prognosis.

Gillison ML, Koch WM, Capone RB, et al. Evidence for a causal association between human papillomavirus and a subset of head and neck cancers. J Natl Cancer Inst. 2000;92:709-720

Commentary by: *Jan Klozar*

Human papillomavirus (HPV) was first linked to head and neck squamous cell cancer (HNSCC) by Syrjanen et al. in 1983 shortly after the connection of HPV and cervical cancer was described. In the following years, most of the research regarding HPV tumor etiology concerned gynecological cancers. This was due mainly to the much higher prevalence of HPV presence in cervical carcinoma than in HNSCC. Another reason was the fact that cervical cancer has frequent and well-defined precancerous lesions that were routinely examined and followed in a build up clinical infrastructure in most of the developed countries. Thus, adding HPV testing to the spectrum of examinations enabled epidemiological studies, which relatively quickly led to interesting results. This was not the case in HNSCC, and before 2000, only a few papers dealt with HPV in connection with head and neck tumors.

The paper "Evidence for a Causal Association Between Human Papillomavirus and a Subset of Head and Neck Cancers" by Gillison et al., published in 2000, was the first publication of a large group of cases showing that HPV-positive oropharyngeal cancers are a distinct clinical and molecular entity, which is very probably causally associated with HPV. In fact, this paper mentioned 13 years ago the majority of the questions on which we have worked in this field of research until today. The study group consisted of 253 HNSCC patients; 60 of them had oropharyngeal tumors. HPV presence was detected by different methods including consensus L1 PCR, E7 type-specific PCR, sequencing of a part of *E6* gene, Southern blot hybridization, and *in situ* hybridization. The authors also analyzed mutations of the *TP53* gene. The question of detection methods is still discussed today. The lack of standardization in HPV detection accounts partially for the differences in HPV prevalence referred to from different parts of the world. The search for a method that would be suitable for clinical practice (invasiveness, difficulty to perform, cost) and at the same time represent the best possible expression of viral involvement in carcinogenesis continues. Recently, the detection of the expression of viral oncogenes E6/E7 has been proposed as the most reliable method capable of distinguishing between the passive presence of the virus and its active form. Other methods and their combination have been shown to be sensitive and specific for the selection of patients with HPV-associated tumors: immunohistochemical detection of p16 protein as a surrogate marker of active viral infection and detection of HPV-specific antibodies.

The authors determined other features of HPV in HNSCC, like type-specific prevalence, the location of HPV-positive tumors, and the impact of HPV presence on prognosis. About 90% of their HPV-positive cases contained HPV 16; this was later confirmed by many other studies. The study also showed much higher HPV prevalence in oropharyngeal cancer than in non-oropharyngeal sites, which is now well documented. The study analyzed survival and stated that the survival advantage of HPV-positive cases was present, particularly in oropharyngeal cancer. The other factors influencing survival in the whole group of patients were nodal involvement, age, and alcohol consumption. Interestingly, smoking habits did not influence survival, and there was no difference found in the smoking habits between the patients with HPV-positive and -negative tumors.

With this study, Gillison and coworkers opened several directions for further research. Since the time of the publication of this study, intense work has been done by many teams, particularly in North America but also in Europe and in other parts of the world. However, many questions remain un answered. It is widely accepted that the presence of HPV infection is a risk factor for the development of oropharyngeal cancer. Nevertheless, in the near absence of precancerous lesions in oropharynx and because of the low prevalence of oropharyngeal tumors, routine HPV testing is not performed. This limits our knowledge about the natural history of HPV in the oral cavity/oropharynx. Regarding epidemiology, we have several pieces of information. The incidence of oropharyngeal cancer increases sharply in contrast to tobacco-related tumors like laryngeal cancer. Also, the proportion of HPV-positive tumors among oropharyngeal cancers has increased in recent years. It is now accepted that sexual behavior plays a decisive role in the worldwide spread of HPV infection. The sexual transmission of HPV has been documented. Many, particularly American, studies have shown differences in sexual behavior between HPV-positive and -negative cases. Nevertheless, several European studies did not find any dissimilarity in sexual habits in case-case studies. This can be due to methodological differences but also to the fact that patients in European cohorts later changed their sexual behavior and subsequently the spread of HPV infection touched this continent later. Actually, HPV prevalence in oropharyngeal tumors was lower 20 years ago in Europe, and the sharp increase in the proportion of HPV-positive tumors occurred in Europe over the last decade, so that the prevalence is now similar in both North America and Europe. Many epidemiological issues still remain unclear. No explanation, for example, exists for the male preponderance in HPV-positive oropharyngeal cancer.

The most important feature of HPV presence from a clinical point of view is its impact on prognosis. The majority of evidence testifies to better survival for patients with HPV-positive tumors. The prognostic advantage is probably independent of the treatment modality. The impact of HPV status on prognosis can outweigh other well-known prognostic factors like smoking or nodal status. All these data suggest that HPV could be used in clinical decision-making. At present, HPV status is an obligatory stratification factor in clinical studies, but it is not included in the clinical guidelines for treatment of head and neck cancer. However, markers of HPV infection would be available for selecting patients for different treatment management. The treatment intensity could probably be reduced in HPV-positive cases, resulting in less toxicity. Whether or not this can be done without compromising the so far very good survival rates is still unclear. Another important clinical aspect is the possibility of vaccination against high-risk HPVs. The efficacy of the HPV vaccine in the prevention of oropharyngeal cancer is still unknown but seems probable. Primary prevention could eliminate the currently existing adverse epidemiological development in oropharyngeal cancer.

In summary, the paper of Gillison and colleagues took an important step towards our understanding of the role of HPV in oropharyngeal cancer. However, many questions regarding this role still remain a subject of intense research.

TRANSORAL ROBOTIC SURGERY FOR ADVANCED OROPHARYNGEAL CARCINOMA

Gregory S Weinstein, Bert W O'Malley, Marc A Cohen, et al.

Objectives: To determine the oncologic and functional outcomes in patients undergoing primary transoral robotic surgery followed by adjuvant therapy as indicated with a minimum of 18-month follow-up for advanced oropharyngeal carcinoma.

Design: Prospective single-center cohort study.

Setting: Academic university health system and tertiary referral center.

Patients: Forty-seven adults with newly diagnosed and previously untreated advanced oropharyngeal carcinoma.

Intervention: Transoral robotic surgery with staged neck dissection and adjuvant therapy as indicated.

Main Outcome Measures: Margin status, recurrence disease-specific and disease-free survival, gastrostomy tube dependence, and safety and efficacy end points.

Results: In the 47 patients enrolled with stages III and IV advanced oropharyngeal carcinoma, mean follow-up was 26.6 months. There was no intraoperative or postoperative mortality. Resection margins were positive in 1 patient (2%). At last follow-up, local recurrence was identified in 1 patient (2%), regional recurrence in 2 (4%), and distant recurrence in 4 (9%). Disease-specific survival was 98% (45 of 46 patients) at 1 year and 90% (27 of 30 patients) at 2 years. Based on pathologic risk stratification, 18 of 47 patients (38%) avoided chemotherapy, and 5 patients (11%) did not receive adjuvant radiotherapy and concurrent chemotherapy in their treatment regimen. At minimum follow-up of 1 year, only 1 patient required a gastrostomy tube.

Conclusions: This novel transoral robotic surgery treatment regimen offers disease control, survival, and safety commensurate with standard treatments and an unexpected beneficial outcome of gastrostomy dependency rates that are markedly lower than those reported with standard nonsurgical therapies.

Weinstein GS, O'Malley BW Jr, Cohen MA, Quon H. Transoral robotic surgery for oropharyngeal carcinoma. Arch Otolaryngol Head Neck Surg. 2010;136:1079-85.

Commentary by: *Eric J Moore*

Ten years ago, Parsons et al. published a review of 51 studies reporting on 6,400 patients with oropharyngeal (OP) squamous cell carcinoma (SCCA) treated with surgery with or without radiation therapy (RT) or primary radiation with our without neck dissection at North American academic medical institutions. The majority of these patients underwent either open surgical resection with mandibulotomy, complete (radical) neck dissection during their primary surgical therapy or after their primary non-operative therapy, and external beam radiation therapy without intensity-modulated radiation therapy (IMRT), as these were the standards for therapy during the 3 decades prior to this review. Most of the patients had a strong history of tobacco and alcohol use, as this was the most common risk factor for OP SCCA during the 3 decades prior to this review. The cumulative 5-year survival in these reviews was 47% for patients undergoing surgery +/- RT and 43% for RT +/- neck dissection. The severe complication rate was 23% in the primary surgery group and 6% in the primary RT group, leading the authors to conclude that "nonoperative therapy was preferable to operative therapy for OP SCCA regardless of stage". During the decade prior to this publication, many practitioners were arriving at a similar conclusion. Chen et al. demonstrated that primary chemoradiation therapy (CRT) for OP SCCA at all institutions in the US doubled between 1985 and 2001, while both primary RT and primary surgical therapy were employed with rapidly decreasing frequency.

While this alteration in treatment recommendations was occurring, several other peripheral changes were occurring that would profoundly affect both the treatment recommendations and outcomes for patients with OP SCCA. For one, the disease was metamorphosizing from a relatively uncommon tumor affecting predominantly tobacco and alcohol abusing elderly men to an increasingly common cancer mediated by a sexually transmitted human papillomavirus (predominantly HPV 16) that many healthy adults were at least exposed to at some period of their lives. This alteration has had far-reaching implications for not only the younger population at risk that was now paying close attention to the cancer, but also the treatment outcomes and behavior of the cancer. Secondly, technology has altered the delivery of operative and nonoperative therapy. Computerized planning and delivery of radiation was changing the treatment course and, most would argue, altering the morbidity of radiation therapy. In surgery, neck dissection was becoming more selective and head and neck surgeons were finding that they could achieve the same goals of pathologic staging and therapeutic neck metastasis removal without resecting the "normal" neurovascular structures removed with a "radical" neck dissection. Also, a few select centers were utilizing techniques perfected in laser laryngoscopy to resect tumors in other head and neck sites transorally, thereby decreasing the number of mandibulectomies, pharyngotomies, and "open" resections that they were doing. Finally, technological advances in endoscopes and robotic instrumentation culminated in the DaVinci surgical robot (Intuitive Surgical, Sunnyvale, California), which was being employed for minimally invasive surgery in multiple areas outside of the head and neck region. This was the historical landscape when Weinstein et al. published "Transoral Robotic Surgery for Advanced Oropharyngeal Carcinoma".

At the time, very few physicians treating advanced OP cancer were considering surgery as a viable option. While the tonsillar fossa portion of the oropharynx lends itself quite well to transoral surgery, as the location of the tumor proceeds distally in the oropharynx to the base of tongue (BOT), transoral exposure and tumor excision becomes more complicated. For centuries, successful surgery has depended on the fundamentals of wide exposure and control of bleeding with hand-held instruments. This is why BOT tumors were treated surgically with mandibulotomy; the mandible precluded the surgeon from seeing the BOT directly through the mouth, and most surgeons could not get their hand in the mouth to manipulate the tumor and control the bleeding during removal. Transoral laser surgery confronts this problem by using a micromanipulator or fiber-guided laser to allow the surgeon to cut tumor at a distance from their hand, but transoral laser microsurgery for BOT tumors is challenging; it requires specific training, patience, hard-earned experience, and it does not translate to the talents or personality of every head and neck surgeon.

These challenges were the inspiration for adopting robotic surgery to transoral surgery of the OP. Surgical robots were designed with the diverse goals of enabling remote telesurgery and eliminating human factors such as tremor, but the DaVinci surgical robot primarily gained its strongest foothold in the minimal access surgical market.

In 2005, Neil Hockstein, then an otolaryngology resident at the University of Pennsylvania, took on this challenge of adapting the configuration of the robot to "fit" the transoral approach. He described the feasibility of transoral robotic surgery utilizing the camera and two of the instrument arms of the DaVinci robot first on a robot, then on a cadaver, and finally on an animal model. The field was set for clinical trials of transoral robotic surgery, and they followed quickly. Greg Weinstein and Bert O'Malley from the University of Pennsylvania published the earliest series of transoral robotic surgery outcomes. Tumors of the oropharynx, particularly the base of tongue are the leading targets of transoral robotic surgery, primarily for anatomic reasons. The dimensions of the robotic arms require that the mouth be held open and the tumor exposed through with sizeable retractors. Tumors of the larynx and hypopharynx are prime candidates for transoral surgery, but they are so far inferior to the oral opening and around the curvature of the tongue base that access with the currently available robot can be difficult or impossible. The base of tongue and tonsil can nearly always be accessed with the robot, and the angled telescopes, wide field of view, and wristed instruments do confer a surgical advantage in this area.

While the combination of chemoradiation therapy has improved the cure rates of OP SCCA, the swallowing-related morbidity of this treatment can be substantial. Weinstein showed that the functional outcomes of patients undergoing transoral robotic surgery on the oropharynx were substantially better compared to historical benchmarks of open surgery, and that the oncologic results could rival any other treatment. In 2009, largely through the work of Weinstein, the FDA granted approval for transoral robotic surgery for select malignant tumors of the "throat and voice box". The body of work in robotic surgery for cancer of the oropharynx produced by Weinstein et al. has created a renaissance of surgery as a treatment option for this disease. Patients who were once recommended to undergo only chemoradiation therapy are now being presented with options for treatment again. Some patients are able to be treated completely in a single episode of care rather than a 6–7 week "course" of treatment, and patients who were routinely treated with chemotherapy can now undergo operative therapy and "de-escalated" postoperative therapy. National randomized head and neck cancer trials are being designed with transoral surgery as a treatment arm, and hundreds of head and neck surgeons around the world are "rediscovering" transoral surgery as a treatment for OP cancer. While the credit for this also belongs to a long lineage of transoral laser surgeons, the changing face of HPV-related OP cancer, and other pioneers in robotic surgery, it is unlikely that transoral surgery would have risen to its current level of prominence so quickly or definitively if Weinstein and his colleagues had not pushed the development of transoral robotic surgery and definitively demonstrated its efficacy.

HUMAN PAPILLOMAVIRUS AND SURVIVAL OF PATIENTS WITH OROPHARYNGEAL CANCER

K Kian Ang, Jonathan Harris, Richard Wheeler, et al.

Background: Oropharyngeal squamous-cell carcinomas caused by human papillomavirus (HPV) are associated with favorable survival, but the independent prognostic significance of tumor HPV status remains unknown.

Methods: We performed a retrospective analysis of the association between tumor HPV status and survival among patients with stage III or IV oropharyngeal squamous-cell carcinoma who were enrolled in a randomized trial comparing accelerated-fractionation radiotherapy (with acceleration by means of concomitant boost radiotherapy) with standard-fractionation radiotherapy, each combined with cisplatin therapy, in patients with squamous-cell carcinoma of the head and neck Proportional-hazards models were used to compare the risk of death among patients with HPV-positive cancer and those with HPV-negative cancer.

Results: The median follow-up period was 4.8 years. The 3-year rate of overall survival was similar in the group receiving accelerated-fractionation radiotherapy and the group receiving standard-fractionation radiotherapy [70.3% vs 64.3%, $P = 0.18$, hazard ratio for death with accelerated-fractionation radiotherapy, 0.90, 95% confidence interval (CI), 0.72 to 1.13], as were the rates of high-grade acute and late toxic events. A total of 63.8% of patients with oropharyngeal cancer (206 of 323) had HPV-positive tumors, these patients had better 3-year rates of overall survival (82.4% vs 57.1% among patients with HPV-negative tumors. $P < 0.001$ by the log-rank test) and, after adjustment for age, race, tumor and nodal stage, tobacco exposure, and treatment assignment, had a 58% reduction in the risk of death (hazard ratio, 0.42; 95% CI, 0.27 to 0.66). The risk of death significantly increased with each additional pack-year of tobacco smoking. Using recursive partitioning analysis, we classified our patients as having a low, intermediate, or high risk of death on the basis of four factor; HPV status, pack-years of tobacco smoking, tumor stage, and nodal stage.

Conclusions: Tumor HPV status is a strong and independent prognostic factor for survival among patients with oropharyngeal cancer.

Ang KK, Harris J, Wheeler R, et al. Human papillomavirus and survival of patients with oropharyngeal cancer. N Engl J Med. 2010;363:24-35.

Commentary by: *Robert L Ferris*

This commentary on the report from Ang et al. summarizes the landmark report of the largest prospective, homogenously treated cohort of oropharyngeal squamous cell carcinoma (OPSCC) patients and the prognostic value of human papillomavirus (HPV) infection as an etiologic agent in OPSCC. The RTOG trial was a randomized phase III assessment of conventional cisplatin chemoradiation (CRT) versus accelerated fractionation radiation with cisplatin chemotherapy. In the accelerated CRT arm, 72 Gy was given over 6 weeks with 2 cycles of cisplatin chemotherapy every 21 days. The conventional CRT arm entailed 70 Gy given over 7 weeks with 3 cycles of cisplatin chemotherapy, each given every 21 days. There were no significant differences between the arms. Concomitant CRT was given between the two arms, and thus the main comparison was shortening the duration of radiation therapy and eliminating the third cycle of chemotherapy.

From a clinical endpoint aspect, there was no difference between the arms, and thus RTOG 0129 has been viewed as a "negative" study. However, one can also conclude that RTOG 0129 was an incremental clinical advance, since it enabled the patient to shorten their treatment to 6 weeks instead of 7 weeks, and shortening the treatment meant that one did not have to give the third cycle of chemotherapy with all of its associated toxicities. Other studies have demonstrated that accelerated fractionation CRT did not benefit patients, but in RTOG 0129 this finding, that patients who were healthy enough could avoid the third cycle of chemotherapy, could permit reducing the number of visits required for radiation even further to improve practicality of completion of therapy.

While the clinical results of this trial were not revolutionary, RTOG 0129 was a landmark trial because it demonstrated that the presence of HPV infection in patients' tumors, directly determined by HPV DNA *in situ* hybridization (ISH) or indirectly determined through p16 overexpression using immunohistochemistry (IHC), conferred approximately 25% improvement in progression free survival (PFS) and overall survival (OS). This trial was the first large randomized phase III trial ($\geq$ 700 patients enrolled) that demonstrated that two different diseases comprise OPSCC etiologically. Thus, the main finding of this study was actually that of a correlative prognostic biomarker of HPV status, rather than the primary endpoint comparing altered fractionation or cisplatin doses. This indicated to the field that we needed to conduct separate trials for HPV+ patients, who need similarly effective therapy with reduced intensity of chemotherapy or radiation therapy. On the other hand, RTOG 0129 demonstrated to the head and neck oncologic community that HPV-negative OPSCC patients fare so badly with our current standard of care (concomitant cisplatin CRT) that we need to effectively intensify or target therapy more efficaciously in order to improve oncologic outcomes. Indeed, based on this philosophy, the Eastern Cooperative Oncology Group (ECOG) designed the first HPV-specific clinical trial of de-intensified therapy for this subset of OPSCC. In addition, the RTOG 0129 trial results led to the launch of the RTOG HPV-specific trial (RTOG 1016), which replaced cisplatin with cetuximab, using 70 Gy of radiation in both arms. This RTOG 1016 trial would not have taken place without the findings from RTOG 0129, proving the beneficial prognostic impact of HPV-positive OPSCC and the need to reduce the chemotherapy or radiotherapy for these patients and its associated toxicity.

Prior to this trial report, the first prospectively treated cohort for whom the prognostic beneficial improvement and outcome was determined came from the ECOG 2399 clinical trial of induction chemotherapy followed by chemoradiation (Fakhry, JNCI J Natl Cancer Inst (2008) 100(4):261-269). The ECOG 2399 trial indicated that HPV+ OPSCC patients survived approximately 25% more frequently at 2 years than HPV- OPSCC and HPV- laryngeal cancer patients. This trial was small (n = 90 patients) and required a separate independent validation cohort, as was provided by the results of RTOG 0129. For this reason, the major value of RTOG 0129 was to validate the preliminary and intriguing findings of ECOG 2399 on the beneficial prognostic impact of HPV-induced OPSCC. In addition, RTOG 0129 specimens were tested for both HPV DNA through ISH and P16 IHC. Thus, in addition to validating the prognostic value of HPV status, RTOG 0129 defined a surrogate biomarker of HPV infection, strongly positive (> 70% positive) p16 expression by IHC, a simple and reproducible test that could be performed in most clinical laboratories, instead of the labor intensive and subjective ISH HPV DNA test. Specific results from the RTOG 0129 trial based on the HPV analysis found that OPSCC patients with HPV-positive tumors had a survival rate of 82.4% versus 57.1% in patients with HPV-negative tumors. The researchers also segregated the subsets with a history of tobacco smoking, demonstrating that tobacco exposure was independently associated with survival for both groups of patients (HPV positive and HPV negative). The risk of death in cancer progression increased by 1% for each pack-year of tobacco smoking. Drs Kian K Ang and Maura L Gillison reported in this study that the biological behavior of HPV-positive tumors may be altered by tobacco use, and potentially genetic alterations induced by tobacco-associated carcinogens may make HPV-positive tumors less responsive to non-surgical cancer therapy.

As pack-years of tobacco smoking increase, survival decreased. Thus, the RTOG 0129 trial defined different strata of risk for OPSCC: high-risk (HPV negative), low-risk (HPV positive never smoker less than 10 pack-year), and intermediate-risk HPV positive with a smoking history greater than 10 pack-years or N2b or greater neck disease). Interestingly, tumor p16 over-expression by IHC demonstrated an even better prognostic impact of p16 positivity then HPV DNA positivity itself. Thus, RTOG 0129 demonstrated that p16-positive patients had the best prognostic and dominated the low-risk group. In this study, p16-positive HPV-negative tumors occurred 19% of the time, whereas HPV-positive but p16-negative tumors occurred only 4% of the time. Thus, concordance with p16 IHC and HPV DNA ISH test was very strong (96% concordances of the 2 tests). The rate of HPV DNA negativity in the p16-positive cohort (19% with the patients) is likely comprised of patients whose tumors had low frequency of HPV DNA and fell below the threshold of ISH positivity. A small subset may have also had HPV subtypes not tested in the RTOG 0129 trial analyses. RTOG 0129 did also demonstrate that HPV type 16 is responsible for the majority of HPV-infected OPSCC, comprising 96% of the HPV-positive patients that were also p16 positive.

In summary, RTOG 0129 was a randomized phase III study with no survival difference between the arms receiving accelerated fractionation CRT or standard conventional CRT, with 2 versus 3 doses of cisplatin chemotherapy. However, the main value of this landmark paper was to validate the beneficial prognostic value of HPV infection and OPSCC, as well as even better prognostic value of p16 IHC. The latter turned out to be a better predictor of good prognosis disease than HPV DNA (by ISH). Furthermore, Ang and Gillison demonstrated that different risk stratification of OPSCC was present, laying the groundwork for intensification therapy for "high-risk" (HPV-negative OPSCC). For good prognosis, HPV+ OPSCC, this trial permitted the design of reduced-dose chemotherapy or radiotherapy in non-surgical clinical trials for the "low-risk" (HPV-positive with smoking less than 10 pack-year history), or in some situations "intermediate-risk" (HPV positive, advanced nodal disease and/or greater than 10 pack-year tobacco smoking exposure). The definition of two separate etiologic diseases in OPSCC was solidified by RTOG 0129 and strongly supports the collection of tissue and other specimens from prospective clinical trials to shed light on the biology of carcinogenesis and response to therapy as a compelling way to move the field of head and neck oncology forward, even when a trial's primary endpoint is not met.

Chapter 9

Hypopharynx and Esophagus

THE SURGICAL TREATMENT OF CARCINOMA OF THE HYPOPHARYNX AND THE ESOPHAGUS

Harold Wookey

A discussion of the surgical treatment of carcinoma of the esophagus must necessarily include lesions involving the pharynx, or at least a portion of the pharynx. There is no essential difference in these two structures and, generally speaking, most malignant lesions of the pharynx and of the esophagus are of the same type—epidermoid carcinomata.

Some of the tumors in the pharynx, however, are structurally different, and to these the terms of transitional-cell carcinoma and lympho-epithclioma have been applied. These tumors are highly anaplastic and do not form cell-nests or become keratinized. They are very malignant and are generally regarded as being radio-sensitive, whereas the epidermoid carcinomata grow more slowly and are definitely radio-resistant. The so-called transitional-cell carcinoma is commonly found in the nasopharynx and rarely in the hypopharynx, and, in our experience, not at all in the esophagus.

In this paper, only that part of the pharynx lying below the epiglottis (generally known as the hypopharynx) and the esophagus are being considered, for I believe that lesions in the nasopharynx and oral pharynx are not amenable to surgical treatment and may respond favorably to radiation. For convenience of description, the subject will be divided into three parts: first, the lesions involving the hypopharynx and upper end of the esophagus; second, those occurring in the middle of the esophagus; and, third, those involving the lower end of the esophagus.

Wookey H. Surgical treatment of carcinoma of the hypopharynx and esophagus. Brit J Surg. 1948;56: 95-103.

Commentary by: *Patrick J Bradley*

Wookey is credited with describing the use of the quadrilateral neck skin flap to repair the circumferential hypopharyngeal defect following pharyngolaryngectomy for a malignant tumor by the use of a two-layered skin tube neopharynx. This flap had been described previously and used by Wilfred Louis Trotter, London (Trotter Flap, 1932) for the repair of partial pharyngeal defects, which had been approached via a lateral pharyngotomy. Previous surgeons, prior to Wookey, had described techniques using cervical skin flaps to reconstruct pharyngeal defects with variable success.

This article published in the *British Journal of Surgery* in 1948 was based on a Hunterian Lecture presented at the Royal College of Surgeons England by Dr Harold Wookey from Toronto General Hospital, Canada on September 1947. He reviews his experience as Head of the Division of General Surgery on the surgical management of hypopharyngeal and oesophageal cancers, dividing the discussion into three segments; the hypopharynx and upper esophagus, the middle esophagus, and the lower end of the esophagus.

He comments that surgical operations devised for the removal of malignant growths in the hypopharynx or esophagus should always include methods of reconstruction. The fate of the individual who is left with an esophageal fistula in the neck and a gastrostomy in the abdomen is a most unhappy one. Wookey divides his discussion on the surgery and reconstruction on the hypopharynx and upper esophagus into three categories; (1) lesions occurring in the piriform fossa or anterior wall of the pharynx, involving the back of the larynx—if surgery is undertaken, the larynx needs to be sacrificed; (2) lesions confined to the retro-cricoid area, and does not involve the larynx or immediate surrounding; and (3) the true cancer of the upper end of the esophagus. In the latter two sited lesions, in selected cases he suggests the larynx may be preserved.

He described this flap as one requiring a wide base, and that it must include the subcutaneous fat and the platysma. He suggested that the upper half of the sternocleidomastoid muscle should be preserved because of the important blood supply through the muscle to the skin. On completion of the pharyngolaryngectomy, having preserved as much of the pharynx and upper esophagus as possible, the flap of skin is brought across the midline so as to lie on the prevertebral fascia. The upper border of the skin flap is sutured to the margin of the upper posterior wall of the oropharynx. Having reached the margin of the pharynx, the line of suture is continued anteriorly. In a similar way, the cut end of the esophagus is sutured to the lower margin of the skin flap. After completion of this maneuver, the remainder of the skin flap is used to cover, as far as possible, the rest of the wound and is secured in position by a few sutures. This raw surface remaining is then covered by a skin graft. After a period of about 5 weeks, collateral circulation of the skin flap should be established, allowing for closure of the longitudinal sulcus. Incision and undercutting of the free margin of the flap and the flap base allows for the margins of the skin tube to be sutured closed. In this way, an adequate tube of skin has replaced the pharynx and is now completely buried. When the wound has completely healed, usually not before 3 weeks, the feeding tube is removed and the patient is allowed fluids and, later, other types of food.

Wookey also described a similar technique to repair circumferential defects when the tumor is located in the retro-cricoid area and upper esophagus, when it is considered that the larynx can be preserved. He recommends that a margin of 1.5 inches below the tumor is sufficient when dividing the esophagus. He warns that "one has been agreeably surprised to find that strictures have not occurred at the suture line between the skin and esophagus, before closing the lateral fissure in the neck one should make certain that this has not occurred". These skin tubes will function satisfactorily, and some cases, which have been followed for several years, are able to take all types of food. Operation on lesions of the hypopharynx and upper esophagus should not be undertaken in advanced cases or where there are metastatic nodes. If this rule is not followed, one will be disappointed to find early recurrences, usually in the nodes of the neck and the mediastinum.

Wookey's article, when published, was one of the first attempts to describe the excision and repair of a circumferential hypopharyngeal defect in two stages using local flaps. Since that time, restoration of pharyngeal continuity after pharyngolaryngectomy for hypopharyngeal cancer has remained a problem for surgeons. Prior to Wookey's description of hypopharyngeal repair by local skin flaps, patients who had undergone a pharyngolaryngectomy were left with an orostome and an esophagostome, and as described, the "fate of the individual was a most unhappy one".

In 1942, Wookey reported successful results in 4 patients following treatment. By 1960, his surgical colleague Robert A Mustard reported his own and Wookey's combined experience with 44 patients (5-year survival rate of 24%, and "satisfactory reconstruction achieved in most patients"). Numerous modifications of the "Wookey Operation" were described and reported subsequently, but despite advances, there were inherent shortcomings using skin as a repair technique, including "partial necrosis of the flap often delayed reconstruction for prolonged intervals, during which inability to eat and constant aspiration of saliva combined to produce a miserable situation". It was realized over time and experience that this procedure could only be used in selected patients who had small tumors, as the flap was only predictably effective to replace short segments. As newer flaps were developed, the use of the "Wookey Procedure" for primary reconstruction was discontinued by most head and neck surgeons.

Following on from Wookey, many surgeons lost their enthusiasm for using local or cervical neck skin, and other skin donor areas were sought, such as distant skin flaps from the chest (Deltopectoral flap) and myocutaneous flaps (Trapezius and Pectroralis Major). During this time, because of the likely occurrence of pharyngocutaneous salivary fistula formation, which increased the likelihood of resulting pharyngeal stenosis and loss of skin flaps, prosthetic stents and other devices were advocated. Again, because of a surgeon's unease with the use of foreign materials in a situation in which anastomotic leaks can be fatal, alternative methods of primary repair were attempted using other parts of the alimentary tract–pedicled colon or jejunum and the stomach transposition. Ultimately, with the introduction of the free vascularised tissue transfer–initially the use of the free jejunum became very popular in the 1960s. Over the past few decades, a plethora and a multitude of differing tissues and structures have been recommended and advocated by surgical enthusiasts for the one stage repair of hypopharyngeal defects following pharyngolaryngectomy.

The ultimate goal of surgery is to resect enough tumor to effect an adequate curative resection while removing as little normal tissue as possible, aiming to reduce morbidity and mortality. This optimum balance can only be achieved when the surgeon appreciates the pathological behavior of the malignancy. This behavior in hypopharyngeal cancer includes the early and high propensity of metastases to the cervical nodes and extensive submucosal tumor spread. Submucosal tumor extension must be taken into account during surgery so that adequate tumor removal can be achieved. The distance of submucosal tumor extension along a longitudinal axis, as reported, can range from 10 mm to 20 mm.

While cure from hypopharyngeal cancer is the agreed upon and combined primary aim and priority of the treating physician team and the patient, the maintenance of speech and swallowing functions are equally of paramount importance to a patient's quality of life after surgery. The ultimate goals of such surgery include concomitant or synchronous, single-stage excision and reconstruction to restore these functions to a high degree and to minimize donor site morbidity. In the current era, the "multidisciplinary team" approach for the management of patients with cancer is crucial to achieve the best results and maintain or improve functional results. The selection of appropriate modalities is crucial to achieve the optimal treatment for each patient. Should primary or salvage surgery be offered to patients with hypopharyngeal cancer, the reconstructive method selected should be appropriate to the type of the defect created, which is dependent on the site and behavior of the tumor. The reconstructive procedure should fit the defect, and not vice versa.

At the present stage and state of knowledge on excisional and reconstructive techniques, there is currently no "ideal tissue or viscus" that will fulfill all of the criteria as a suitable substitute for the original organ. Thus, the current trend of primary surgery has shifted to an initial preference for a non-surgical treatment for the majority of hypopharyngeal cancers, with the aim of "organ preservation"—emphasizing the preservation of laryngeal and hypopharyngeal functions. There continues to be an urgent need to compare non-surgical and surgical treatment options for hypopharyngeal cancer, not only by the traditional oncologic outcome measures (alive or dead) but the functional outcomes (larynx and hypopharynx) as well as the longitudinal documentation of a patient's quality of life. In the past, hypopharyngeal cancer patients were recruited into the "laryngeal preservation trials", which mainly included patients with advanced laryngeal cancer. There is a need to separate patients into hypopharyngeal and laryngeal cancers and study each group separately and in greater detail. This will allow for the accumulation of more objective evidence on quantity and quality of life, and with this information presented to patients with hypopharyngeal cancer, they may be more reasonably able to select their "individualized care plan" with greater confidence and knowledge of their likely longevity and qualitative outcome.

PHARYNGOGASTRIC ANASTOMOSIS AFTER ESOPHAGO-PHARYNGECTOMY FOR CARCINOMA OF THE HYPOPHARYNX AND CERVICAL ESOPHAGUS

Guan B Ong, Thomas C Lee

The result of surgical treatment of carcinoma of the hypopharynx and cervical esophagus is so poor that it should be considered as a form of palliation. Sweet (1954) stated that only in the earliest cases should surgery be considered, and in his series there was not a single 5-year survival. Raven (1952) believed that for some patients surgery may be the only form of treatment, although there may be metastasis in the lymph-nodes. Whether the growth be early or late, the aims of treatment should be a rapid reconstruction of the pharyngogastric continuity. The classical methods advocated and practised by Trotter (1912), Wookey (1940), and Raven (1954) have left much to be desired. Reconstruction of the pharynx with skin tubes is often made difficult by the tendency to form stricture or fistula at the sites of anastomosis. This will require secondary plastic procedures and thus very often it will be months before patients can swallow normally. Occasionally the patient dies of metastasis before the final reconstruction can be completed.

Ong GB, Lee TC. Pharyngogastric anastomosis after esophago-pharyngectomy for carcinoma of the hypopharynx and cervical esophagus. Br J Surg. 1960;48:193-200.

Commentary by: *Manjit S Bains*

Surgical treatments of cancers involving the hypopharynx and the cervical esophagus have been challenging. Major problems in these patients have been in the area of reconstruction, not only to restore function but to provide cosmesis for social acceptance. In their 1960 article entitled "Pharyngogastric Anastomosis after Esophago-Pharyngectomy for Carcinoma of the Hypopharynx and Cervical Esophagus", which was published in the *British Journal of Surgery*, Ong and Lee presented a novel technique that provided the following:

• Single-stage reconstruction
• Ability to swallow effectively
• Low morbidity and mortality
• Acceptable cosmetic outcome.

The first recorded pharyngoesophageal reconstruction was done in 1877 by Czerney; and the first successful cervical esophageal reconstruction was done in 1886 by Mikulicz. Numerous variations in using the skin tubes for the reconstruction of the defects following resection of the hypopharynx and/or cervical esophagus have been used since then. However, the techniques required multi-stage procedures often associated with a high rate of complications and left patients unable to swallow comfortably and with a high frequency of salivary aspiration. These procedures usually required the creation of a pharyngostoma and esophagostoma. Wookey had reported a technique of performing a skin tube from the anterior neck skin in a staged manner to provide a conduit for the cervical esophagus. There was often compromised viability of the cervical skin flaps, especially in patients who had previous radiation therapy.

In 1965, Bakamjian popularized a two-stage reconstruction with a delto-pectoral flap that was based on blood supply medially from the perforating branches of the internal mammary artery. It was clearly more successful than the Wookey skin tube and became a standard for reconstruction of the defects of the hypopharynx and cervical esophagus. Improvement in the use of other skin flaps was met with some degree of success, but postoperative complications including anastomotic stricture formation was common.

The authors reviewed some of the techniques employed to bridge the gap left after resection of the pharynx and cervical esophagus and then presented the technique of pharyngogastric anastomosis that they employed in 3 patients. Their 3 patients came through the procedure well. The second patient, however, required rehospitalization for a "breakdown of the wound in the neck". It was noted: "There is induration extending down into the root of the neck and he died suddenly. No autopsy was performed".

The technique described by the authors was a major milestone in the treatment, especially for the reconstruction of the defects left after resection, of cancers of the hypopharynx and the cervical esophagus. It had the advantage of a single-stage procedure, provided continuity of the GI tract, and with no compromise to swallowing. In all 3 patients, a thoracotomy was performed for the mobilization of the thoracic esophagus. Mobilization of the intra-thoracic esophagus can be carried out without a thoracotomy and only through laparotomy and cervical incisions. Mobilization of the stomach and the intrathoracic esophagus can in most cases be done while resection of the tumor at the primary site is being undertaken. The stomach is an ideal conduit for the replacement of the esophagus, since it has a rich blood supply and it can easily reach the pharynx. It requires only a single anastomosis, and the patient's hospital stay is short. Most patients start oral intake of diet in less than a week.

Complications related to the procedure are few. Since the majority of the patients are in the older age group, cardiac arrhythmias are not uncommon but are easy to control. Intraoperative pneumothorax is a common finding, and most patients do require placement of unilateral or bilateral chest tubes. Anastomotic leaks can occur but are rarely serious. Patients can experience regurgitation, especially when they are straining or bending forward.

In the rare circumstances when the stomach is not available, a segment of the colon can be used for reconstruction. The use of the colon in an isoperistaltic fashion based on the left colic vessels is preferable. On rare occasions, supercharging the colon can be considered by doing a microvascular anastomosis in the neck.

Defects that are limited to the neck can be reconstructed by using revascularized jejunal autografts, the first of which were described in 1958. Functionally, jejunal autografts are likely to work better compared to a colon that has larger caliber and the muscular components are patulous. The down side of either of these two procedures is the need for a laparotomy, and on rare occasions, necrosis of the transposed organ.

In my opinion, Ong and Lee introduced a technique that heralded a major landmark in the reconstruction of the defects created by the resection of the hypopharynx and cervical esophagus. It provided a single-stage procedure, short hospital stay, with uncompromised ability to swallow and no cosmetic deformities, allowing the patient to resume his/her lifestyle. The use of the stomach has proven to be of advantage, since the blood supply to it is excellent, and it can stretch easily to the pharynx.

LARYNX PRESERVATION IN PYRIFORM SINUS CANCER: PRELIMINARY RESULTS OF A EUROPEAN ORGANIZATION FOR RESEARCH AND TREATMENT OF CANCER PHASE III TRIAL

Jean-Louis LeFebvre, Dominique Chevalier, Bernard Luboinski, et al.

Background: As a general rule, surgery whenever possible, followed by irradiation is considered to be the standard treatment for cancer of the hypopharynx, thus sacrificing natural speech. In most patients, surgery includes removal of the larynx.

Purpose: A prospective, randomized phase III study was conducted by the European Organization for Research and Treatment of Cancer (EORTC) starting in 1990 to compare a larynx-preserving treatment (induction chemotherapy plus definitive, radiation therapy in patients who showed a complete response or surgery in those who did not respond) with conventional treatment (total laryngectomy with partial pharyngectomy, radical neck dissection, and postoperative irradiation) in previously untreated and operable patients with histologically proven squamous cell carcinomas of the pyriform sinus or aryepiglottic fold, but free of other cancers.

Methods: Patients were randomly assigned to one of two treatment arms: (1) immediate surgery with postoperative radiotherapy (50–70 Gy) or (2) induction chemotherapy [cisplatin (100 mg/m^2) given as a bolus intravenous injection on day 1, followed by infusion of fluorouracil (1000 mg/m^2 per day) on days 1–5]. An endoscopic evaluation was performed after each cycle of chemotherapy. After two cycles, only partial and complete responders received a third cycle. Patients with a complete response after two or three cycles of chemotherapy were treated thereafter by irradiation (70 Gy); nonresponding patients underwent conventional surgery with postoperative radiation (50–70 Gy). Salvage surgery was also performed when patients relapsed after chemotherapy and irradiation. The trial was designed to test the equivalence of the two treatment arms; i.e. the induction chemo-therapy treatment would be judged equivalent to immediate surgery if the relative risk of death for induction chemotherapy compared with immediate surgery was significantly less than 1.43 using a one-sided hypothesis test at the .05 level of significance.

Results: Two hundred two patients entered the trial and were randomly assigned; only 194 were eligible for treatment (94 in the immediate-surgery arm and 100 in the induction-chemotherapy arm). In the induction-chemotherapy arm, complete response was seen in 52 (54%) of 97 patients with local disease (primary tumor) and in 31 (51%) of 61 patients with regional disease (involvement of the neck). Treatment failures at local, regional, and second primary sites occurred at approximately the same frequencies in the immediate-surgery arm (12%, 19%, and 16%, respectively) and in the induction-chemotherapy arm (17%, 23%, and 13%, respectively). In contrast, there were fewer failures at distant sites in the induction-chemotherapy arm than in the immediate-surgery arm (25% versus 36%, respectively; P = .041). The median duration of survival was 25 months in the immediate-surgery arm and 44 months in the induction-chemotherapy arm and, since the observed hazard ratio was 0.86 (log rank test, P = .006), which was significantly less than 1.43, the two treatments were judged to be equivalent. The 3- and 5-year estimates of retaining a functional larynx in patients treated in the induction-chemotherapy arm were 42% (95% confidence interval = 31%-53%) and 35% (95% confidence interval = 22%-48%), respectively.

Conclusions and Implications: Larynx preservation without jeopardizing survival appears feasible in patients with cancer of the hypopharynx. On the basis of these observations, the EORTC has now accepted the use of induction chemotherapy followed by radiation as the new standard treatment in its future phase III larynx preservation trials.

LeFebvre J-L, Chevalier D, Luboinski B, et al. Larynx preservation in pyriform sinus cancer: Preliminary results of a European Organization of Research and Treatment of Cancer Phase III trial. J Natl Cancer Inst. 1996;88:890-899.

Commentary by: *Arlene A Forastiere*

Investigations of combined modality therapy that includes chemotherapy for initial curative treatment of head and neck cancer began in the late 1970s and continue today. The purpose then and now is two-fold, to improve survival and to improve quality of life, the latter through the preservation of function of organs involved in speech and swallowing, e.g., the larynx, the hypopharynx, and the base of the tongue. Clinical investigations that integrated chemotherapy into treatments previously limited to surgery and adjuvant radiotherapy required the collaboration of leaders in the three disciplines—surgery, radiation oncology, and medical oncology—and very importantly, a cytotoxic regimen with a demonstrated high level of anti-tumor activity. The rapid reduction in tumor observed when cisplatin was combined with infusional 5-fluorouracil (5-FU) led to multi-center randomized controlled trials in the United States and in Europe. The key, in my opinion, to the success of these early trials was the leadership and championing of such investigations by pre-eminent head and neck surgeons without whom it would have been impossible to accrue the necessary patients for statistically valid comparisons in rigorously designed and conducted trials.

The EORTC trial 24891 led by Professor Jean-Louis Lefebvre from the Centre Oscar Lambret in Lille, France, evaluated induction chemotherapy followed by radiotherapy to preserve the larynx of patients with locally advanced pyriform sinus cancer. First reported in 1996, this randomized controlled trial is of seminal importance. Under Professor Lefebvre's leadership, the collaborating head and neck cancer specialists in France, Italy, The Netherlands, Switzerland, and individuals at the EORTC coordinating center in Brussels designed and carried out the most definitive organ preservation trial in patients with cancer of the hypopharynx reported to date. The outcomes of the trial remain relevant nearly two decades later.

In 1986, when the trial was initiated in two EORTC institutions, there was on the one hand excitement about the possibility of preserving laryngeal function but on the other hand a reluctance to deviate from the standard surgical approach, total laryngectomy with partial pharyngectomy, for fear of jeopardizing overall survival. The US Veterans Administration Laryngeal Cancer Study Group (VALCSG) had successfully undertaken a randomized controlled trial of induction cisplatin and 5-FU in patients with stages III and IV cancer of the glottis and supraglottis that required total laryngectomy. The VALCSG (led by Dr Gregory T Wolf and Dr Waun Ki Hong) showed that preservation of the larynx (reserving laryngectomy for poor responders to induction chemotherapy or later recurrence) could be safely accomplished in 62% of patients without compromise in survival and with good laryngeal function. There was, therefore, precedent for the approach taken by the EORTC; but while the organ being preserved was the same, cancer of the hypopharynx is biologically different, with considerably worse survival outcome and a risk of distant dissemination second only to nasopharyngeal cancer. The very poor prognosis of cancer of the hypopharynx and the negative impact of surgery on quality of life underscored the need for alternative and improved treatments and provided the rationale for embarking on this clinical trial. The morbidity of induction chemotherapy and 70 Gy of radiation, and the feasibility of salvage surgery were important questions that needed to be addressed separately from cancer of the larynx. In 1990, after the first 100 patients were enrolled, the trial was broadly expanded to include other institutions within the EORTC.

The trial design and major outcomes are described in the abstract of the *Journal of the National Cancer Institute* 1996 publication of the 3-year and 5-year survival estimates. The investigators sought to demonstrate equivalence or non-inferiority of an organ preservation approach (induction cisplatin and 5-FU followed by radiotherapy in those achieving complete response) compared to immediate surgery in patients with cancer of the pyriform sinus, stages T2-4, N0-2b or N3, M0. With a total of 194 randomized eligible patients and after a median follow-up of 51 months, the trial objective was met and statistical hypothesis of equivalence demonstrated to be true. Moreover, not only was the experimental non-surgical treatment not inferior to the standard of care of immediate surgery but the 3-year survival estimate was better for the group receiving induction chemotherapy, 57% (95% CI, 42%–72%) versus 43% (95% CI, 27%–59%), and the median survival time was 44 months versus 25 months, respectively (HR, 0.86 [95% CI, 0.50–1.48]). There was no difference in rates of local or local-regional control, and chemotherapy did appear to reduce the risk of distant metastases [HR, 0.59 (95% CI, 0.27–1.27)]. This contrasted with the VALCSG trial comparing induction cisplatin and 5-FU in larynx cancer to immediate total laryngectomy. In that trial, while the distant metastatic rate was lower in the chemotherapy-treated group, local control was worse, and the non-significant difference in overall survival was largely attributed to the effectiveness of salvage laryngectomy. It is likely that the EORTC trial design also influenced the result. The EORTC investigators required a clinical complete response of the primary and recovery of larynx mobility in response to a maximum of 3 cycles of induction chemotherapy in order to proceed with radiotherapy and the opportunity for preservation of the larynx. A complete response was achieved in 54% of patients and resulted in a preservation rate of a functioning larynx (no tracheotomy or feeding tube, and no local disease) of 42% (95% CI, 31%–53%) at 3 years. This is a highly impressive outcome considering the stringent response criteria. Left unanswered was whether the approach could also be successful for partial responders to induction chemotherapy. While later trials loosened this criterion to include both complete and partial responders, the studies were not powered to address this question directly, nor has there been another trial limited to cancer of the hypopharynx and with a surgery control arm. Based on the results, the EORTC adopted induction cisplatin and 5-FU followed by radiotherapy as the control arm for a subsequent series of randomized organ preservation trials that included a mix of larynx and hypopharynx primary site cancers.

This work was also notable for its consideration of the larynx preservation endpoint. First, the investigators used a surrogate of function—the absence of a tracheotomy or feeding tube. Secondly, they required an intact larynx and freedom from local progression/recurrence. Thus, patients with local recurrence or progression (either alive or dead) and those with a nonfunctioning larynx constituted treatment failures (statistical events). The confusing composite endpoint of laryngectomy-free survival, that does not account for patients with a functioning larynx who die from causes unrelated to the primary cancer, was intentionally avoided. The most informative endpoint definition remains an issue of controversy today, but logic would suggest that these investigators had it right.

While today concomitant chemoradiation is a standard organ preservation approach for cancers of the oropharynx and larynx, induction chemotherapy followed by radiation alone continues to be recommended in oncology practice guidelines (e.g. National Comprehensive Cancer Network 2013) for managing locally advanced cancer of the hypopharynx, including the requirement for a clinical complete response to induction chemotherapy. This is because it is the only treatment paradigm for hypopharynx cancer that has level 1 evidence, and secondly, because of the higher risk of serious late toxicity to the hypopharynx and surrounding tissues after concomitant chemoradiation. The complication of cervical esophageal stricture leading to gastrostomy tube dependence is well documented, as are high complication rates with attempted salvage surgery. The risk of complications may be reduced with advances in conformal radiation techniques. EORTC trial 24891 showed that neither radiation nor surgery following induction chemotherapy was compromised. The approach was feasible and safe.

Professor Lefebvre and the EORTC conducted a seminal trial that established fundamental principles for the treatment of locally advanced, operable cancer of the hypopharynx to preserve a functioning larynx that are still recommended today. Finally, the non-inferiority overall survival result of larynx preservation compared to immediate surgery (total laryngectomy and partial pharyngectomy) was maintained in the long-term, 10-year follow-up analysis published in 2012 in the *Annals of Oncology*. The median overall survival was 2.1 years (95% CI, 1.8–4.2) for the surgery control arm and 3.7 years (95% CI, 2.3–4.7) for the chemotherapy arm [HR, 0.88 (95% CI, 0.65–1.19)], favoring induction chemotherapy. Larynx preservation was successful, and over half of the surviving patients retained a functioning larynx at 5 and 10 years after treatment.

Chapter 10

Larynx

CONSERVATIVE SURGERY OF CANCER OF THE LARYNX

Justo M Alonso

When we have to treat a patient suffering from cancer of the larynx we feel that the two principal objectives to be striven for are, first, the preservation of the life of the patient and, second, the preservation, if possible, of the function of the organ of speech.

Two methods of attempting to secure these ends are available: surgery and radiation therapy. Surgery provides a greater percentage of lasting cures, but it often causes mutilation. Radiation therapy preserves the function of the organ, but is not so successful in achieving lasting "cures" and the results are sometimes misleading and contradictory. The roentgenologists, however, are constantly trying to better their apparatus and technic.

Alonso JM. Conservative surgery of cancer of the larynx. Trans Am Acad Ophthalmol Otolaryngol. 1947;51:633-642.

Commentary by: *Harvey M Tucker*

This landmark communication was presented in Chicago, IL, on October 18, 1946, at the 51st annual meeting of the American Academy of Ophthalmology and Otolaryngology (AAOO). It outlined Dr Alonso's experience and understanding of the concept that subtotal laryngectomy might be successfully undertaken in circumstances which, at the time, had been thought to require either total laryngectomy or radiation therapy for attempted cure. The obvious advantages of possible preservation of a stoma-free airway and preservation of voice were his main reasons for having attempted such operations, at a time when surgery of any type carried greater risks of infection, bleeding, and other complications than they do today.

He described the need for complete extirpation of the pre-epiglottic space in most supraglottic cancers, as well as the tendency for such lesions to spare the glottis and to present with involved neck nodes on the same or both sides. His technique generally was carried out in two stages, since he was uncertain that these resections could be closed or reconstructed in a single operation.

All of this was relatively new and was not readily accepted by most practicing otolaryngologists, at least partly because many of them did not clearly understand the embryological grounds upon which subtotal resections of the supraglottic larynx could succeed in extirpating disease. Although no citations appeared with the article, Dr Alonso made reference to previous communications, largely case reports like this one, and there was a brief discussion by several of the recognized leaders of laryngology.

The fact that this report is now included in a list of the 100 most important articles in Head and Neck Surgery is not surprising, because this and Alonso's subsequent work led directly to that of Som, Ogura, and others who were able to develop our modern understandings of conservation (not conservative) surgery for malignancies in the head and neck, while improving upon his two-stage technique. Since Dr Alonso was from a relatively small Central American country, rather than from one of the "major" centers in the US or Europe, and because all of this experience had been gained up to and during World War II, it is particularly remarkable that his work was received, understood, and carried forward to such an extent.

AN ENDOSCOPIC TECHNIQUE FOR RESTORATION OF VOICE AFTER LARYNGECTOMY

Mark I Singer, Eric D Blom

Reports of restoration of voice after total laryngectomy include diversion of exhaled pulmonary air through planned or spontaneous fistulae with a variety of modified tracheal cannulas and valves. Limitations of these techniques include aspiration, scar closure of the shunts, would complications, and failure to achieve voice consistently. We report a two-year experience with an endoscopic method using a unique valved prosthesis eliminating complicated surgical reconstructions, aspiration, and stenosis. Fifty-four of 60 patients (90%) achieved fluent voices with one deglutition problem. Radiation therapy preceded voice restoration in 63% of the patients and radical neck dissection in 72%. The endoscopic procedure, hospitalization and period of speech therapy are short and constitute a cost-effective voice rehabilitation program. The results of this simple method and lack of complications are encouraging.

Singer MI, Blom ED. An endoscopic technique for reconstruction of voice after laryngectomy. Ann Otol Rhinol Laryngol. 1980;89:529-533

Commentary by: *Frans JM Hilgers*

In medical literature, in my perception there are two types of landmark papers. First there are the global landmark papers, which are publications that constitute a milestone on a certain topic, have a worldwide impact, and often initiate a significant change in our thinking and clinical practice. Then there are personal landmark papers, which are publications that not only alter one's view on a certain topic, but also redirect one's personal clinical research focus. Not too often there is a paper that embodies both qualifications. Such a combination of constituting both a global and a personal milestone publication is the paper by Mark Singer and Eric Blom: "An Endoscopic Technique for Reconstruction of Voice after Laryngectomy", published in the November issue of the Annals in 1980.

For me, however, this milestone was erected roughly half a year earlier. In May 1980, accompanied by my wife and our two and a half-year-old daughter, I traveled for the first time to the USA to attend the two annual head and neck meetings, that of the Society of Head and Neck Surgeons in San Francisco, and that of the American Society for Head and Neck Surgery in New York some 10 days later. In San Francisco one of the many presentations I attended, and in hindsight for me the most relevant one, was given at the last session on one of the afternoons by Mark Singer. He presented the results of a secondary endoscopic tracheoesophageal puncture (TEP) technique for prosthetic voice restoration after total laryngectomy. Over the preceding 2 years he and speech language pathologist Eric Blom had explored this technique, which with the one-way shunt valve (called a duckbill prosthesis) they had developed, allowed pulmonary driven speech again. I remember that I was impressed about the fact that the presented patient series, with 60 patients followed for a period of between 2 and 23 months, was unusually large for such an innovation. The reported success rate was high, with 54 (90%) of 60 patients developing fluent speech. The 10% failures were probably caused by a too high tonus in the pharyngeal musculature, which blocked the flow of pulmonary air and thus the development of sound through mucosal vibrations in the pharynx. The reported complication rate was low, with some 10% peri-prosthetic leakages, mostly solved with cautery of the TEP tract to induce narrowing. The average life expectancy of the one-way shunt valve, based on the observation of a total of 6,960 patient-days, was 60 days. The main drawback was that 28% of the patients experienced inadvertent dislodgment of the device, requiring dilatation of the TEP tract, or even a repeated TEP. Nevertheless, the overall impression I got from Mark Singer's presentation was that it was a straightforward technique with a high success rate and a solution for potential aspiration problems. For me, that was an eye-opener, because a year earlier, in the Netherlands Cancer Institute we had started with the primary surgical voice fistula procedure according to Staffieri, which had been published shortly before.

By the time of Mark Singer's presentation, we had operated on 11 patients, who all rapidly developed a surprisingly good voice. However, as many colleagues at that time experienced as well, most of them had some aspiration issues, which were not all that easy to handle. Also, Mark Singer, as he later told me, had started with a comparable surgical procedure, the Asai technique, with similar good voice results and similar aspiration problems. For him and Eric Blom that experience was the main reason to develop the non-indwelling one-way shunt valve to overcome the aspiration issues all surgical methods had and still have to some extent. Based on our own Staffieri results, I thought I had to speak to the presenter, since this device might be the solution for our leaking surgical voice fistulas. But there were already at least 10 more attendants lining up to talk to him and I was somewhat in a hurry, because my wife and daughter were waiting for me in the hotel. Fortunately, I did not leave and did wait for my turn. Finally, I got to speak to him, and after explaining our experiences with the Staffieri proce-dure, Mark Singer spontaneously invited me to visit him in Indianapolis. And my decision to do that was one of the best of my professional life. After having arrived in New York, I convinced my wife to stay a few days behind, bought a return ticket to Indianapolis, and spent 2 days with Mark Singer and Eric Blom who happened to be great hosts. I was able to observe whatever was needed to be observed, i.e., secondary TEP procedures and several already rehabilitated patients, and returned happily to New York and thereafter to Amsterdam with a bag full of duckbill prostheses. We immediately used those to salvage our leaking Staffieri voice fistulas and subsequently for secondary TEP. That was the beginning of surgical prosthetic voice restoration at our Institute, like it happened in many clinics worldwide. But it also was the start of a long line of clinical research projects on various postlaryngectomy rehabilitation aspects at our Institute. Thus, my verdict that this paper deserves both a global and personal landmark status is undisputable.

Great thoughts often arise simultaneously at different places in this world. At the time Singer and Blom presented their prosthetic tracheo-esophageal voice rehabilitation method, others were working on this topic as well. Some years earlier, professor Mozolewski from Poland had published in the Polish ENT journal (1973) and had given a presentation in Boston (1978) on a voice prosthesis he had developed and successfully applied. Also in 1980, colleagues of the ENT department of the Groningen University Hospital at a National ENT meeting in the Netherlands presented an indwelling voice prosthesis, which could be inserted both primarily at the time of laryngectomy and secondarily at a later date (published in 1982). Nevertheless, the real starting point of this global move towards surgical prosthetic voice restoration is formed by Singer and Blom's landmark paper. This publication immediately stimulated a worldwide clinical research wave. One of the first issues addressed was the suboptimal retention of the first non-indwelling Blom-Singer duckbill prosthesis. Already in the same year (1980) Bill Panje introduced his voice prosthesis, which had a retention collar at the esophageal side, subsequently also implemented in the Blom-Singer line of prostheses, which turned out to be helpful in decreasing the number of inadvertent prosthesis losses Singer and Blom had reported. This dislodgment problem then was virtually eliminated with the introduction of the inherent sturdier flanges of indwelling devices, making these prostheses for many clinicians the preferred TEP appliance.

Another reason the Singer-Blom publication is a true landmark paper is that the authors also have put in huge efforts into teaching numerous head and neck surgeons and SLPs over several decades now. Doing innovative clinical research and writing a concise paper about the outcomes seldom is enough to achieve the status of landmark paper. Continued research and relentless and passionate teaching often form the real keys to reach this status. And with 602 citations (mid-October 2012; http://www.harzing.com/pop.htm: "Publish or Perish"), an annual average of 18.24 citations, this is a true landmark paper indeed. And its status as a personal landmark paper is underlined by the fact that I probably have contributed at least 5% to this total with my own publications on prosthetic voice rehabilitation.

While re-reading this paper after 32 years, I realized how surprisingly complete the authors already pictured all the major aspects of prosthetic vocal rehabilitation, even with their description of their first automatic speaking valve (ASV) for re-establishing hands-free speech. The paper did not contain many tables, and there were no statistical analyses of any significance, as presently would be required by any editor, but all clinical relevant issues were already presented:

- Spasm-hypertonicity of the pharyngeal musculature, which a few years later Singer and Blom unraveled and found the first solution for with their partner in the following years, Ron Hamaker;
- Description of the air-insufflation test, being a relative guide for patient selection;
- Patient motivation as a selection factor (e.g. the ability to care for prosthesis and stoma), obviously especially important in secondary TEPs, which they started out with;
- The suggestion that there should be a suitable disease-free interval, something that more or less has become irrelevant, however, after primary TEP has become the norm now;
- Patient dexterity/ability to occlude the stoma as an important factor for success, something that has become less relevant in the Western world, however, after the introduction of heat and moisture exchangers and better functioning ASVs;
- And last but not least, the importance of teamwork by the head and neck surgeon and SLP: "The surgeon and the speech pathologist work as a team for the selection and rehabilitation of the laryngectomy patient. It is this interdisciplinary approach to the communication-impaired patient that forms the cornerstone of this voice restoration method".

Re-reading this global and personal landmark paper brought back great memories about those pioneering years, realizing the enormous progress that has been made since by these authors and many others stimulated by this paper, and a feeling of satisfaction that since then prosthetic voice rehabilitation has become the method of choice for restoring oral communication after total laryngectomy. This is especially important in view of the present dispute about the optimal (organ sacrificing or organ preservation) treatment for advanced larynx and hypopharynx cancer, for which the dilemma fortunately no longer is "to talk or not to talk".

INDUCTION CHEMOTHERAPY PLUS RADIATION COMPARED WITH SURGERY PLUS RADIATION IN PATIENTS WITH ADVANCED LARYNGEAL CANCER
The Department of Veterans Affairs Laryngeal Cancer Study Group

Background: We performed a prospective, randomized study in patients with previously untreated advanced (Stage III or IV) laryngeal squamous carcinoma to compare the results of induction chemotherapy followed by definitive radiation therapy with those of conventional laryngectomy and postoperative radiation.

Methods: Three hundred thirty-two patients were randomly assigned to receive either three cycles of chemotherapy (cisplatin and fluorouracil) and radiation therapy or surgery and radiation therapy. The clinical tumor response was assessed after two cycles of chemotherapy, and patients with a response received a third cycle followed by definitive radiation therapy (6600 to 7600 cGy). Patients in whom there was no tumor response or who had locally recurrent cancers after chemotherapy and radiation therapy underwent salvage laryngectomy.

Results: After two cycles of chemotherapy, the clinical tumor response was complete in 31 percent of the patients and partial in 54 percent. After a median follow-up of 33 months, the estimated 2-year survival was 68 percent (95 percent confidence interval, 60–76 percent) for both treatment groups (P = 0.9846). Patterns of recurrence differed significantly between the two groups, with more local recurrences (P = 0.0005) and fewer distant metastases (P = 0.016) in the chemotherapy group than in the surgery group. A total of 59 patients in the chemotherapy group (36 percent) required total laryngectomy. The larynx was preserved in 64 percent of the patients overall and 64 percent of the patients who were alive and free of disease.

Conclusions: These preliminary results suggest a new role for chemotherapy in patients with advanced laryngeal cancer and indicate that a treatment strategy involving induction chemotherapy and definitive radiation therapy can be effective in preserving the larynx in a high percentage of patients, without compromising overall survival.

Induction chemotherapy plus radiation compared with surgery plus radiation in patients with advanced laryngeal cancer. The Department of Veterans Affairs Laryngeal Cancer Study Group. N Engl J Med. 1991;324:1685-1690.

Commentary by: *Jean-Louis LeFebvre*

In 1991, Gregory T Wolf, under the auspices of the Department of Veterans Affairs Laryngeal Study Group, reported the first randomized trial on larynx preservation. This trial has had a tremendous impact on the daily practice and on subsequent clinical research on larynx preservation.

For decades, the treatment of locally advanced laryngeal cancers has been based on two different approaches: either total laryngectomy with postoperative irradiation or definitive irradiation with salvage surgery if required. In the absence of a prospective randomized comparison of both attitudes, the indication for either of these options was based on national or institutional policies. For example, Northern Europe favored radiation while Southern Europe, Italy and Spain, favored upfront surgery.

At the turn of the 70s–80s, new chemotherapy regimens based on the combination of cisplatinum and 5-fluorouracile were able to provide impressive response rates in previously untreated patients. If the use of induction chemotherapy failed to demonstrate a significant improvement in survival, it appeared that tumors responding to induction chemotherapy were also responding to a subsequent irradiation. This was the rationale of the discussion on organ preservation. Induction chemotherapy was considered as a possible tool to separate two groups of patients: poor or good candidates for irradiation. As the total removal of the larynx has an obvious impact on quality of life (but it is a very efficient treatment), logically the larynx was the first primary site included in organ preservation clinical research.

The concept of this randomized trial was to compare the conventional treatment (total laryngectomy and postoperative irradiation) and an experimental arm starting with induction chemotherapy followed in good responders by irradiation or by surgery and postoperative irradiation in poor responders. A quite large number of patients were enrolled in the trial (332 in total, 166 patients in each arm), allowing valid statistical comparison tests. There was no significant difference in overall survival between both arms, and the larynx could be preserved in nearly two-thirds of the patients in the experimental arm. Similar trials were conducted in Europe (GETTEC, EORTC 24891, and GORTEC 2000–01) either on larynx or hypopharynx cancers using induction chemotherapy (cisplatin + 5-fluorouracil, and more recently, cisplatin + 5-fluorouracil + docetaxel). These trials concluded that the concept could be validated as survival was not compromised (but also not improved) in the induction arm, while a substantial number of larynges could be preserved. To this extent, the Veterans trial is an important milestone in the treatment of laryngeal cancers and must be acknowledged as such. However, this trial also generated several discussions:

1. What would have been the results of irradiation alone in such cases?
2. How does concurrent chemoradiotherapy compare with induction chemotherapy-based approaches?
3. What about the function of the preserved larynx, and does quality of life improve after such protocols?
4. Are all the data from larynx preservation trials comparable?
5. Are such protocols translatable into daily practice (i.e., outside the frame of clinical trials)?

A North American trial (RTOG 91–11) aimed to answer the first two questions, showing the superiority of concurrent chemoradiotherapy in terms of larynx preservation but not in laryngectomy-free survival or overall survival. A European trial (EORTC 24954) failed to find any difference between induction chemotherapy before irradiation and alternating chemo-radiotherapy.

The question of laryngeal function remains unsolved as the definition of larynx preservation varies in different trials. In addition, the side effects of non-surgical treatments may improve or worsen over time, and the quality of function may subsequently change with time.

A comparison between the trials is also problematic as the inclusion criteria were somewhat different. From a logical point of view larynx preservation should be considered as an alternative to a total laryngectomy (without compromising disease control and survival). When properly indicated and performed, partial larynx surgery is able to control the disease and to preserve satisfactory laryngeal function. In the European trials, the main eligibility criterion was "larynx cancer patients for whom a total laryngectomy is indicated". In the VA trial, the eligibility criterion was "stages III and IV, disease according to the 1985 AJCC staging system", and around one tenth of the patients had T1 and T2 disease. Due to such discrepancies, comparisons of published results may be misleading. Gregory T Wolf participated in an experts meeting defining recommendations for future trials (*Int J Radiat Oncol Biol.* 2009;73:1293-303).

This is probably the main concern. The gold standard for treating a cancer patient (and the only gold standard) is a multidisciplinary discussion with evidence-based rationale. This being said, the highest level of evidence-based medicine comes from large randomized trials. These randomized trials are conducted on highly selected groups of patients with clear eligibility criteria, with precise treatment and follow-up protocols. In daily practice, patients may be less selected. Clearly, all candidates for a total laryngectomy are not candidates for a larynx preservation approach. Eligibility criteria in daily practice must follow exactly those of randomized trials, as well as the treatment and follow-up protocol.

Larynx preservation is a challenging approach. Selected patients may benefit from these new protocols. The Veterans Affairs Laryngeal Study Group trial has opened this important clinical research.

CONCURRENT CHEMOTHERAPY AND RADIOTHERAPY FOR ORGAN PRESERVATION IN ADVANCED LARYNGEAL CANCER

Arlene A Forastiere, Helmuth Goepfert, Moshe Maor, et al.

Background: Induction chemotherapy with cisplatin plus fluorouracil followed by radiotherapy is the standard alternative to total laryngectomy for patients with locally advanced laryngeal cancer. The value of adding chemotherapy to radiotherapy and the optimal timing of chemotherapy are unknown.

Methods: We randomly assigned patients with locally advanced cancer of the larynx to one of three treatments: induction cisplatin plus fluorouracil followed by radiotherapy, radiotherapy with concurrent administration of cisplatin, or radiotherapy alone. The primary endpoint was preservation of the larynx.

Result: A total of 547 patients were randomly assigned to one of the three study groups. The median follow-up period was 3.8 years. At two years, the proportion of patients who had an intact larynx after radiotherapy with concurrent cisplatin (88 percent) differed significantly from the proportions in the groups given induction chemotherapy followed by radiotherapy (75 percent, P = 0.005) or radiotherapy alone (70 percent, P < 0.001). The rate of locoregional control was also significantly better with radiotherapy and concurrent cisplatin (78 percent, vs 61 percent with induction cisplatin plus fluorouracil followed by radiotherapy and 56 percent with radiotherapy alone). Both of the chemotherapy-based regimens suppressed distant metastases and resulted in better disease-free survival than radiotherapy alone. However, overall survival rates were similar in all three groups. The rate of high-grade toxic effects was greater with the chemotherapy-based regimens (81 percent with induction cisplatin plus fluorouracil followed by radiotherapy and 82 percent with radiotherapy with concurrent cisplatin, vs 61 percent with radiotherapy alone). The mucosal toxicity of concurrent radiotherapy and cisplatin was nearly twice as frequent as the mucosal toxicity of the other two treatments during radiotherapy.

Conclusions: In patients with laryngeal cancer, radiotherapy with concurrent administration of cisplatin is superior to induction chemotherapy followed by radiotherapy or radiotherapy alone for laryngeal preservation and locoregional control.

Forastiere AA, Goepfert H, Maor M, et al. Concurrent chemotherapy and radiotherapy for organ preservation in advanced laryngeal cancer. N Engl J Med. 2003;349:2091-2098.

Commentary by: *Jatin P Shah*

Observations from the landmark Veterans Administration trial of larynx preservation clearly documented that adding chemotherapy to radiotherapy enhanced the response of radiation in controlling laryngeal cancer and demonstrated that 64% of stage III and IV laryngeal cancer patients were able to preserve their larynx with induction chemotherapy followed by radiotherapy. However, the optimal timing of chemotherapy remained unknown. To address this particular issue the RTOG, under the leadership of Dr Arlene Forestiere and her colleagues, embarked upon a randomized trial of induction chemotherapy with cisplatin and 5-FU followed by radiotherapy compared to radiotherapy with concurrent administration of cisplatin, vs radiotherapy alone, in patients who would have required laryngectomy. This trial accrued 547 patients, and the initial follow-up period reported was 3.8 years. The rationale for the second group of concurrent chemotherapy with radiation was based on the enhancement of radiation effects on tumor cells with concurrent administration of cisplatin. The primary objective of the trial was to compare the rates of laryngeal preservation associated with the three treatment arms. Although the primary endpoint of the study was preservation of the larynx, the authors also investigated and reported on disease-free survival, local control, local/regional control, time to distant metastases, and laryngectomy-free survival. In addition, patients were required to fill out a quality of life questionnaire. This was the first such trial comparing induction versus concurrent chemotherapy with radiation in head and neck cancer. The authors are to be complimented for embarking upon this study, whose outcomes would significantly impact the management of advanced laryngeal cancer in the subsequent two decades.

The total rates of severe toxic effects for all phases of the study were 81% in the group that was assigned to induction chemotherapy, 82% in the group assigned to receive concurrent cisplatin, and 61% in the group receiving radiotherapy alone. The rates of laryngeal preservation at 3.8 years was 84% in the concurrent chemotherapy arm, 72% in the induction chemotherapy arm, and 67% in the radiotherapy alone arm. The 2- and 5-year overall survival estimates, however, were comparable in the three groups. The rates of local control were 64% in the induction arm, 80% in the concurrent arm, and 58% in the radiotherapy alone arm. The rates of distant metastases at 2 years were 9% in the induction arm, 8% in the concurrent arm, and 16% in the radiotherapy alone arm. The overall survival was 75% at 2 years. An important observation in this trial supported the concept that 91% of patients in the induction arm and 92% of the patients in the concurrent arm were metastases free compared to 84% of those who had received radiotherapy alone. Thus, an important observation that adding chemotherapy to radiotherapy reduced the rate of distant metastases was confirmed. Another important observation of the study was that induction chemotherapy followed by radiotherapy compared to radiotherapy alone did not significantly improve the rate of laryngeal preservation or survival. Therefore, the conclusion of the study was that if the aim of treatment is laryngeal preservation, concurrent chemoradiotherapy was the choice of treatment.

This landmark study made significant progress in the concept of organ preservation with concurrent administration of chemotherapy and radiotherapy. The impact of the observations from this trial shifted paradigms and made concurrent chemoradiotherapy the standard of care for laryngeal preservation in advanced laryngeal carcinoma for nearly the next 2 decades. However, as the observation and follow-up period progressed, it became apparent that the acute short-term toxicities and long-term sequelae of concurrent chemoradiotherapy were significantly higher than initially reported. In addition, treatment-related deaths in the long term continue to remain a cause of concern. Nevertheless, this trial significantly shifted paradigms in the management of advanced laryngeal cancer leading to the preservation of larynx in greater than 80% of patients requiring total laryngectomy.

Chapter 11

Neck

EXCISION OF CANCER OF THE HEAD AND NECK WITH SPECIAL REFERENCE TO THE PLAN OF DISSECTION BASED ON ONE HUNDRED AND THIRTY-TWO OPERATIONS

George W Crile

Though signal advances have been made recently in many surgical problems, the treatment of cancer of the head and neck has, it would seem, neither received the attention nor kept the pace of progress in other fields. These unhappy cases are too often regarded as specters at the clinic. The operative treatment is hampered by tradition and conventionality, and the tragic ending of so large a proportion of these cases has held back lay and even professional confidence.

In this paper it is intended to present an outline sketch of the conclusion regarding the surgical treatment of cancer of the head and neck in the curable stage. The etiology, the diagnosis and the pathology will not be considered. It is generally admitted that cancer is primarily a local disease. Each case, then, is presumably at some period curable by complete excision.

Crile GW. Excision of cancer of the head and neck with special reference to the plan of dissection based on 132 operations. JAMA. 1906;47:1780-1786.

Commentary by: *Donald P Shedd*

George Washington Crile (1864–1943) was a very impressive surgeon whose interests extended far beyond medicine. One of his books, entitled *Mechanistic View of War and Peace,* was published in 1915. He was part of the group who founded the American College of Surgeons, and he was also a co-founder of the Cleveland Clinic in Cleveland, Ohio, USA. Crile is credited with being one of the first to employ direct blood transfusion. His contributions to the knowledge of surgical physiology are notable.

The article cited is an account of Crile's surgical experience with cancer of the head and neck. It describes the results from 132 operations for various sites of head and neck cancer, including the lip and skin. Crile's experience led him to the conclusion that the removal of individual involved nodes did not lead to satisfactory results. He concluded that bloc dissection was a more rational approach to the problem.

The reference in the article to the Halsted operation for breast cancer indicates Crile's respect for the concept of the comprehensive removal of definitive zones of lymphatic spread in the surgical care of the cancer patient.

From the total of 132 patients, 36 underwent a complete neck dissection. The author devotes considerable attention to the avoidance of problems and to the details of anesthesia. At that time, 1906, rather than using endotracheal intubation, the anesthesia was administered through two tubes passed through the nostrils to the level of the epiglottis. Gauze packing was utilized to occlude the pharynx around the tubes. Dr Crile employed a compression suit to prevent the problem of shock. He also employed compression of the common carotid artery as a method of reducing bleeding.

The article has excellent detailed drawings of all the technical steps for performing the operation. Potential complications and their avoidance are covered well. It is of interest to note that there is no reference to the thoracic duct. There were 11 deaths among the 132 operations.

A wide variety of modifications have appeared over the years, most notable of which was the development of the composite operation in which the primary tumor is excised in continuity with the radical neck dissection. There have also been a large number of variations in the placement of the skin incisions.

The many patients who have been cured after undergoing operation for head and neck cancer with node involvement owe a large debt to George Crile for his development of a rational surgical approach to the problem.

It is difficult to trace the sequence of events that led to the complete neck dissection becoming a standard procedure in the care of head and neck cancer patients, but it certainly did become that. This first description of the technical details of the operation makes the article clearly of landmark status. Such a statement is supported by the fact that the article was reprinted in the *Journal of the American Medical Association* in 1987 as a landmark article.

BIOPSY BY NEEDLE PUNCTURE AND ASPIRATION

Hayes E Martin, Edward B Ellis

From the Pathological laboratory of the Memorial Hospital of New York
This paper is a presentation of technical procedures employed and results attained
by securing tissue from suspected neoplasms for histological examination by needle
puncture and aspiration.

Martin HE, Ellis EB. Biopsy by needle puncture and aspiration. Ann Surg. 1930;92:169-181.

Commentary by: *Carl E Silver*

In 1889, Dr John Collins Warren Jr. at the Massachusetts General Hospital, in an effort to facilitate earlier diagnosis of tumors requested that his colleague, the neurosurgeon Dr Samuel J Mixter, devise an instrument to enable a minimally invasive biopsy of these tumors. Mixter adapted a fine cannula, sharpened on the inner edge, which when rotated between the thumb and finger acted like a trephine. When withdrawn, a plug of tissue obtained from the tumor was extruded by inserting the stylette, and could be processed and examined histologically. Use of this device was vigorously attacked when presented to the American Surgical Association. Moreover, this device, and several similar ones did not find general acceptance by the surgical community. The main limitation was in preparation and interpretation of the minute specimens. Recognizing this, Warren employed a dedicated histologist, present on all operating days, for this purpose. Lack of availability of such assistance, as well as fear of bleeding, rupture of tumor capsule, implantation of tumor along the needle tract, and incorrect diagnosis relegated needle biopsy to a medical curiosity.

In the 1920s, Dr James Ewing was Chief of Pathology at the Memorial Hospital for Cancer and Allied Diseases in New York City. Dr Hayes Martin, who was at that time a young surgeon and part-time radiotherapist, was unwilling to treat patients with metastatic disease without a tissue diagnosis. Ewing objected to incisional biopsy because he believed it led to spread of cancer. As a compromise, Martin, with the help of Ewing's technician, Edward Ellis, began to experiment with aspirations of palpable tumors using an 18-gauge needle attached to a large syringe.* The first aspirates were performed on cadavers. The pathologic material was interpreted by Dr Fred W Stewart, who published papers in 1933 and 1936 on some of the problems of the method—such as interpretation of scanty specimens or specimens from lesions difficult to classify, particularly tumors of the thyroid.

Although it is difficult to ascertain sensitivity and specificity of the method from the paper itself, it appears that in 60% of the 65 reported cases

---

*These events were related by Dr Leopold Koss, my colleague and co-author, with myself, of a 1985 monograph on the subject. Dr Koss was former Chief of the cytopathology service at Memorial Hospital, and attributed the story to Dr Fred W Stewart, Ewing's successor.

the authors were able to positively confirm the needle biopsy results with paraffin section on larger specimens obtained by open biopsy or excision. The authors also noted that the needle biopsy was of value in detecting benign lesions, although they kept no record of these cases. The early Memorial Hospital experience was extended to bone tumors, and to lung lesions—although fluoroscope guided transthoracic needle biopsy was associated with a high incidence of pneumothorax. This simple and effective method of tissue diagnosis was practiced at Memorial Hospital continuously from the initial reported series of patients to the present time—and was in use long before the procedure achieved general acceptance by the medical community. I believe that major issues involved in the lack of acceptance outside of Memorial Hospital were related to the caliber of needle that was used. Even with the relatively large (by today's standards) 18-gauge needle, most of the "tissue" obtained was in the form of a smear of whole cells, requiring cytologic analysis. While some material was embedded in paraffin to produce histologic sections, this material was often too scant to allow a reliable diagnosis. Most pathologists could not interpret cytologic smears at that time. Consequently, when required, large bore "core" needle biopsies were performed, which yielded more satisfactory histologic material, but were subject to all the complications enunciated above, such as bleeding and tract implantation. Thus "needle biopsy" remained unpopular, and the advantages of aspiration biopsy through finer needles went unrecognized.

However, the Memorial Hospital experience was noticed and discussed in European countries. Modifications of the method began to attract attention, principally in the Netherlands and Sweden. In Delft and Leiden, Paul Lopes Cardozo began to implement aspiration cytology on a large scale in the 1940s. In Sweden, Nils Söderström began experimenting with thin needle aspirates at about the same time. In 1968, Sixten Franzén, at the Radiumhemmet in Stockholm developed a single grip syringe that was initially designed to facilitate prostate biopsy and subsequently adapted to other targets. The writings of Franzén and his co-workers of the Stockholm group had a profound influence on the development of aspiration biopsy in Europe. By the mid 1970s, evidence of the utility and safety of this procedure crossed the Atlantic to regain the interest of American surgeons and oncologists.

In 1970, Dr Leopold Koss, former Chief of Cytology Services at Memorial Hospital came to our institution as Chairman of Pathology. In response to encouragement by his group, we began performing routine needle biopsies of thyroid nodules. Prior to this, aside from clinically obvious cancers, the only objective criteria employed in selection of thyroid nodules for surgery were relatively poor concentration of radioiodine in the nodule—or failure to respond to a regimen of thyroid hormone. The overall incidence of cancer in nodules selected for surgery was 16%. Thyroid nodules present a particular problem, because even histologic sections of follicular lesions are often difficult to interpret. We found that the results of fine needle aspiration could be classified into positive, negative and indeterminate groups, with regard to the presence of cancer. Recommending surgery for lesions with positive and indeterminate biopsies as well as for obviously benign goiters because of their size or mechanical factors increased the yield of cancer to approximately 35% of lesions selected for surgery. Recalling Warren's experience, our paper was vigorously attacked when presented to a regional meeting in 1982.

Fine needle aspiration proved quite accurate in the diagnosis of neck masses—particularly enlarged cervical nodes. Metastatic squamous cell carcinoma can be diagnosed with almost complete accuracy, without the disadvantages associated with open biopsy. Aspiration biopsy proved less accurate in diagnosis and classification of lymphoma, but knowledge of the lymphoid nature of the lesion served as an indication for open biopsy of the mass. Salivary gland lesions can be identified as such with extreme accuracy, with high sensitivity and specificity for malignancy, and with reasonable dependability for exact diagnosis. These results, obtained over a 20-year period on our service, are consistent with those reported by many others.

The key factor in fine needle aspiration biopsy is that the method produces primarily a cytologic rather than histologic specimen for interpretation. Small chunks of material extruded on the slide should be retrieved, embedded in paraffin, and sectioned for histologic examination. The residual contents of the needle and syringe are flushed and centrifuged to produce a cell block for histologic section. Nevertheless, the majority of biopsy material is smeared, fixed in alcohol, and stained either with Papanicolau stain or with hematoxylin and eosin. Modern cytologic techniques can achieve a level of diagnostic accuracy that approaches conventional histologic sectioning. Material can be submitted for immunochemical and genetic analysis. Very fine needles—22–25 gauge—have supplanted the larger 18-gauge needle previously employed. The finer needles actually produce superior specimens because of the lack of contamination with blood. In years of experience, there have been no reported instances of needle tract implantation or tumor spillage. Significant bleeding rarely occurs. Pneumothorax may occur occasionally after transthoracic biopsy, but most resolve without intervention. Modern imaging techniques permit a much higher degree of accuracy in biopsy by guiding the placement of the needle into deep seated lesions, or into the most suspicious areas of a tumor mass. Ultrasound guidance is extremely effective in biopsy of cervical lymph nodes, thyroid and parotid nodules. CT and MRI are effective modalities for biopsy of deeper lesions, particularly in other parts of the body. Modern technology has permitted the development of almost equally fine needles for "core" biopsy, so that both cytology and histology are available to the modern physician.

During my residency and early years of practice, numerous patients underwent surgical exploration of various body cavities only to find inoperable and/or metastatic disease. Other patients had lesions that were "watched" to see if they enlarged, while their malignant tumors grew. Still others underwent major resections of masses in the chest or abdomen, only to find they were benign. The widespread use of fine needle aspiration biopsy, in combination with modern methods of imaging, has rendered these practices essentially extinct.

EL PROBLEMA DE LAS METASTASIS LINFÁTICAS Y ALEJADAS DEL CÁNCER DE LARINGE E HIPOFARINGE (THE PROBLEM OF LYMPHATIC AND DISTANT METASTASES IN CANCER OF LARYNX AND HYPOPHARYNX)

Osvaldo Suarez

En el estado actual de los estudios oncológicos malignos, no es posible tratar por separado el problema del tumor en si, y el del territorio ganglionar, ya que constituye una única entidad nosológica: el llamado complejo órgano ganglionar.

(In the current state of malignant cancer studies, it is not possible to treat separately the problem of the tumor itself, the lymph node and territory, as it is the single disease entity: the so-called nodal complex organ).

Suarez O. El problema de las metastasis linfáticas y alejadas del cáncer de laringe e hipofaringe. (The problem of the lymphatic and distant metastases). Rev Otorhinolaryngol. 1963;23:83-89.

Commentary by: *Jesus E Medina*

What a pleasant task it is to comment on Dr Oswaldo Suarez's paper entitled "El Problema de las Metastasis linfáticas y alejadas del cáncer de laringe e hipofaringe" (The Problem of the Lymphatic and Distant Metastases). Since the first time I read this paper many years ago, I have found it fascinating to follow the observations and reasoning that led an astute and courageous surgeon to the performance and description of a novel surgical technique: the functional neck dissection. Today, I have the opportunity to attest that the work of Dr Suarez, described in this paper, was truly seminal; it strongly influenced later developments in the surgical treatment of cervical lymph node metastases.

First, the work and the reasoning: The main premise of Dr Suarez's paper is that the study of the lymphatic system is of vital importance in oncology. He set out to study from an oncological viewpoint the lymphatics of the larynx and hypopharynx in 1,318 cases with neoplasms, on whom he performed 532 therapeutic neck dissections and 271 "prophylactic" neck dissections. The results of his observations, described with exquisite detail, are organized into four areas: the origin of the lymphatic vessels, the collecting lymphatic network, the "satellite" lymph nodes, and the circulation of lymph in the neck.

After presenting what is arguably the most detailed description of the lymphatics within the larynx and hypopharynx, he describes one of his fundamental observations. He noted that in their extralaryngeal course, the collector lymphatic vessels "never traversed the musculature per se, neither the suprahyoid nor the infrahyoid, nor the sternocleidomastoid muscle, instead they are located and run within the connective tissue". He also observed that these lymphatics are not within the fascia that envelops muscles like the sternocleidomastoid muscle or glands like the submandibular gland. They are found, however, within the parotid gland. Another key observation regarding collector vessels and cervical lymph nodes pertains to their relationship with neighboring vessels, particularly veins. He describes it as a relationship of "vicinity" and notes that they are not a part of the adventitia, but are located outside of it. Following these observations he points out that these characteristics of the lymphatic system of the neck are of "capital importance in the functional surgical treatment of lymphatic metastases and constitute one its foundations".

He goes on to discuss the distribution of lymph node metastases, pointing out that they frequently involve the jugular, transverse cervical and spinal accessory nodes and the fact that in cancers of the supraglottic larynx and hypopharynx, nodal metastases are often bilateral. Therefore, if the neck nodes are to be treated surgically, as most surgeons of his time recommended, the ideal treatment would include bilateral lymph node dissection. As he puts these facts in the context of his experience with unpleasant complications of bilateral radical neck dissections, mainly marked facial edema and increased risk of carotid rupture, he justifies his quest: to develop a "type of technique that would allow us to eliminate completely the lymph node containing tissues of the neck in conjunction with the primary and respecting noble structures".

He finishes his 16-page paper with a 2-page description of such a surgical technique and called it "functional dissection" as it "eliminates all the areolar tissue, fascia and lymph nodes and leaves the muscles, great vessels and noble parts without mutilation".

Now, to the influence of Dr Suarez's work: There is no doubt that the main reason why Dr Suarez's work had such an influence in the treatment of the neck in patients with head and neck cancer in general and cancer of the larynx in particular, is its solid anatomical and clinical foundations. Dr Suarez did not report specific outcomes, but he indicated in this paper that he obtained good results with the technique he described. However, as the functional neck dissection was adopted and popularized in America and in Europe in particular, the oncologic and functional results reported by several clinicians were excellent in the treatment of both the N0 and the N+ neck. The concept made sense and its feasibility and effectiveness were validated by others. For several decades since, the functional neck dissection remained the mainstay of the surgical treatment of the neck in patients with larynx cancer in Europe, South America, and to a lesser extent, the United States.

I know that the concept put forth by Dr Suarez influenced open-minded clinicians at the MD Anderson Cancer Institute like Ballantyne, Jesse, Byers and Lindberg who, in addition, noted that metastases were more likely to occur to certain lymph nodes in the neck, depending upon the location of the primary tumor. These observations led to the development of the selective neck dissections, which are the most common neck dissections performed today in patients with cancers of the head and neck.

I have no doubt that the readers of this commentary would agree with me in that the selection of "El Problema de las Metastasis Ganglionares y Alejadas" by Oswaldo Suarez as one of the seminal works in head and neck oncologic surgery in the last century is well deserved.

THE EXTRACAPSULAR SPREAD OF TUMORS IN CERVICAL NODE METASTASIS

Jonas T Johnson, E Leon Barnes, Eugene N Myers, et al.

Extracapsular spread (ECS) of lymph node metastases is believed to be an indicator of poor prognosis. In general, it has been thought that ECS was limited to large "fixed" nodes. To test the validity of the assumption that nodes less than 3 cm in diameter do not have ECS, the specimens from 177 radical neck dissections were reviewed retrospectively with regard to ECS. Sixty-five percent of the nodes that were 2.9 cm or less in diameter were found to demonstrate ECS. We found no substantial difference in the number of patients who had no histologic disease in their necks when compared with a second group of patients who had metastasis confined to the lymph node. The patients whose lesions had ECS had statistically significantly reduced numbers of survivors. Other factors, e.g., tumor differentiation and the number of malignant nodes, had no prognostic importance. The impact of ECS on staging, the reporting of retrospective reviews, and therapy are discussed.

Johnson JT, Barnes EL, Myers EN, et al. The extracapsular spread of tumors in cervical node metastasis. Arch Otolaryngol. 1981;107:725-729.

Commentary by: *Michiel WM van den Brekel*

Since the end of the 1970s, extranodal tumor spread (ENS), or transcapsular spread, has been recognized as a poor prognostic feature. The article by Jonas Johnson and the Pittsburgh team from 1981 was one of the first articles from that era to address and confirm the importance of ENS for prognosis in head and neck cancer. It showed that this was an independent factor from many other clinical factors.

As combinational treatment using surgery and radiotherapy was gaining popularity at the end of the 1970s, there was a search for clinical and pathological features to select patients that could benefit from this combination. Furthermore, there was controversy as to whether radiotherapy should be employed before or after surgery. Initial reports had shown that ENS had relevance to predict prognosis, but many questions remained on the correlation between the number and size of lymph node metastases and the presence of ENS. It had to be proven that ENS was an independent prognostic factor and really an indication for postoperative radiotherapy. As ENS could only be diagnosed after surgery, this was an important argument for the use radiotherapy after surgery.

As all studies were in those days, it was a retrospective study, looking at outcome of head and neck cancer patients in relation to histopathologic features. Unfortunately, they did not select for a specific tumor site or stage but included all head and neck cancer patients who had undergone a radical neck dissection. In 5 years, 161 patients underwent a neck dissection, and 89 of these actually had lymph node metastases. In those days, even for the N0 neck, a radical neck dissection was common practice, as selective neck dissections were not described yet. In the study, Johnson showed that patients with ENS had a significantly poorer survival compared to those without ENS. There was no difference in survival between patients with lymph node metastases without ENS and those with a pathologically negative neck. This finding had later been argued but also confirmed by several authors and is probably caused by the effect of postoperative radiotherapy. In larger series, however, it has been shown that those with lymph node metastasis without ENS have an intermediate risk and those without lymph node metastasis have a low risk. Furthermore, other features, such as level of metastases and volume, have repeatedly been shown to be of prognostic importance. It was also shown that the extent of ENS (microscopic or macroscopic) is a prognostic feature as well.

The article by Johnson et al. was the first to show that even corrected for tumor stage, number of involved lymph nodes or tumor differentiation, ENS was an independent prognostic feature. ENS was frequently found in limited neck disease. As radiotherapy was employed in the majority of patients and especially those with stage IV disease or ENS and there was no control group or any randomization, this study could not really prove that ENS was an indication for postoperative radiotherapy. It was, however, shown that most recurrences were regional in the ENS group, and this was used as an argument that ENS indeed was an indication for the most aggressive treatment possible. Later studies have confirmed that ENS is the most important prognostic feature and is independent of other features. However, no study has ever randomized between postoperative radiotherapy and surgery alone. So all our arguments to use radiotherapy are based on retrospective studies.

In this study, some striking statements were made. First, it was postulated that ENS was not a feature of mere tumor progression, but rather a sign of a biologically more aggressive tumor or a deficient immune response. In fact, this would mean that there is no real biologic or prognostic difference between microscopic and macroscopic ENS. This issue is not clarified yet, and although there have been some reports on the fact that macroscopic ENS is more important than microscopic ENS, this remains a controversial issue. Only very few studies have found a correlation between ENS and other biological markers that could substitute ENS. Progression in the field of gene expression analyses is slow.

Until now, unfortunately, we have not been able to find markers for aggressive tumor behavior that are as strong as ENS. Although we can detect ENS on MRI or CT in about 50% of the cases (Lodder W, et al. in press), we need surgery to assess this criterion. The authors make a strong plea to

Neck **171**

use ENS in the UICC and AJCC staging system. This is a realistic proposal, and we know that histopathological features are more and more incorporated in the current staging system. In melanoma, for example, the number of mitoses and the presence of micrometastases lead to different subcategories. Furthermore, ENS is currently the most important prognostic feature available, and recently, it has been shown that it has therapeutic consequences. In two randomized trials, it was shown that patients with ENS have a better outcome when treated with postoperative chemoradiation compared to radiation alone. However, ENS has not yet been incorporated into the head and neck staging system. A possible explanation is that ENS is not a straightforward criterion and there is considerable variation in diagnosing ENS among pathologists.

In conclusion, this paper by the Pittsburg group was one of the earlier papers stressing the importance of ENS as a prognostic criterion. Although their plea to incorporate it into the staging system was never heard, it still is one of the few predictive features that has survived the test of time and has even led to more personalized therapy.

FUNCTIONAL NECK DISSECTION: AN EVALUATION AND REVIEW OF 843 CASES

Oreste Pignataro, Ettore Bocca, Cesare Oldini, et al.

After briefly reviewing the principles, indications, and merits of functional neck dissection, the results of 1200 neck dissections performed on 843 patients in the period 1961–1979 are presented. They compare very favorably with those reported for classic (radical) neck dissection by other leading authors; however, a retrospective analysis of data derived from material of different origin is hardly possible and has a disputable value. Therefore, we decided to compare our data on functional neck dissections (FND) with those of classic neck dissections (CND) performed by the same surgical team at the same clinic in the period 1948–1960.

The clinical material was largely the same in both cases, and the data were collected and analyzed using the same criteria. In both series, neck dissections were divided into elective and curative. It could be demonstrated that the number of neck recurrences observed in the dissected necks is the same for FND and CND in curative dissections, while it is considerably lower for FND in elective neck dissections. This of course does not prove improved radicality in FND, but only proves that a systematic bilateral elective neck dissection in No cases affords improved cancerological safety.

This radical bilateral approach to regional lymph nodes is made possible routinely by FND which avoids the problems of unnecessary mutilation.

The figures produced speak in favor of a wider adoption FND especially for expanding the indications to elective treatment of regional lymph nodes in cancer of the head and neck. Elective neck dissection is made practically harmless by this newer technique and averts the dreadful appearance of late metastases in N0 cases.

Pignataro O, Bocca E, Oldini C, Cappa C. Functional neck dissection: an evaluation and review of 843 cases. Laryngoscope. 1984;94:942-945.

Commentary by: *Javier Gavilán*

This paper constitutes one of the major steps in the history of neck dissection. It could be considered the "official" introduction of functional neck dissection (FND) in the English literature. Before this paper, FND was very popular in Southern European countries, such as Italy and Spain, as well as other countries in South America, such as Argentina or Uruguay.

If we look at this paper with scientifically critical eyes, a large number of methodological flaws could be mentioned. The article is based on a retrospective study of patients included in two different time periods, different N stages are included on every arm of the study, and heterogeneous series from other centers are used as comparisons. However, an important message emerged above these faults: *"we have a huge experience with functional neck dissection (843 patients, 1,500 operations) and the procedure works in our hands as well as in those of surgeons in our environment".* This was basically what Bocca and his team wanted to state.

As a consequence of this paper, FND began to be known among American surgeons as "Bocca's procedure", something I have always disapproved of. In fact, if I had to criticize something in this article, it would have to be the minimal recognition made by the authors to the origin of the operation. On previous and subsequent papers, Bocca and coworkers usually gave more credit to Oswaldo Suárez as the father of FND.

The rationale for FND was proposed in the 1960s by Oswaldo Suárez, an otolaryngologist and anatomist from Córdoba, Argentina. The main goal of the "functional" approach to neck dissection proposed by Suárez was the removal of the lymphatic tissue in the neck, preserving the remaining neck structures. This may be achieved by using the fascial planes of the neck that surround most cervical structures and separate them from the adjacent lymphatic tissue.

The paper by Bocca et al. includes a table on the first page that details all the concepts that constitute the rationale of FND. Unfortunately, this table was overlooked by most readers. As a consequence, FND was accepted by American surgeons as another modification to the classic radical neck dissection described by Crile and popularized by Hayes Martin. This was reflected in the name used for FND in the English literature: *"Modified Radical Neck Dissection"*. FND is not a modification of previous operations. FND was a new procedure with its own rationale, anatomical basis, and surgical technique. Bocca et al. made this clear in their paper.

Why was the name of the operation changed in the United States? It is difficult to say, but possible explanations include the late arrival of the operation to American surgeons—more than a decade after it was introduced in Europe—and the fact that it did so through the experience and words of third parties. Thus, part of the message vanished in the process of adaptation to the new environment. Unfortunately, the part missing was the philosophical element of the message—supposedly the less important piece of information, but in reality the core of the new procedure.

What happened later belongs to the recent history of neck dissection. Selective operations took over the classic procedures and what initially was considered "too little" for some head and neck tumors (FND) suddenly became "too much" for most patients. Again, the philosophy of FND was misunderstood, giving the operation the meaning of "comprehensive" neck dissection, when in fact it is just a surgical approach to the neck through fascial planes and spaces. The extent of the resection does not change the concept of FND.

In conclusion, Bocca should be credited as the man who introduced FND to non-Spanish speaking surgeons. The paper included in this commentary is only one of a large list of articles published by him and his group emphasizing the oncologic radicalness and the functional advantages of the operation when compared to radical neck dissection. He was able to introduce a new operation for head and neck surgeons, with excellent oncologic and functional results. Even if the conceptual aim of the procedure was lost on the way, the operation has been accepted as a safe procedure for the management of the neck in head and neck cancer patients.

RATIONALE FOR ELECTIVE MODIFIED NECK DISSECTION

Robert M Byers, Patricia F Wolf, Alando J Ballantyne

A retrospective study was conducted to give surgeons direction in deciding which type of modified neck dissection is proper elective treatment for the patient with a clinically negative neck. The medical records of 428 previously untreated patients (seen between January 1, 1970, and December 31, 1979) whose necks (i.e. N0) were electively dissected and who had had a primary squamous carcinoma of the oral cavity, oropharynx, larynx, or hypopharynx were included. The three major types of modified neck dissections studied were the supraomohyoid, the anterior, and the functional. Sixteen percent (70 of 428) of the patients had multiple positive nodes and 6% (28 of 428) had evidence of extracapsular invasion. A unilateral supraomohyoid dissection was most often used for primaries of the oral cavity. Bilateral anterior dissection was common for cancers of the larynx and hypopharynx, and functional neck dissection was equally distributed among the primary sites. None of the patients with primaries of the larynx or hypopharynx had pathologically positive nodes in the submental or submaxillary triangles. Advanced T-stage was generally associated with a greater incidence of subclinically positive nodes. Thirty percent of the patients received postoperative radiotherapy. The total number of nodes removed, the number of positive nodes with or without extracapsular invasion, and the anatomic location of the positive nodes were correlated with the type of dissection, the stage and site of the primary cancer, the degree of histological differentiation of the primary cancer, the use of postoperative radiotherapy, the regional (neck) failure, and survival. An elective modified neck dissection appeared to be an appropriate part of the initial surgical treatment for patients with primaries of the oral tongue, floor of the mouth, retromolar trigone, pharyngeal wall, base of the tongue, pyriform sinus, and glottic and supraglottic larynx, Adjunctive postoperative radiotherapy appeared to have a statistically significant effect for only those patients who had pathologically multiple positive nodes and extracapsular invasion.

Byers RM, Wolf PF, Ballantyne AJ. Rationale for elective modified neck dissection. Head Neck Surg. 1988;10:160-167.

Commentary by: *C René Leemans*

We must realize that findings we take for granted today, were very novel and controversial when they were first presented, and courage and perseverance were surely needed on the part of those who pointed others in the right direction.

The original and influential article by Byers RM et al. on the "Rationale for Elective Modified Neck Dissection" from 1988 is noteworthy, since it not only should be seen as an important and indispensable step in our thinking from radical and comprehensive elective neck dissections to the more selective neck dissections we perform today in the clinically negative neck, but also since it attempted to relate the type of selective (modified as it was named at the time of this article) to the site of the primary tumor and its T-stage.

With a direct line from Crile to Martin, the radical neck dissection, removing all 5 nodal levels, remained largely unchallenged until the 1960s. In his 1951 paper on prophylactic neck dissection, Martin failed to see a role for routine elective nodal dissection, mainly based on practical arguments. This is understandable from the point of view of the relatively large impact that neck dissection, especially bilateral, had with respect to morbidity after surgery.

Because more sparing procedures became available, such as those preserving the spinal accessory nerve, many surgeons subsequently performed elective nodal dissections using these procedures. The reason was the relatively high incidence of occult nodal disease in the cN0 neck in an era when imaging was virtually non-existent for this indication, which seemed to influence prognosis when not treated timely.

Suarez is generally regarded as the first to describe the functional neck dissection (removing all 5 nodal levels, while preserving non-lymphatic structures), a procedure we would now call a modified radical neck dissection type III, which yielded similar results to the original radical neck dissections while resulting in diminished morbidity. This operation was later popularized by Bocca. Suarez' paper can be seen as the beginning of a shift towards the neck dissections (selective and modified radical) we perform today. At MD Anderson, Houston, Texas, Jesse and Ballantyne together with Byers were instrumental in developing these procedures. These surgeons used the information of the radiation oncologist Lindberg, who in 1972, described the distribution of pathologically positive nodes in neck dissection specimens. They not only performed these procedures, but also provided the scientific basis for the safety in doing so, at a time when many were opposed to any compromise as to the radicality and comprehensiveness of the neck dissections.

The basis of modern selective neck dissection lies in a sophisticated understanding of the relatively orderly lymphatic drainage patterns from head and neck squamous cell cancers, later meticulously described by Shah et al. in his series from Memorial Sloan-Kettering Cancer Center, New York, NY.

The classic study by Byers, Wolf, and Ballantyne gave surgeons direction in deciding which type of modified neck dissection is proper elective treatment for the patient with a clinically negative neck. The study included the medical records of 428 previously untreated patients (seen between January 1, 1970 and December 31, 1979) whose necks (i.e. N0) were electively dissected and who had had a primary squamous carcinoma of the oral cavity, oropharynx, larynx, or hypopharynx. The three major types of modified neck dissections studied were the supraomohyoid, the anterior, and the functional, but also the suprahyoid and combinations. Supraomohyoid dissections removed, according to current terminology, level I through III nodes together with the upper and middle posterior cervical (level V) nodes. This is therefore different compared to what would be removed today in selective (I–III) neck dissection. Anterior dissections removed level I through III nodes [selective (II–IV) neck dissection], whereas the functional dissections removed all nodal groups (I through V; i.e. modified radical neck dissection).

Sixteen percent (70 of 428) of the patients had multiple positive nodes, and 6% (28 of 428) had evidence of extranodal spread. A unilateral supra-omohyoid dissection was most often used for primaries of the oral cavity. Bilateral anterior dissection was common for cancers of the larynx and hypopharynx, and functional neck dissection was equally distributed among the primary sites. None of the patients with primaries of the larynx or hypopharynx had pathologically positive nodes in the submental or submandibular triangles. Advanced T-stage was generally associated with a greater incidence of subclinically positive nodes. Thirty percent of the patients received postoperative radiotherapy. The total number of nodes removed, the number of positive nodes with or without extranodal spread, and the anatomic location of the positive nodes were correlated with the type of dissection, the stage and site of the primary cancer, the degree of histological differentiation of the primary cancer, the use of postoperative radiotherapy, the regional failure, and survival.

The important and landmark conclusion of this paper was that an elective modified neck dissection appeared to be an appropriate part of the initial surgical treatment for patients with primaries of the tongue, floor of the mouth, retromolar trigone, pharyngeal wall, base of the tongue, pyriform sinus, and glottic and supraglottic larynx. Adjuvant radiotherapy appeared to have a statistically significant effect for only those patients who had pathologically multiple positive nodes and extranodal spread.

It was probably foreseeable that the paper by Byers et al. when first published would also be met by some critics. Contrary to the later papers by Shah et al. in the MD Anderson series, often not all 5 nodal levels were dissected, and thus a true incidence of nodal presence per level was somewhat difficult to generate. Also, the terminology used at the time this paper was published generated some confusion and pointed to the unclear nomenclature and the wide variety of names given to different types of neck dissections in the past. Goepfert and Suen, and others pointed to this issue, which was later tackled by Robbins et al. on behalf of the American Academy of Otolaryngology—Head and Neck Surgery.

Any article cited more than 100 times can be regarded as very influential. Byers' paper is truly seminal, since to date it has been cited more than 260 times in the head and neck literature. It is, therefore, one of the works in head and neck cancer treatment that changed the practice of our predecessors and our current practice.

PATTERNS OF CERVICAL LYMPH NODE METASTASIS FROM SQUAMOUS CARCINOMAS OF THE UPPER AERODIGESTIVE TRACT

Jatin P Shah

A consecutive series of 1,081 previously untreated patients undergoing 1,119 radical neck dissections (RNDs) for squamous carcinoma of the head and neck was reviewed to study the patterns of nodal metastases. Primary tumors were located in the oral cavity in 501 patients, in the oropharynx in 207 patients, in the hypopharynx in 126 patients, and in the larynx in 247 patients. Lymph node metastases were confirmed histologically in 82% of 776 therapeutic neck dissections, and micrometastases were discovered in 33% of 343 elective RNDs. Lymph node groups in the neck were described by levels (I to V). Predominance of certain levels was seen for each primary site. Levels I, II, and III were at highest risk for metastasis from cancer of the oral cavity, and levels II, III, and IV were at highest risk for metastasis from carcinomas of the oropharynx, hypopharynx, and larynx. Supra-mohyoid neck dissection (clearing levels I, II, and III) for N0 patients with primary squamous cell carcinomas of the oral cavity and anterolateral neck dissection (clearing levels II, III, and IV) for N0 patients with primary squamous cell carcinomas of the oropharynx, hypopharynx, and larynx are recommended.

Shah JP. Patterns of cervical lymph node metastasis from squamous carcinomas of the upper aerodigestive tract. Am J Surg. 1990;160:405-409.

Commentary by: *Eugene N Myers*

The pathway to the current status of neck dissection spans three centuries. The giants of late 19th century surgery in Europe, von Langenbeck, Billroth, von Volkmann and Kocher, described several different ways of removing cervical lymph nodes involved with cancer. Sir Henry Butlin, in England, conceived the idea of elective neck dissection in his patients with cancer of the oral cavity. In 1880, the Polish surgeon Jawdynsky described in detail the first successful en bloc neck dissection. However, it was not until Dr George Crile's report in 1906 that the first significant series of en bloc radical neck dissections caught the attention of the medical world. His milestone paper, "Excision of Cancer of the Head and Neck. With special reference to the plan of dissection based on one hundred and thirty-two operations" (JAMA 1906;47:1780-6), established the basis for the effective treatment of cancer of the head and neck, delineating a systematic en bloc resection of the cervical lymphatic bearing tissue removed either in continuity with the primary tumor or as a secondary operation for subsequent metastasis. Crile's publication in the *Journal of the American Medical Association* produced a widespread response and transformed the radical neck dissection from a surgical curiosity into a useful reproducible procedure that revolutionized the treatment of cancer of the head and neck.

A half century later, the second milestone was an important paper entitled "Neck Dissection", published in 1951 by Dr Hayes Martin, Chief of the Head and Neck Service at Memorial Hospital in New York. This was a detailed analysis of 1,450 neck dissections performed from 1928 to 1950, including 490 cases in which a unilateral radical neck dissection was combined with the excision of the primary lesion en bloc in one stage. Information obtained in this study included: the site of the primary lesion, chronology of cervical metastasis, the number of lymph nodes in the surgical specimen, and postoperative recurrence. The authors categorically insisted that the spinal accessory nerve, the internal jugular vein, and sternocleidomastoid muscle should be removed in the presence of cervical lymph node metastasis. He emphasized that "any technique designed to preserve the spinal accessory nerve should be condemned unequivocally", since it did not allow for the complete removal of lymph nodes in the posterior triangle. Dr Hayes Martin pronounced the Memorial Hospital's Division of Head and Neck Surgery's unwavering adherence to the therapeutic radical neck dissection and stated that, "routine prophylactic neck dissection is considered illogical and unacceptable for cancer of the oral cavity". The results of this very large series of cases established the basis of treatment in the management of patients with cancer of the head and neck for the second half of the 20th century.

After WWII, the introduction of antibiotics, blood banking, and improved anesthesia techniques propelled the field of head and neck surgery into an entirely new era of treating cancer of the head and neck surgically instead of with radiation therapy. But by the early 1960s, there were several groups of surgeons who felt that it was not always necessary to do a radical neck dissection. By the latter part of that decade, neck dissections done by Alando J Ballantyne of the MD Anderson Hospital in Houston and by Ettore Bocca and Oreste Pignataro in Italy spared the non-lymphatic structures, such as the spinal accessory nerve, sternocleidomastoid muscle and the internal jugular vein. In patients who are staged N0 and often N1, there is no compelling need to remove the non-lymphatic structures unless they are invaded by tumor.

The oncologic safety of these operations has been proven by the very low recurrence rate both with the functional neck dissection, and more recently, the selective neck dissection. Bocca and Pignataro noted that the functional neck dissection is an anatomical operation that is as effective as a traditional radical neck dissection from an oncologic point of view for these stages of the disease. In fact, in Dr Bocca's first 100 functional neck dissections, no regional recurrence was noted. In another milestone article in 1984, entitled "Functional Neck Dissection: An Evaluation of 853 Cases", Bocca et al. provided further support for their concept when they evaluated

1,200 functional neck dissections performed on 843 patients from 1961 to 1979, with very few recurrences and an important improvement in quality of life. Our own experience here at the University of Pittsburgh and other institutions worldwide has proven the validity of these findings.

The rationale for the functional neck dissection was introduced in the early 1960s by an Argentinian, Professor Oswaldo Suarez. Suarez was said to be an excellent otolaryngologist and superb surgeon as well as a fine anatomist at the University of Cordova Medical School in Argentina. Bocca had the privilege of observing Suarez in the operating theater in 1962 and later in 1969 at the Department of Otolaryngology at LaPaz Hospital in Madrid. Suarez's dual identity as an anatomist and otolaryngologist conferred on him a privileged position, since he was very familiar with the anatomical details of the neck and a thorough knowledge of cancer of the head and neck. Bocca and his coworkers popularized the functional neck dissection, but if one reads carefully Bocca's articles on functional neck dissection, the name of Suarez is always mentioned, since Bocca correctly attributes the origin of this technique of neck dissection to Suarez. The principles of this technique are based on a most careful anatomical and physiological investigation on the site and drainage of lymph vessels and lymph nodes in the neck. On the grounds of these studies and the classical works of Truffert and Rouviere on the anatomy of the cervical lymphatics, Suarez elaborated a surgical method that was said to be a "masterpiece of precision and of oncologic validity". He stated that "if we remove the superficial and middle deep cervical fascia from the base of the skull to the pleural dome we shall have removed practically the entire lymphatic system of the neck without injury to the vascular, nervous, and muscular structures, e.g., spinal accessory nerve, internal jugular vein, cervical roots, brachial plexus, carotid artery and sternocleidomastoid muscle".

The selective neck dissection constitutes the next step in the evolution of neck dissection. Gavilan emphasized that selective neck dissections are only a modification of a functional neck dissection based on the better knowledge of the pattern of spread to the cervical lymph nodes from head and neck squamous cell carcinoma.

We must acknowledge the pivotal role that the milestone article in 1990, entitled "Patterns of Cervical Lymph Node Metastasis from Squamous Carcinomas of the Upper Aerodigestive Tract" (JP Shah, MD, FACS, New York), played in the development of selective neck dissection and its impact in advancing the field. Shah studied 1,119 radical neck dissections and analyzed the lymph node levels at high risk for metastasis from a variety of anatomical sites. The information derived from this study has been invaluable in guiding surgeons to determine exactly which lymph node groups should be removed based on the site of the primary cancer.

Now that we have more than two decades of experience with selective neck dissections in our Department, we have found that oncologically the results compare very favorably with the use of the radical and the selective neck dissection for patients with N0 and N1 and N2 necks. Dr Shah stated that with the classical radical neck dissection "although anatomical clearance of lymph node groups at all triangles of the neck is achieved with this operation, the rational for excision of all the regional lymph nodes has not been established".

The objectives of Dr Shah's study were to analyze the distribution of metastatic nodes in the neck in previously untreated patients undergoing either elective or therapeutic but complete radical neck dissection for a primary tumor in the upper aerodigestive tract. He felt that the data on the patterns of neck metastasis would then provide a basis for advocating limited neck dissection and planning future prospective trials to evaluate the role of limited neck dissection in the management of squamous cell carcinoma of the upper aerodigestive tract. The results of his study provided the clinical correlate of the observations of the classical analysis of the cervical lymphatics of Rouvier and Truffant.

These important observations now allow us to create an algorithm for treating the neck in patients with squamous cell carcinoma of the head and neck:

- *Oral Cavity*: The majority of metastatic lymph nodes in cancer of the oral cavity were present at Levels I, II, and III. Levels IV and V were involved infrequently.
- *Oropharynx*: The majority of the metastatic nodes were present in Levels II, III, and IV; again with Levels I and V seldom involved.
- *Hypopharynx*: The metastatic lymph nodes were confined to Levels II and III.
- *Larynx*: The majority of metastatic lymph nodes were present at Levels II, III, and IV, with Levels I and V involved only in individuals who had advanced metastatic cancer at Levels II, III, and IV.

Dr Shah, however, obviously felt that good oncologic results could be obtained with a form of surgery less mutilating than that described by Dr Martin and those who followed him imbued with the Memorial Hospital legacy. I personally have to commend Dr Shah, who spent almost his entire career at Memorial Hospital, an institution that is admired as the most famous cancer hospital in the world. However, this was at the time when the legacy of Hayes Martin who was adamantly opposed to the so-called "prophylactic neck dissections" still prevailed. It appears that the results published in this paper and the appointment of Dr Shah as Chief of the Division of Head and Neck Surgery were contemporaneous and no doubt made the transition away from Dr Martin's philosophy possible.

Thanks to the precise information provided by Dr Shah's study, and in spite of the absence of multi-institution prospective controlled clinical trials, evidence has been accumulated that demonstrates the effectiveness of the selective neck dissection in the treatment of squamous cell carcinoma of the head and neck. Our department in 1990 began to use selective neck dissection for the N0 neck and later N1 and N2 necks and have validated the oncologic effectiveness and safety of this procedure by analyzing our own data. We found that by using the excellent road map provided by Dr Shah, we have served well the needs of thousands of patients. Using this experience as a multiplier worldwide, we must admire Dr Shah's contributions even more. He has stood on "the shoulders of giants" at Memorial Hospital and contributed the important piece of evidence missing in Dr Hayes Martin's study.

END RESULTS OF A PROSPECTIVE TRIAL ON ELECTIVE LATERAL NECK DISSECTION VS TYPE III MODIFIED RADICAL NECK DISSECTION IN THE MANAGEMENT OF SUPRAGLOTTIC AND TRANSGLOTTIC CARCINOMAS

Ricardo R Brentani, Luiz P Kowalski, Jose F Soares, et al.

Background: Either modified type III radical neck dissection (MRND) or lateral neck dissections (LNDs) are considered valid treatments for patients with laryngeal carcinoma with clinically negative neck findings (N0). The object of this prospective study was to compare complications, neck recurrences, and survival results of elective MRND and LND on the management of laryngeal cancer patients.

Patients and Methods: This prospective randomized study began in 1990, and patient accrual was closed on December 1993. A total of 132 patients was included in the trial. All patients had previously untreated T2-T4 N0 M0 supraglottic or transglottic squamous cell carcinoma. No significant imbalance was found between groups with respect to demographic, clinical, pathologic, and other therapeutic variables. Seventy-one patients were given MRNDs (13 bilateral) and 61 were given LNDs (18 bilateral).

Results: The false-negative rate was 26%, and most positive nodes were sited at levels II and III. Complications and period of hospitalization were similar in both groups. There were 6 ipsilateral neck recurrences (4 in the MRND group, and 2 in the LND group). The 5-year actuarial survival calculated by Kaplan-Meier method was 72.3% in the MRND group and 62.4% in the LND group (log-rank test p = .312).

Conclusions: The rate of false-negative nodes in supraglottic and transglottic carcinomas was 26%, and most positive nodes were at levels II and III. The rates of 5-year overall survival, neck recurrences, and complications were similar in both groups. These results confirm the efficacy of lateral neck dissection in the elective treatment of the neck in patients with supraglottic and transglottic carcinomas.

Brazilian Head and Neck Cancer Study Group. End results of a prospective trial on elective lateral neck dissection vs type III modified radical neck dissection in the management of supraglottic and transglottic carcinomas. Head Neck. 1999;21:694-702.

Commentary by: *Ashok R Shaha*

This manuscript represents and reports a prospective trial on elective lateral neck dissection against the type III modified radical neck dissection in the management of patients with supraglottic and transglottic carcinomas. The information collected by the authors in a prospective, randomized fashion from a multi-institutional study group in Brazil is interesting. There are very few randomized, prospective studies in head and neck surgery. The majority of the prospective studies are related to radiation therapy or chemotherapy, primarily through RTOG, ECOG, or EORTC. This study represents one of the few surgical trials in head and neck cancer management. The authors have divided patients with N0 neck in supraglottic and transglottic carcinomas who underwent surgical treatment and neck dissection. They divided the patients into elective modified radical neck dissection and lateral neck dissection. The modified neck dissection included levels I-V, while the lateral neck dissection included levels II, III, and IV. They concluded the study in 3 years with a collection of 132 patients on the trial. All of the patients had 2-T4 supraglottic or transglottic squamous cell carcinoma. The next status was N0 based on clinical evaluation or CT scan. Seventy-one patients underwent modified radical neck dissection, while 61 underwent lateral neck dissection. The positivity rate in the neck dissection was 26%. Interestingly, the majority of the positive nodes were at levels II and III. The 5-year overall survival, neck recurrence, and complications were similar in both groups. This study clearly confirms the efficacy of lateral neck dissection in elective treatment of neck in patients with supraglottic and transglottic carcinomas.

One of the most important prognostic features in squamous cell carcinoma of the head and neck is stage of the disease and presence of nodal metastasis. Once the patient presents with clinically apparent nodal metastasis, the survival drops by almost by 50%, a major and important prognostic feature. The classical radical neck dissection for metastatic carcinoma in the neck started with a large experience by George Crile with his landmark publication in 1906 in *JAMA*. Interestingly, in the same article Crile mentioned preserving the accessory nerve if there was no gross disease around the nerve. It appears that this information was not passed on, and the radical neck dissection became the standard of care for more than half a century.

The modified neck dissection, initially called the functional neck dissection, was popularized by Oswaldo Suarez from Argentina. His landmark publication in Spanish rationalized the role of the functional neck dissection based on the facial envelope and containment of the metastatic disease to various regions in the neck. Interestingly, the leading head and neck surgeons from Europe, Ettore Bocca and Javier Gavilan from Madrid, learned the technique from Oswaldo Suarez and practiced functional neck dissection mainly for laryngeal cancer. The results were excellent, and they gave due credit to Oswaldo Suarez for his innovative and rational approach to neck metastasis. Clearly, Bocca used this operation mainly for laryngeal cancer in which the incidence of metastatic disease was quite low. The patterns of nodal metastasis are very well described in two landmark publications from MD Anderson by Robert Lindberg and from Memorial Sloan-Kettering Cancer Center by Shah et al. Both publications describe the location of the regional metastasis based on the primary tumor in the head and neck area. Clearly, there was a distinction in the location of the metastatic disease from the oral cavity, oropharynx, or laryngopharyngeal area. The majority of oral cavity metastasis was located at levels I, II and III, while metastatic disease from the oropharynx was limited generally to levels II and III, and from the laryngopharyngeal area to levels II, III and IV.

Several publications subsequently re-emphasized similar findings. This brought in the biological understanding of patterns of metastatic disease and its application in the modification of neck dissection. The classical radical neck dissection had direct functionality issues primarily related to shoulder dysfunction with direct impact on quality of life. Bilateral radical neck dissection, if performed simultaneously, had a mortality rate of approximately 17%.

In the United States, Jesse, Ballantyne and Byers from the MD Anderson Cancer Institute popularized the modified neck dissection. Several different modified neck dissections were proposed, and an effort was made by the American Academy of Otolaryngology Head and Neck Surgery to standardize the nomenclature as reported by Robbins et al. Memorial Sloan-Kettering Cancer Center divided the regions of the neck from level I to level V, which was universally accepted and used all around the world as the locations of metastatic disease in the neck region. The American Academy of Otolaryngology re-visited the issue through the neck dissection committee and modified the high levels to 7 levels, with levels I, II and V divided into A and B. Even though this system appears slightly complicated compared to the Memorial classification, the multiple levels and sub-leveling are biologically sound in relation to the patterns of nodal metastasis. Nodal metastasis at levels Ia and Ib is quite rare. Similarly, metastatic disease at level Va is quite rare. This information is important, especially in thyroid cancer; clearly, the attention will now focus more on the modified neck dissection or selective neck dissection rather than classical radical neck dissection. Also around this time, postoperative radiation therapy came into practice for patients presenting with positive nodal disease.

The authors have reported 26% positivity in the neck dissection and recommended elective neck dissection in patients undergoing treatment for supraglottic or transglottic carcinomas. From the time of the presentation in 1999, imaging has become an integral part of the evaluation of the neck along with ultrasound and occasionally PET scan. The ultrasound is extremely popular in Europe along with ultrasound-guided needle biopsy. The role of PET scan in N0 continues to be controversial, and there are no definitive studies indicating its strong applicability. The authors did use postoperative radiation therapy in positive nodal disease. They also used postoperative radiation therapy for positive margins or positive lymph nodes. The authors reported conversion from lateral neck dissection to modified neck dissection with accessory nerve preservation if the frozen section was confirmatory of metastatic disease.

The reported medium number of lymph nodes in the modified neck dissection was reported to be 30, while in lateral neck dissection it was 22. The authors reported no significant difference in depth or complication rates in both groups. The most frequent complications were flap necrosis, wound infection, and fistula. The authors have discussed the elective neck treatment used over the last four decades. They also discussed the role of elective neck irradiation. However, the decision regarding the neck dissection or irradiation depended mainly on the type of treatment offered to the primary tumor. The lateral neck dissection became routine in a significant number of institutions, because it is anatomically and oncologically a sound procedure based on the probability of metastasis. There were no published prospective, randomized trials comparing elective lateral neck dissection to modified radical neck dissection. The main objective of the authors' study was to report the results of a cooperative, prospective randomized trial design to compare complications, recurrences, and survival rates after elective lateral neck dissection versus modified neck dissection in the treatment of T2–T4 N0 supraglottic and transglottic squamous cell carcinoma. The authors have referred to other publications of level IV metastatic disease as separate skip metastasis in transglottic tumors.

As mentioned before, this manuscript represents one of the few randomized, prospective control studies in the surgical approach to the N0 neck. Clearly, the lateral neck dissection has become standard practice now. The neck dissection depends mainly on the patterns of nodal metastasis and the highest likelihood of presence of nodal disease in the selected group of lymph nodes. This brought in the classical supraomohyoid neck dissection, which is primarily performed for N0 patients with oral cavity cancer for staging purposes; for the oropharyngeal and laryngopharyngeal areas, the jugular node dissection or lateral node dissection has become a common practice; while the posterior lateral neck dissection is reserved mainly for patients with recurrent nasopharyngeal cancer or melanoma or skin cancers of the occipital area. The senior author, Kowalski, has taken a major leadership role in prospective studies in Brazil and clearly has shown that such studies can be undertaken.

I do hope that more and more prospective well-controlled surgical studies will be performed to enhance the best possible surgical approaches to head and neck cancer.

IMAGING-BASED NODAL CLASSIFICATION FOR EVALUATION OF NECK METASTATIC ADENOPATHY

Peter M Som, Hugh D Curtin, Anthony A Mancuso

Objective: This study was undertaken to create an imaging-based classification for the lymph nodes of the neck that will be readily accepted by clinicians, result in consistent nodal classification, and be easily used by radiologist.

Subjects and Methods: Over an 18-month period, the necks of 50 patents with cervical lymphadenopathy were scanned with CT, MR imaging, or both. Imaging anatomic landmarks were sought that would create a nodal classification of these necks similar to the clinically based nodal classifications of the American Joint Committee on Cancer and the American Academy of Otolaryngology-Head and Neck Surgery. Each nodal level was defined to ensure consistent nodal classification and eliminate areas of confusion existing in the clinically based classifications.

Results: Necks were classified using the imaging-based classification and then compared with the classification of the same necks using the most common clinically based classifications. The imaging- based nodal classifications of the superficial nodes were the same as the clinically based classification; however, the deep nodes of eight patients were found only by imaging. The anatomic precision and the level definition afforded by sectional imaging allowed the radiologists to use the imaging-based classification in a consistent manner.

Conclusion: This imaging-based classification has been endorsed by clinicians who specialize in head and neck cancer. The boundaries of the nodal levels were easily discerned by radiologists and yielded consistent nodal classifications. The reproducibility of this classification will allow it to become an essential component of future classifications of metastatic neck disease.

Som PM, Curtin HD, Mancuso AA. The imaging based nodal classification for evaluation of neck metastatic adenopathy. AJR Am J Roentgenol. 2000:174:837-844.

Commentary by: *Lawrence E Ginsberg*

On the occasion of the Centennial of the Head and Neck Service at Memorial Sloan-Kettering Cancer Center, Dr Shah and the IFHNOS leadership have seen fit to include in this monograph the accompanying landmark article by Drs Peter M Som, Hugh D Curtin and Anthony A Mancuso, among the foremost luminaries in the field of head and neck imaging.

The paper first appeared in the *Archives of Otolaryngology-Head and Neck Surgery* (currently *JAMA Otolaryngology-Head and Neck Surgery*). The impact was quick and highly positive, so much so that the *American Journal of Roentgenology* requested its own version, and in 2000, with minor variation, primarily more radiographic images, essentially a re-publication made the material more widely available to the radiology community.

This re-classification of cervical lymph nodes was envisioned as a way to take greater advantage of the high-quality cross-sectional imaging, which had become routine in staging head and neck cancer, and bridge a perceived terminology gap in a way that would facilitate better communication between clinicians and radiologists involved in the care of those patients. The classification was a highly successful attempt to simplify, clarify, and make more reproducible among different medical specialists the nodal staging of head and neck cancer. The work evolved from Dr Peter Som's experience in treating patients with his Head and Neck Surgery colleagues at the Mt Sinai School of Medicine in New York City, and he enlisted as collaborators his long-time colleagues Drs Hugh Curtin from the Massachusetts Eye and Ear Infirmary and Anthony Mancuso from the University of Florida College of Medicine in Gainesville.

While addressing discrepancies and shortcomings of the primarily palpation-based prior classifications, the re-classification was immediately accepted by the clinical and radiologic communities because it was *easy to learn* and readily adapted into one's practice. Within a very short time frame, and I remember this from personal experience, my clinical colleagues and me began speaking to each other in the same language; *we were on the same page.*

How appropriate that the authors of this work were who they were— among the foremost authorities in head and neck radiology. Indeed, the occasion of this Centennial is an appropriate opportunity to pay tribute to these individuals who have contributed so much to the joint goal of treating patients with head and neck disease.

Peter Som literally descended from Otolaryngology; his father Max was a pioneer head and neck surgeon in New York City. After radiology training at Mount Sinai and a brief stint in the US Army, Dr Som spent his entire professional career practicing head and neck radiology at Mt Sinai. Among his 270+ peer-reviewed publications are many directly linked to the imaging of head and neck cancer, or provided innovative observations that served the head and neck cancer radiologist directly. Many of Dr Som's publications are considered landmarks in the field. From the days of plain film tomography through PET/CT, Dr Som has contributed to our understanding of head and neck disease, and the head and neck cancer community has been immeasurably enriched by his efforts.

Hugh Curtin, Professor of Radiology at the Massachusetts Eye and Ear Infirmary and Harvard Medical School, did his post-graduate training at the University of Pittsburgh where he spent much of his career. Dr Curtin has contributed significantly to the head and neck imaging literature, and from the time I entered the field in 1988 has been considered an international authority on the imaging of laryngeal cancer, skull base neoplasms, and endless additional subjects pertaining to head and neck cancer, to which his 225+ publications proudly attest. In addition to serving as the president of both the American Society of Head and Neck Radiology (ASHNR) and

North American Skull Base Society (of which he was a founding member), Dr Curtin was Head and Neck Associate Editor of the *American Journal of Neuroradiology (AJNR)* and held many other important leadership positions in organized radiology. He is widely known and respected in ENT-Head and Neck Surgery circles and is very familiar at their gatherings. Along with Dr Som, Dr Curtin co-edits the "bible", or leading textbook of head and neck imaging, currently in its fifth edition.

Anthony (Tony) Mancuso is Professor and Chair of Radiology at the University of Florida College of Medicine, Gainesville. After training in California, Tony spent nearly his entire career in Gainesville. Along with his well-respected mentor, Dr William N Hanafee, Dr Mancuso made major contributions to the head and neck cancer literature, particularly describing the early CT-era findings of sinonasal, nasopharyngeal and laryngeal malignancy, and metastatic cervical lymphadenopathy. Tony went on to conduct very important investigations through his collaboration with William M Mendenhall in the field of imaging and radiation treatment of head and neck cancer. Dr Mancuso has been a mainstay of important radiology and ENT symposia for a generation, and is highly valued as an educator. I confess that just meeting Drs Som, Curtin, and Mancuso was an early highlight of my career, and to count them as my colleagues and friends is indeed an honor.

In conclusion then, the nodal classification included in this monograph was the natural product of three lives and careers devoted to a single purpose —the improvement of head and neck cancer imaging, and was an inevitable, enormous accomplishment. Literally, from these three distinguished individuals, who were very much in a class of their own, a monumental work sprang forth, quite literally, a classification of their own.

Chapter 12

Thyroid and Parathyroid

THE OPERATIVE STORY OF GOITER
THE AUTHOR'S OPERATION

William S Halsted

The extirpation of the thyroid gland for goiter typifies, perhaps better than any operation, the supreme triumph of the surgeon's art. A feat which today can be accomplished by any really competent operator without danger of mishap and which was conceived more than one thousand years ago might appear an unlikely competitor for a place in surgery so exalted.

Halsted WS. The operative story of goiter: the author's operation. Johns Hopkins Hospital Reports. 1920;19:71-257.

Commentary by: *Gregory W Randolph*

Thyroid and parathyroid surgery has traveled a long and dusty road through the last 200 years. Even when first recognized, thyroid and parathyroid disorders were misunderstood; Graves' disease was considered a cardiac condition, hypothyroidism a neurologic and dermatologic disorder, and hyperparathyroidism a primary bone disease. In fact, one of the earliest surgical attempts at thyroidectomy in 1600 led to the imprisonment of a thyroid surgeon.

It is William Halsted (1852–1922), the author of "*The Operative Story of Goiter*", to whom we owe a debt of gratitude. After graduating from Yale in 1879, because of a desire to improve his knowledge in thyroid disease and surgery, he undertook additional training for a period of several years outside of the US, in Europe, studying with both Kocher and Billroth. Billroth, who was described as a rapid operator, published in 1862 a 40% mortality rate at thyroid surgery mainly from uncontrollable hemorrhage at surgery as well as postoperative sepsis. Kocher on the other hand, in the year of his death, at the 1917 Swiss Surgical Congress reported an 0.5% mortality rate in a series of 5,000 thyroidectomies. Interestingly, although the physiologic underpinnings were not clear to Halsted at the time, he noticed in Billroth's clinic that after bilateral thyroidectomy, cachexia struma priva or postoperative myxedema was infrequent but tetany was common, whereas in Kocher's clinic the opposite was true, after bilateral thyroidectomy, myxedema was common but tetany was rare. Halsted observed that "a greater advance was made in the operative treatment of goiter in the decade from 1873 to 1883 than any in the foregone years and I may say all the years that have followed... during which period the art of operating for goiter by Billroth and Kocher and men of this school had been almost perfected with relatively minor problems remain to be solved".

Halsted's masterwork published in 1920 "*The Operative Story of Goiter*" provides a sweeping and detailed historical narrative of advances made in thyroid surgery from the earliest days to the revolutionary work of Billroth and Kocher whose techniques he held in great esteem. Halsted starts this tome with the now famous quote "the extirpation of the thyroid gland for goiter better typifies perhaps than any other operation the supreme triumph of the surgeons art". Halsted follows: "and further is there any problem in surgery having required for its solution such intrepid... and prolonged striving of the world's greatest surgeons which has yielded results so bountiful and so adequate?" Halsted chronicles the history of thyroid goiter surgery from Albucasis who in 500 AD performed perhaps the first goiter excision with hemorrhage control through ligature and use of a hot iron. He documents the trials and tribulations of early thyroid surgeons with quotes from Dieffenbach (1848)—"the operation for goiter is one of the most thankless and most perilous undertakings which if not altogether prohibited should at least be restricted to certain varieties of malady". Gross (1866) notes that "no sensible man will ...attempt to extirpate a goiter of the thyroid gland.... every step he takes will be environed with difficulty every stroke of his knife followed by a torrent of blood and lucky will it be for him if his victim live long enough to enable him to finish his horrid butchery .... No honest or sensible surgeon it seems to me would ever engage in it!" Succinctly, Mutter (1846) notes "it [goiter surgery] is a proceeding by no means to be thought of".

Slowly though, Halsted notes that hot irons, setons, caustics, turpentine, struma amputation, voice loss, respiratory embarrassment, vascular insults of all kinds including carotid artery division, and sepsis slowly give way through the history of goiter surgery to hemostatic clips, the understanding of recurrent laryngeal nerve and parathyroid anatomy and physiology as thyroidectomy emerges as a safe anatomically based surgical procedure. Interestingly, Halsted notes that Lister's anti-septic techniques while initially readily accepted in Germany were accepted in England and the US "very tardily". Halsted notes that numerous workers thought that the symptoms of postoperative hypothyroidism after total thyroidectomy were due to postoperative tracheal and oxygenation changes or due to cerebral blood flow alterations rather than to thyroid hormone deficiency. Halsted also interestingly reviews the work of Wolfler in describing contralateral vocal cord compensation, the setting of vocal cord paralysis: "...this increase in speech which is noted in paralysis of the recurrent laryngeal nerve...

is not due to restoration in so short a time of the function of the paralyzed vocal cord but to the healthy cord...[approximating]...the paralyzed one effecting an almost complete closure of the glottis.... This improvement in voice is why so few authors have thought it necessary to make an examination of the vocal cords after extirpation of a goiter".

In this work, Halsted notes that he first became interested in thyroid surgery reading the work of Wolfler, an assistant to Billroth, when Halsted served in Billroth's surgical laboratory in 1880. He discusses the slow evolution in the understanding of thyroid and parathyroid physiology and pathophysiology including the work of Gley and Vassale in which excision of a millimeter fragment of canine parathyroid precipitated lethal tetany.

Halsted adopted Kocher's meticulous thyroid surgical technique and introduced these to the US, blending these surgical techniques with knowledge of antisepsis and the use of modern hemostatic forceps. In 1881, in New York, Halsted assisted Dr Harry Sand of Roosevelt Hospital with resection of a right thyroid mass with the patient awake in the dental chair with a rubber bag tied around his neck to catch the blood. The two hemostats available at the hospital at that time were both used for this case; these hemostats Halsted writes were of the "mouse-tooth" and "bulldog" varieties. In 1881, Halsted wrote that "the confidence acquired from masterfulness in controlling hemorrhage gives the surgeon the calm which is so needed for clear thinking and orderly procedure at the operative table". Halsted in turn disseminated Kocher's surgical techniques to numerous prominent US surgeons including the Mayo Brothers, Lahey, and Crile. Through Halsted's instruction, thyroidectomy became a safe and even triumphant treatment form. Early American successful medical clinics such as the Mayo Clinic, Lahey clinic and Crile clinic were initially financially fueled by high-volume goiter surgery made possible through Halsted's techniques.

Halsted helped to found the auspicious Johns Hopkins Hospital, where he was named the first Johns Hopkins Professor of Surgery. There, he introduced surgical residency training and trained many surgeons including Cushing, Dandy and Reed and a number of respected thyroid surgeons including Charles Horace, Frank Lahey, and George Crile. Halsted's early work was not without peril. While experimenting with local infiltration anesthetic agents, Halsted became addicted to cocaine. His treatise "*The Operative Story of Goiter*" is a testament to one man's ability to collect, analyze, and present definitively the important surgical topic of thyroidectomy, and represents an epic case study in modern surgical evolution.

RELATIONSHIP OF THE AGE OF THE PATIENT TO THE NATURAL HISTORY AND PROGNOSIS OF CARCINOMA OF THE THYROID

George Crile Jr., John B Hazard

Although the rate of growth and the presence of cervical or distant metastases are clinical features of some value in separating tumors of the thyroid into two great classes of papillary and non-papillary carcinoma, the most important clinical feature is simply the age of the patient. Most cancers of the thyroid in persons under 40 years of age will behave like papillary carcinomas, even if they are predominantly alveolar. This feature of the natural history of thyroid tumors is of importance to the surgeon who often must operate without benefit of frozen section diagnosis and to the pathologist who often faces difficult problems of classification when called on to interpret frozen sections and who also may find difficulty in locating papillary areas in certain variants of papillary carcinoma, even when permanent sections are available.

Crile G Jr, Hazard JB. Relationship of the age of the patient to the natural history and prognosis of carcinoma of the thyroid. Ann Surg. 1953;138:33-38.

Commentary by: *Ashok R Shaha*

George Crile Jr. and Hazard did a fantastic job some 60 years ago publishing their experience with papillary carcinoma of the thyroid, and more importantly, in dividing thyroid cancer into papillary and non-papillary forms while also implying the importance of age as a prognostic factor. In their series, the survival in patients below the age of 45 was excellent, while the survival in patients above the age of 60 was miserably poor. Also, patients above the age of 60 more often had non-papillary thyroid carcinoma. The authors also reviewed their experience with patients between the ages of 40 and 60 as an intermediate prognostic group. It is interesting that 60 years ago these authors came up with prognostic features that hold true today, and a large number of recent publications essentially show similar data.

George Crile Sr. was founder of the Cleveland Clinic, and more importantly, the father of head and neck surgery in the United States. His landmark article on neck dissection is familiar to every head and neck surgeon in the world. The senior author in this manuscript, George Crile Jr, has been a major advocate of conservative surgery and preserving quality of life. His pioneering work in conservative surgery of the breast is well known, and similarly, he was a strong proponent of lobectomy only in patients with well-differentiated thyroid cancer, which are intrathyroidal. The authors also mention performing a modified neck dissection and not sacrificing the vital structures, such as the sternomastoid muscle, the jugular vein, and accessory nerve. These structures were commonly sacrificed in patients with papillary carcinoma of the thyroid in the past, with considerable morbidity and long-term sequelae. The authors also reviewed the histological prognostic features in great detail, distinguishing between papillary and non-papillary thyroid cancer and adding other histologies such as alveolar type, undifferentiated, and they also use a term, sarcoma, which is probably consistent more with anaplastic thyroid carcinoma than sarcoma of the thyroid *per se.*

The incidence of thyroid cancer has almost quadrupled over the last 25 years. In 1975, we used to see approximately 8,000 new patients with thyroid cancer in the United States, while today the number exceeds 56,000. Interestingly, the mortality from thyroid cancer has essentially remained unchanged. The majority of patients who die of thyroid cancer generally die of more aggressive form of thyroid cancer or the high-risk thyroid cancer. Byers et al. from France were one of the early groups to discuss the prognostic features of thyroid cancer. The Mayo Clinic and Lahey Clinic popularized the prognostic features such as Ages (age, grade of the tumor, extrathyroidal extension, and size of the tumor). While the Lahey Clinic popularized the aims (age, distant metastases, extrathyroidal extension, and size of the tumor), the nodal metastasis has not been a major prognostic feature in patients with papillary carcinoma of the thyroid. As a matter of fact, the microscopic metastatic disease is well known in papillary thyroid cancer and is seen in approximately 50% of the individuals. However, the biology of the thyroid cancer is so unique that the presence of nodal metastasis has very little prognostic implication in the long-term outcome however recently various publications have shown some impact of nodal metastasis especially when there is bulky nodal disease, or gross extranodal extension or aggressive histology. The prognostic features described by Mayo clinic and Leahy clinic are similarly also described in various other publications including Dgroot, Memorial Sloan-Kettering Cancer Center and other institutions with large series of patients with papillary thyroid cancer. The histologic distinction from papillary to anaplastic thyroid cancer, with progression of the disease from papillary to tall cell, to insular, to poorly differentiated and undifferentiated thyroid cancer has been described in the recent literature. Rosai et al initially described the importance of analyzing the histological variations in great details. The Mayo clinic with their large experience of patients with well differentiated thyroid cancer came up with a new prognostic features in 1994 implying Maci's as a group of prognostic factors where completeness of resection was the most important prognostic feature. Satisfactory surgical resection with all extrathyroidal extension and removal of the adjuvant involved structures is the basis of adequate treatment in well differentiated thyroid cancer. Age continues to be a most important prognostic feature in patients with thyroid cancer. As a matter of fact, this is the only human cancer where age has been included in the staging system of AJCC and UICC. There is no stage III and IV thyroid cancer in patients below the age of 45 implying the best outcome in this group of patients. The overall survival in patients below the age of 45 exceeds 98% a remarkable human malignancy with best outcome based on age alone as an important prognostic factor. Recently, there has been considerable interest in molecular biology of thyroid cancer with special emphasis on ploidy and BRAF mutation. Even though the experience is limited, the information appears quite promising and in future I'm sure we'll be studying well-differentiated thyroid cancer in greater details based on these molecular features. However, it's implication in the clinical practice at this time appears to be of limited significance. Interestingly, the BRAF mutation is commonly seen in more aggressive thyroid cancer or high-risk thyroid cancer. Based on the prognostic features in well differentiated thyroid cancer, the Mayo and Leahy clinic divided their patients into low and high risk groups based on the age, the size of the tumor, grade of the tumor, extrathyroidal extension and distant metastases. Almost 80% of the patients in both the cities belong to the low risk group while 20% belong to the high risk group with poor prognostic features.

The Memorial Sloan Kettering Cancer Center divided their patients into low, intermediate and high-risk groups. The low risk group included young patients, smaller tumors and good histology. While the high risk group included older patients, larger tumors, gross extrathyroidal extension and aggressive histology. While the intermediate risk group included young patients with aggressive thyroid cancer or older patients with smaller or intrathyroidal tumors, the prognosis in these four groups is different based on the risk group analysis. The mortality in the high-risk group exceeds 45% which is directly related to local recurrence in the central compartment of the neck and distant metastases. It is interesting that the authors in this manuscript have discussed about gross extrathyroidal extension and adequacy of the surgical resection some 60 years back. The information, which has become more critical in recent years for best local control. They also reported surgery alone as the best treatment choice and they have not used radioactive iodine or external radiation therapy in their series. Our recent experience shows limited use of radioactive iodine in selected patients and extra radiation therapy reserved only for aggressive histology or gross residual tumor. Crile and Hazard deserve special compliments and congratulations for this fine manuscript the information of which continues to hold true even today.

PAPILLARY THYROID CARCINOMA: A 10-YEAR FOLLOW-UP REPORT OF THE IMPACT OF THERAPY IN 576 PATIENTS

Ernest L Mazzaferri, Robert L Young

Data from 576 patients with papillary thyroid cancer were retrospectively analyzed. With a median follow-up of 10 years and three months, there were six deaths from, and 84 recurrences of, thyroid cancer. Of the latter, 16 (19 percent) could not be eradicated. Death from thyroid cancer occurred only in those 30 years of age or over at the time of diagnosis and only in patients with primary tumors larger than 1.5 cm in diameter. Locally invasive tumor was associated with a poor prognosis. Cervical lymph node metastases found at initial surgery were associated with higher recurrence rates but not higher mortality rates. Treatment with total thyroidectomy, postoperative radioiodine and thyroid hormone resulted in the lowest recurrence and mortality rates except in those patients with small primary tumors (< 1.5 cm diameter) in whom less than total thyroidectomy and postoperative therapy with thyroid hormone alone gave results which did not differ statistically from those achieved with more aggressive therapy. No important differences in outcome were observed when cervical lymph node metastases were simply excised or more aggressively treated by neck dissection. External radiation used as initial adjunctive therapy adversely influenced outcome.

Mazzaferri EL, Young RL. Papillary thyroid carcinoma: a 10-year follow-up report of the impact of therapy in 576 patients. Am J Med. 1981;70:511-518.

Commentary by: *Ashok R Shaha*

This is one of the landmark publications from Ernie Mazzaferri, one of the legends in thyroid cancer management. His contributions in the field of endocrinology are extremely well recognized, and his leadership and mentorship is appreciated by all his colleagues and trainees. Unfortunately, Dr Mazzaferri passed away recently and there continues to be a great void in the endocrine world.

This is the second publication by Dr Mazzaferri on 576 patients with thyroid cancer he had retrospectively analyzed. The earlier publication was in *Medicine*, published in 1977. This is a review of 576 patients treated in the United States Air Force by multiple surgeons in different institutions, which clearly leads to some concerns about the collection of data and the interpretation of the available information; however, the information provided by Dr Mazzaferri is very important in relation to the prognostic factors in thyroid cancer. He reported that there was no mortality in patients with tumors less than 1.5 cm in a 10-year follow-up. Only 6 individuals died; however, 84 patients developed recurrent disease. He reported locally invasive tumor as a sign of poor prognosis. Patient's presenting initially with cervical lymph node metastasis had a high incidence of recurrence in the neck; however, there was no higher mortality rate. The information provided and conclusions made are very important. A total thyroidectomy, postoperative radioiodine and thyroid hormone were the hallmarks of treatment with the lowest risk recurrence and mortality rates. However, in patients with tumors less than 1.5 cm, the radioactive iodine ablation was not indicated. They have strongly recommended total thyroidectomy followed by postoperative radioiodine and thyroid hormone suppressive therapy in tumors 2.5 cm or greater, multifocal, or locally invasive or metastatic tumors. The authors did consider local excision of the lymph node metastasis compared to formal neck dissection. The lymph node metastasis was noted to be present in 46% of the patients. The authors have elaborated on individual prognostic factors such as sex, age, size of the primary tumor, local tumor invasion, cervical lymph node metastasis, extent of thyroidectomy, and lymph node surgery in great details in this manuscript. Even though the information about age does not appear to be strongly described in this manuscript, the authors do mention about differences of outcome and excellent prognosis in children compared to adults.

This is one of the important earlier publications in the field of management of thyroid cancer and various prognostic factors. This is probably one of the most quoted papers in thyroid cancer. Clearly, the information provided in this manuscript is extremely important in the evaluation of patients with thyroid cancer as well as long-term outcome and management choices.

Subsequently, various authors have published the prognostic factors in well-differentiated thyroid cancer, such as Hei from the Mayo Clinic, Cady from the Lahey clinic, and Shaha from Memorial Sloan-Kettering Cancer Center. The important prognostic factors defined in various publications include patient age, the grade of the tumor, the size of the tumor, extrathyroidal extension, and the presence of distant metastases. Based on these prognostic factors at Memorial Sloan-Kettering Cancer Center, we have divided our patients into low-, intermediate-, and high-risk groups. The Mayo Clinic and the Lahey clinic divided their patients into low- and high-risk groups in which 80% of the patients belong in the low-risk group and 15–20% belong in the high-risk group. The classification popularized from Sloan-Kettering Cancer Center is extremely critical in the evaluation of patients with thyroid cancer, and their overall prognosis and treatment choices based on the risk group analysis. The low-risk group includes young patients with smaller tumors, generally less than 4 cm. The survival rate in this group exceeds 99%. The high-risk group includes patients above the age of 45, with tumors generally larger than 4 cm, high-grade histology, or gross extrathyroidal extension. The average survival rate in this group is approximately 60%. The intermediate group includes young patients with more aggressive thyroid cancer or older patients (above the age of 45) with smaller tumors. The treatment decisions are generally based on individual risk group analysis. In the low-risk group, adjuvant treatment such as radioactive iodine ablation is generally not recommended. Decisions for the intermediate-risk group are generally based on tumor factors rather than the age of the patient alone, while in the high-risk group, in which the mortality is quite high, one would be extremely aggressive surgically, with radioactive iodine ablation and appropriate suppressive therapy. Certain individual patients in the high-risk group may require external radiation therapy, those with gross residual tumor or tumor in the critical area, which is shaved off the trachea of the cricoid, and the chances of future recurrences are quite high. Even though the role of external radiation therapy is always controversial in the management of thyroid cancer, in high-risk thyroid cancer it has shown better local control. The risk group stratification popularized into low-, intermediate-, and high-risk groups is now used by the American Thyroid Association in their guidelines. The factors mainly considered by the American Thyroid Association are tumor-related factors based on the pathology report. The grade of the tumor appears to also be one of the important features; however, there could be considerable variations among different pathologists. Recently, there has been considerable interest in the tall cell variety of thyroid cancer. Clearly, we need to distinguish between the tall cell variant and tall cell tumors. The presence of tall cells in papillary thyroid carcinoma is well recognized; however, papillary carcinoma is recognized as tall cell variant if the percentage of tumor cells is greater than 50%.

These tumors with either tall cell variety or poorly differentiated variety are generally radio resistant and are hypermetabolic in PET scans. These patients are best followed and evaluated in the follow-up with a PET scan. The issues over neck node metastasis continue to generate considerable debate and controversy. There used to be strong opposition to doing preoperative CT scan with contrast; however, recently with palpable nodal disease in the neck, generally most surgeons would recommend preoperative CT scan with contrast for better evaluation of the parapharyngeal, retropharyngeal, paratracheal and superior mediastinal lymph nodes. Over the last 10 years, there has been a major debate in the field of management of thyroid cancer related to prophylactic (elective central compartment dissection versus no dissection). The majority of surgeons believe that elective nodal dissection is not indicated in patients with papillary thyroid carcinoma; however, it should be considered in larger tumors, high-grade tumors, or tumors with gross extrathyroidal extension. The complication rate is considerably high in relation to temporary and permanent hypoparathyroidism and temporary and permanent recurrent laryngeal nerve injury in individuals undergoing elective or prophylactic central compartment nodal dissection. The extent of nodal dissection in the central compartment remains quite unclear as to (1) medial to the recurrent laryngeal nerve or lateral to the recurrent laryngeal nerve, (2) unilateral or bilateral, and (3) lowermost extent of the disease. Interestingly, the staging system now divides superior mediastinal on level VII nodes as N1b, which puts the patients above the age of 45 into stage IV compared with other patients without level VII nodal metastasis as Stage III. This issue probably requires further detailed analysis of the data and review of the literature.

Overall, this is one of the important contributions in the field of management of thyroid cancer, and the contributions of Dr Mazzaferri will be remembered for years to come. We will wholeheartedly miss Ernie!

OPERATIVE MONITORING OF PARATHYROID GLAND HYPERFUNCTION

George L Irvin III, Victor D Dembrow, David L Prudhomme

With a 20-year experience of more than 700 parathyroidectomies, our persistent hypercalcemic postoperative failure rate of 7% has remained constant. Reasons for failure have been misdiagnosis or inability of the surgeon to detect and excise all hypersecreting glands. We have modified a commercially available immuno-radiometric assay for intact parathyroid hormone (PTH) resulting in a 15-minute turnaround time. Since intact PTH has half-life measured in minutes, whole blood samples taken 10 minutes after gland excisions were monitored intraoperatively to confirm significant changes in circulating hormone. Quantitative evidence that all hyperfunctioning parathyroid tissue had been ablated during operation was obtained in 19 of 21 patients. Less than four glands each were identified in 53% of these patients. The PTH "quick" test correctly pointed to an inadequate excision requiring further parathyroid ablation in two patients, made bilateral neck exploration unnecessary in two patients who had previously undergone parathyroidectomy, and predicted persistent hypercalcemia in two patients with complications.

Irvin GL III, Dembrow VD, Prudhomme DL. Operative monitoring of parathyroid gland hyperfunction. Am J Surg. 1991;162:299-302.

Commentary by: *Martha A Zeiger*

Dr George L Irvin III truly revolutionized the way in which endocrine surgeons operate on patients with primary hyperparathyroidism and, as a result, dramatically improved the overall surgical outcomes of patients with this disease entity. With the introduction of intraoperative PTH (IoPTH) monitoring and the increase in minimally invasive parathyroidectomy (MIP) procedures, patients experience significantly less pain, enjoy smaller surgical incisions, and undergo shorter operations; furthermore, the procedure incurs significantly less cost than the traditional bilateral neck exploration. In the early 1990s Dr Irvin, with tenacious persistence, perfected the use and interpretation of IoPTH measurements. He tirelessly investigated the intraoperative use of the immunoradiometric assay (IRMA) for measuring intact parathyroid hormone introduced to us by Dr Samuel R Nussbaum in 1988. Over the ensuing years, Dr Irvin regaled us with stories of his sentinel operative event, namely, the surgical failure and then ultimate success on his operating room nurse who had primary hyperparathyroidism, about how he transported radioactive materials from one hospital to another in Florida to test the use of IoPTH, and about the time he gathered endocrine surgeons in a hotel room in order to demonstrate the "Quick PTH" assay at the Association of Endocrine Surgeons' (AAES) meeting in Miami in 1992.

Prior to this significant change in parathyroid surgery, endocrine surgeons generally believed that all four parathyroid glands needed to be identified and either biopsied if they were normal or removed if they were enlarged;

in other words, every patient needed to undergo a four-gland exploration. Sestamibi (technetium-99) had also been introduced in the 1980s and soon replaced the less sensitive and less specific thallium-technetium subtraction scans used for the localization of parathyroid adenomas, making MIP more feasible. High-definition ultrasound would also soon facilitate better localization of parathyroid adenomas. Before the popularity of MIP took hold, arguments at the AAES annual meetings were comprised of two schools of thought as to the appropriate surgical approach: the first and more conservative group believed that all four glands should be identified at the time of surgery and proven with either excision or frozen section biopsy; the second school of thought put forth that, statistically speaking, if the surgeon identified one adenoma and one normal gland on the same side that further exploration would be very unlikely to reveal a second adenoma, and thus, a unilateral neck exploration would suffice.

Through the ensuing years, the Endocrine Surgery Group at the University of Miami painstakingly developed what is now referred to as the "Miami criteria" to document a successful drop in IoPTH. After the removal of the adenoma, the PTH level must fall, within 10 minutes, below 50% of the pre-incision or post-excision value, whichever is valued higher serving as baseline. Other groups have added criteria, such as within the normal range, within other timeframes, but the "Miami criteria" have stood the test of time, resulting in less false positive and less false negative surgical results.

Before the popularization of MIP, indications for surgery were often more stringent, closely following the NIH Consensus Guidelines and, as a consequence, not affording a patient with more protean or subtle symptoms, the supposed "asymptomatic patient", access to parathyroidectomy that generally would relieve them of their vague signs and symptoms. Arguments against MIP abounded through the years—that false positive drops in PTH would miss a double adenoma, that it was not applicable to four-gland hyperplasia, as examples. Given, however, the worst case scenario, in which the surgeon believed a patient was cured based on IoPTH results only to learn 10 days later that the calcium and PTH were still elevated, re-exploration is much easier technically, simply because the surgeon has only explored one quadrant of the neck and the remainder of the neck around the thyroid gland is virtually untouched.

Dr Irvin and his group at the University of Miami continued to rigorously study, promote, and perfect the use of IoPTH and MIP, carefully scrutinized their outcomes, and successfully applied its use to even redo-parathyroidectomies. Endocrine surgeons are generally reluctant to explore the entire neck in a patient who has undergone prior neck surgery, and the use of localization studies, minimally invasive approaches, and IoPTH have facilitated a more limited surgical approach in these patients who have persistent or recurrent hyperparathyroidism.

In summary, despite resistance, skepticism, and challenges, Dr Irvin and his colleagues, like many quintessential innovators, stayed the course and persisted in perfecting the technique and our results from MIP with the use of IoPTH. Because of his incredible dedication and effort, Dr Irvin truly revolutionized and improved the way in which we now routinely care for patients with primary hyperparathyroidism.

MEDULLARY CARCINOMA OF THE THYROID: CURRENT DIAGNOSIS AND MANAGEMENT

Terry C Lairmore, Samuel A Wells

Medullary thyroid carcinoma (MTC) accounts for 5–10% of thyroid malignancies and occurs in either a sporadic or a familial form. The familial form is inherited in an autosomal dominant pattern, and expressed clinically as multiple endocrine neoplasia (MEN), types IIa and IIb, or as familial MTC alone. This neoplasm is derived from the parafollicular or C-cells, and has the ability to secrete a variety of polypeptide hormones including calcitonin, which serves as a tumor marker for the presence of MTC. The development of a calcitonin radioimmunoassay and the screening of patients at risk for the familial forms of MTC allows the diagnosis of the neoplasm in an occult stage when total thyroidectomy results in virtually 100% cure. We will present our experience with the diagnosis, treatment, and postoperative follow-up of our patients with this interesting neoplasm.

Lairmore TC, Wells SA. Medullary carcinoma of the thyroid: current diagnosis and management. Semin Surg Oncol.1991;7:92-99.

Commentary by: *Herbert Chen, Sara E Murray*

Dr Samuel A Wells' contributions to the field of endocrine surgery throughout his nearly 5-decade career cannot be overstated, and his advances within head and neck oncology are perhaps his most significant. In particular, Dr Wells' research and clinical expertise regarding medullary thyroid cancer (MTC) has greatly influenced the way this disease is diagnosed, treated, and monitored.

As understood, MTC is a neuroendocrine tumor arising from the parafollicular C-cells of the thyroid. Although the majority of MTC occurs in a sporadic fashion, it may present clinically in three familial syndromes — familial MTC (FMTC) and multiple endocrine neoplasia IIa and IIb (MEN-IIa and MEN-IIb). FMTC and the MTC in MEN-IIa or IIb are genetically transmitted in an autosomal dominant pattern, meaning all family members of affected individuals are at risk for the disease and should undergo screening. Identifying an effective screening tool has been one of the major goals of MTC research.

Prior to biochemical testing, ultrasound was the primary method used in screening for MTC. However, because MTC may be small, it is difficult to visualize radiographically on ultrasound. In addition, even very small MTC tumors have been reported to metastasize. Therefore, patients were often diagnosed at advanced stages with local or distant metastases. The discovery of calcitonin and its relationship to MTC provided an innovative diagnostic tool. However, although serum calcitonin levels were found to be elevated in patients with MTC, only those with large tumor burdens had significant calcitonin elevations. Dr Wells' successive work went on to describe the relationship of higher plasma calcitonin levels to a greater extent of disease, emphasizing the importance of early biochemical diagnosis.

Dr Wells' landmark 1991 article entitled, "Medullary Carcinoma of the Thyroid: Current Diagnosis and Management", outlines a protocol utilizing serum calcitonin that distinguishes patients with either C-cell hyperplasia or early MTC to those without disease, as well as accurately identifying recurrence in postoperative patients. The protocol involves the use of provocative testing with pentagastrin or calcium-stimulated calcitonin levels as a diagnostic test for MTC. This pioneering discovery allowed for an early biochemical diagnosis before the disease was clinically evident. The provocative test was very sensitive, allowing for early surgical intervention when necessary, occasionally prior to the development of malignancy. Alternatively, the test was specific enough to identify patients at risk who were unlikely to develop MTC, thus avoiding an unnecessary thyroidectomy.

The ensuing clinical question was how to manage patients with only mild or modest elevations in peripheral plasma calcitonin levels. In reply, Dr Wells' group instituted selective venous catheterization of the inferior thyroid vein in conjunction with provocative testing. This offered a more accurate identification of patients with C-cell hyperplasia or MTC, leading to appropriate surgical management.

The provocative testing for MTC was the standard screening test until recently, when Dr Wells' group introduced genetic testing for mutations in the RET proto-oncogene. This finding revolutionized the screening and diagnosis of MTC, allowing for the identification of a mutated RET allele by DNA analysis in kindred members of individuals with heritable forms of MTC. This discovery led to the characterization of risk in family members, allowing for timely thyroidectomy in those with an inherited mutated RET allele, prior to the development of MTC. Because MTC is the most common cause of death in these familial syndromes, RET mutation screening programs are currently standard in MEN-II and FMTC families.

Within the past few years, Dr Wells and colleagues have been actively involved in molecular targeted therapies for MTC. They recently demonstrated the efficacy of Vandetanib—a tyrosine kinase inhibitor and antagonist of signaling pathways of RET, vascular endothelial growth factor receptor, and epidermal growth factor receptor—against locally advanced or metastatic hereditary MTC. After successful clinical trials, in 2011 Vandetanib became the first drug to be approved by the Federal Drug Administration for treatment of late-stage MTC in adult patients who are not surgical candidates.

In conclusion, Dr Wells has greatly influenced the field of Head and Neck Oncology through his significant advancements in the prevention, diagnosis, and treatment of MTC. No other surgeon has made such lasting contributions to MTC through his pioneering work on early disease recognition, risk profiling, and targeted therapeutic modalities. His early focus on identifying pre-malignant disease, permitting early intervention, has become the benchmark for innovative oncologic screening and has had widespread influence beyond just head and neck cancer. His groundbreaking research and clinical expertise has provided a framework that will continue to be built upon, leading to improved patient outcomes for years to come.

THYROID CANCER AFTER CHERNOBYL

Vasili S Kazakov, Evgeni P Demidchik, Larisa N Astakhova

Sir—We would like to report a great increase in the frequency of thyroid cancer in children in Belarus, which commenced in 1990 and continues. Table 1 shows the incidence of thyroid cancer in children in the six regions of Belarus and Minsk City from 1986 to the end of the first half of 1992. It can be seen that the overall incidence rose from an average of just four cases per year from 1986 to 1989 inclusive, to 55 in 1991 and is projected to be not less than 60 in 1992. This increase is not uniformly distributed across the country: for example, there is no significant increase in Mogilev, Minsk City or Vitebsk, By far the greatest increase is seen in the Gomel region, from one or two cases per year to 38 in 1991, and a less obvious increase is seen in the Brest and Grodno regions.

The occurrence of this increase in thyroid cancer in children within a few years of exposure to radioactive isotopes of iodine is unexpected, but real. It poses both humanitarian and scientific problems, and is placing great strains upon the health services of our new country. It also provides an opportunity, which we hope will not be repeated, to study the consequences of major exposure of a population to isotopes of iodine from fallout. We are collaborating with several international groups and are preparing detailed reports of various aspects of the problem.

Kazakov VS, Demidchik EP, Astakhova LN. Thyroid cancer after Chernobyl. Nature. 1992;359:21-22.

Commentary by: *Daniel Branovan*

The article by Kazakov et al. entitled "Thyroid Cancer after Chernobyl" was published in *Nature* in 1992, about 6 years after the Chernobyl nuclear accident. The Belarus scientists were the first to report the sharp increase in thyroid cancer incidence in the regions of Belarus most affected by radioactive fallout.

At the time, a causal relationship between external radiation and an increased incidence of thyroid carcinoma was best understood through

Table 1: Incidence of thyroid cancer in children in Belarus

Region of Belarus	1986	1987	1988	1989	1990	1991	1992*	Total
Brest	0	0	1	1	6	5	5	18
Vitebsk	0	0	0	0	1	3	0	4
Gomel	1	2	1	2	14	38	13	71
Grodno	1	1	1	2	0	2	6	13
Minsk	0	1	1	1	1	4	4	12
Mogilev	0	0	0	0	2	1	1	4
Minsk City	0	0	1	0	5	2	1	9
Total	**2**	**4**	**5**	**6**	**29**	**55**	**30**	**131**

*Six months of 1992.

work with Japanese atomic bomb survivors. However, prior to the Chernobyl accident, the carcinogenic potential of ingested radioactive iodine was not appreciated. Previous studies had shown that among more than 6,000 children who received known amounts of Iodine-131 (^{131}I) for diagnostic purposes (mean dose, 1 Gy), there was no increased risk of thyroid cancer, but the numbers of children exposed under the age of 10 was small (1, 2, 3). The exposure of 3,440 young children in the 1940s–1950s to fallout from essentially pure ^{131}I from the Hanford nuclear site also did not lead to an increased risk of thyroid cancer at doses on the order of 0.17 Gy (maximum dose, 1 Gy).

The thyroid dose from exposure to ^{131}I during the Chernobyl accident was 1000–2000 times the average annual body dose. In the early period after the accident, it became evident that residents of Southeastern areas of Belarus demonstrated the most thyroid pathology. Unfortunately, reliable information about the accident and the resulting dispersion of radioactive material was initially unavailable to the affected people in what was then the Soviet Union, and remained inadequate for years following the accident. This led to widespread public distrust of official information and the mistaken attribution of many unrelated health disorders to radiation exposure. The early and sharp increase in pediatric thyroid cancer in Belarus after the Chernobyl accident was entirely unexpected. The first reports of a dramatic increase of thyroid cancer cases in children in Belarus were greeted skeptically in the West, US, and Japan. Shigematsu and Thiessen, in remarks to the publication of Kazakov et al. in 1992 noted that "the data provided in these reports are limited and preliminary in that they do not allow one to state whether the suggested increase in thyroid cancer cases is unequivocally attributable to radiation exposure" because there is no screening data, no control group, and no thyroid dose. Only by 1996, did Professor Williams lament: "it was not thought plausible that exposure to radioisotopes of iodine in fallout could lead to such an increase in thyroid cancer with such a short latency". In retrospect, it can be seen that the skepticism was unjustified.

Special epidemiological investigations and large-scale screening studies were organized to ascertain the true rise in thyroid pathology and its radio-induced character. In 1990–1991, the staff of the Research Institute of Radiation Medicine (Belarus) conducted the first screening investigation of thyroid status in Belarus children exposed to Chernobyl fallout in several contaminated areas of the Gomel region. According to the screening study, in Choiniki the prevalence of nodular pathology was 1.24%, among that of thyroid carcinoma—0.62%, adenoma—0.09%, nodular goiter (morphologically verified)—0.27%, and cystic goiter—0.09%. At the same time, in the control group (non-exposed children from the Braslav of Vitebsk region) nodular goiter presented as only cystic nodules in 0.75%. Thyroid cancer was not observed among examined children in the control region. Data obtained by different investigators in screening studies in Belarus during 1990–2008 showed that the prevalence of thyroid carcinoma varied from 0.19% to 0.62%. All studies concordantly demonstrated an extremely high level of thyroid cancer incidence.

The dramatic increase in the incidence of radiation-induced thyroid cancer in subjects exposed to ionizing radiation in childhood is now accepted as the most significant health consequence of the Chernobyl accident in Belarus, the Ukraine, and the Russian Federation. According to radiobiological prognoses, thyroid cancer morbidity is projected to rise, peaking up to 40 years after radiation exposure. The incidence rate of thyroid cancer in Belarus per 100,000 children before the Chernobyl accident was 0.085 in 1986. Based on the Belarusian official health authorities data, the highest crude incidence rate of thyroid cancer in children after the Chernobyl accident was observed in Belarus in 1993—4 per 100,000 (91 cases), and in the Gomel region (most contaminated) in 1996—12.6 per 100,000 (45 cases). The highest number of thyroid cancer cases was registered among adolescents (14–18 years old) in 2001—18.3 (83 cases). The incidence rate of childhood thyroid cancer is likely to continue to decrease (2010—11 cases, 2011—19 cases), while the incidence of thyroid cancer among older age groups of the population has increased, and the tend is likely to persist (1993–484 cases; 2010—1,098 cases; 2011—1,165 cases).

The Belarusian scientists' article also pointed out that tumors detected in children until 1992 had aggressive behavior. Fifty-five of the 131 cases showed direct extension to the perithyroid tissues and six distant metastases. Recent molecular studies of post-Chernobyl thyroid carcinomas have shown that RET-PTC3 is linked to a more aggressive tumor than RET-PTC1, and BRAF mutations have been less common than in unexposed populations. The importance of the correlation of molecular and morphological findings with latency is well shown by studies on Chernobyl-related tumors. When RET-PTC rearrangements were analyzed, the early short latency papillary carcinomas were largely of the solid type, often associated with direct invasion, and showing RET-PTC3 rearrangements. Later tumors showed a high proportion with RET-PTC1 and a classical morphology and less aggressive behavior

The incidence of thyroid cancer has increased over the past three decades not only in Belarus, but also in the United States, Europe, and other developed countries. This fact presents both a scientific dilemma and a reason for concern in the healthcare community. While the incidence of many head and neck cancers in the United States is decreasing, a number of registries have reported that the incidence of thyroid cancer is increasing.

Papillary thyroid cancer in the United States more than doubled over the past 30 years, from 2.7 to 11.9 per 100,000 (2011). The reasons for the increase are not yet understood, and may be multifactorial. A small role in the general statistic can be attributed to a high level of prevalence of thyroid cancer among immigrants from the former Soviet Union (Screening data of "Project Chernobyl" New-York). Some investigators have attributed the increase to environmental radiation, while others have found no obvious source (fallout from nuclear weapon testing, genetic predisposition, history of thyroid diseases, and residence in an endemic goiter area). Recent studies have shown that long-term stimulation of the thyroid gland by thyroid-stimulating hormone can lead to tumor formation. Animal experiments indicate that iodine deficiency is a potent promoter of thyroid carcinogenesis and that iodine excess may play a role in tumor promotion. Also, dietary factors, including cruciferous and goitrogenic vegetables, may play a role in thyroid carcinogenesis.

Recent tragic radiation exposure in Fukushima, Japan, and the rapid, comprehensive response of Japanese scientists to the expected development of thyroid pathology demonstrates the lessons learned from the Chernobyl nuclear accident. Kazakov et al. first sounded the warning bell, and the international medical community has since listened and responded.

LOBECTOMY VERSUS TOTAL THYROIDECTOMY FOR DIFFERENTIATED CARCINOMA OF THE THYROID: A MATCHED-PAIR ANALYSIS

Jatin P Shah, Thom R Loree, Digpal Dharker, et al.

The extent of surgical resection for differentiated carcinoma of the thyroid gland confined to one lobe remains controversial. Although primary tumor size and extra-thyroid extension are associated with a poor prognosis, the presence of multifocal lesions is not associated with an adverse prognosis. Therefore, the role of lobectomy versus total thyroidectomy must be studied in a prospective, randomized trial. Due to the need for long-term follow-up, such a trial has not yet been undertaken. As an alternative to such a trial, we have identified 146 patients from a consecutive series of 931 previously untreated patients undergoing surgical treatment at 1 institution between 1930 and 1980. For this study of matched-pair analysis, 73 patients, aged 45 years or older, were matched in each arm for significant prognostic factors. One group underwent lobectomy, and the other group underwent total thyroidectomy. The 20-year survival rate in the lobectomy group was 82% compared with 73% in the total thyroidectomy group (p = not significant). The patterns of failure in these two groups of patients were examined. A comparison of the patients who underwent lobectomy with an unmatched group of patients who underwent lobectomy showed similar survival rates. On the other hand, unmatched patients undergoing total thyroidectomy had a poorer survival rate than the matched group. This signifies a more aggressive nature of disease in the unmatched group of patient undergoing total thyroidectomy. We therefore conclude that low-risk patients undergoing lobectomy are likely to do as well as those undergoing total thyroidectomy and without the increased risk of the morbidity of total thyroidectomy.

Shah JP, Loree TR, Dharker D, Strong EW. Lobectomy versus total thyroidectomy for differentiated carcinoma of the thyroid: a matched-pair analysis. Am J Surg. 1993;166:331-335.

Commentary by: *Claudio R Cernea, Lenine G Brandão*

This is a landmark paper, produced by a truly iconic institution, on one of the most prevalent tumors treated by the head and neck surgeon: the well-differentiated thyroid cancer (WDTC). It is a true privilege for us to be invited to comment on such an important study. In addition, writing a comment after a nearly 20-year gap enables us to add a historical perspective to this remarkable publication.

The authors addressed a very important controversy concerning the extent of the surgical resection of the thyroid gland in WDTC. In a very efficient way, they tried to circumvent the obvious limitation of being unable to employ the most effective study design to answer a clinical question: the prospective randomized controlled trial. In fact, after nearly 20 years, no such high-evidence level study has been published. The reason is the well-known indolent nature of this disease. In order to reach statistical significance regarding disease-specific survival, this theoretical study would have to include several thousand patients followed for more than 15 or 20 years.

Thus, with all the limitations of a case-control matched-pair analysis, they were able to include two very statistically comparable cohorts of 73 patients with WDTC submitted to total thyroidectomy (TT) or to total lobectomy (TL). There were 31 patients in the TT group who could not be matched to any TL case, obviously because they had more advanced disease. Interestingly, the features of these patients were also reported, in spite of their exclusion. The characteristics of these unmatched patients, as well as their statistically lower survival rates (38% vs 82% matched TL vs 73% matched TT) reflected the clear option for TT in more advanced WDTC. Perhaps a new histopathologic analysis of the specimens of these patients, reviewing the slides and trying to identify the most recently described high-risk subtypes (e.g., tall-cell, columnar cell, etc.) would give further support to this basically clinical therapeutic decision.

It is noteworthy that the authors intentionally chose patients older than 45 years of age, thus *not* in the low-risk category. It would be interesting if they had performed a similar study including only patients in the *low-risk category*. We would be especially curious about the long-term impact of the morbidity in these younger patients, comparing it with the relevance of locoregional recurrence. We believe that the application of QOL instruments would be essential for such analysis. Incidentally, morbidity was not disclosed, as it was not an endpoint of this paper. Evidently, one of the main reasons to perform a unilateral thyroidectomy would be to theoretically reduce by 50% the complication rate concerning laryngeal nerve paralysis and hypoparathyroidism, both temporary and permanent. Nevertheless, it would be interesting to know how relevant this morbidity increment would really be in a scenario of patients treated by such extremely skilled world-class head and neck surgeons. We would guess that, in this scenario, even the morbidity after TT would be negligible.

Most clinical and pathological features did not differ significantly between matched TL and matched TT, but in at least two of them there were differences that maybe would reach statistical significance if the number of patients would be larger. Regarding multifocality (and, again, in this kind of retrospective analysis, it is difficult to realize if this feature was found preoperatively or only at the final pathology report), the proportion was 14% in the matched TL group, compared to 22% in the matched TT group. More strikingly, 44% of the patients in the matched TL group were male, compared to only 33% in the matched TT group (and this difference reached a p = 0.054, which could be considered marginally significant). In our opinion, this is not intuitive, because some authors consider male gender to be a *negative* prognostic factor; hence, the proportion of male patients should be higher in the matched TT group.

The authors did not find any difference concerning local recurrence rates among the patients of both groups, albeit this was not the primary endpoint of this study. This is undoubtedly an argument in favor of their philosophy of performing TL for this low-stage WDTC. However, it is important to emphasize that most recurrences within the thyroid bed are actually central compartment lymph node regional recurrences, instead of recurrences in the contralateral remaining lobe.

Presently, most services around the world recommend TT for the treatment of WDTC, with the argument of facilitating the biochemical and imaging postoperative surveillance. In an era of increasingly sensitive diagnostic tools, the early diagnosis of locoregional recurrence is markedly enhanced, leading to the detection of recurrent/residual disease. One of the resulting dilemmas is how to deal with these very stressful situations both for the patients and for the surgeons. Similar controversy includes the indication for elective central compartment dissection, which now-a-days is the true controversial issue rather than deciding between TL and TT. On the other hand, not all patients with WDTC are going to be operated on by *experienced* surgeons. Thus, although belonging to an institution that historically has been training surgeons and performing TT for all WDTC patients, I recognize the immense contribution offered by this landmark article, emphasizing that TL is an acceptable procedure for selected cases, even in the high-risk age group with small tumors restricted to the thyroid gland.

PATTERNS OF FAILURE IN DIFFERENTIATED CARCINOMA OF THE THYROID BASED ON RISK GROUPS

Ashok R Shaha, Jatin P Shah, Thom R Loree

Background: Risk-group stratification based on prognostic factors is well established in differentiated carcinoma of the thyroid gland. Patients in the low-risk group have an excellent prognosis, whereas there is significant mortality associated with the high-risk group. The purpose of this paper is to analyze the patterns of treatment failure in the various (local, regional, distant, and associated mortality) risk groups.

Methods: In a retrospective review of a consecutive series of 1038 previously untreated patients with differentiated carcinoma of the thyroid during a period of 55 years, various prognostic factors and risk groups were analyzed. Significant prognostic factors were patient's age, presence of distant metastasis, extrathyroid extension, size, and grade of the tumor. Based on these factors, patients were divided into low- (39%), intermediate- (39%), and high- (22%) risk groups.

Results: The overall treatment-failure rates in the low-, intermediate-, and high-risk groups were 13%, 26%, and 50%, respectively, whereas the mortality rates in the same groups were 1%, 10%, and 33%, respectively.

Conclusions: The overall incidence of recurrence rate in the low-risk group is only 13%, compared with 50% in the high-risk group. The incidence of distant metastasis in the low-risk group is only 2%, compared with 34% in the high-risk group. The understanding of the patterns of treatment failure in different risk groups reaffirms the need to direct treatment strategies based on individual risk groups and intraoperative findings.

Shaha AR, Shah JP, Loree TR. Patterns of failure in differentiated carcinoma of the thyroid based on risk groups. Head Neck.1998;20:26-30.

Commentary by: *Christopher McHenry*

One of the major advances in the management of differentiated thyroid cancer has been the development of risk group definitions based on well-defined prognostic factors including age, tumor size, tumor differentiation, local invasion, and distant metastases. Risk group definition has also been important for the assessment of risk of recurrence and mortality from differentiated thyroid cancer. It has also been important in helping to determine the extent of thyroidectomy, the adjuvant use of radioiodine and the extent of thyrotropin (TSH) suppression, postoperatively.

Doctors Shaha, Shah and Loree, in their paper "Patterns of failure in differentiated carcinoma of the thyroid based on risk groups", made an important contribution to risk group stratification for differentiated thyroid cancer. Based on a robust review of 1,038 patients with differentiated thyroid cancer treated at Memorial Sloan-Kettering Cancer Center, with a mean 20-year follow-up, they were able to divide patients into low-, intermediate-, and high-risk groups for recurrence and mortality. Their risk group stratification is unique in that an intermediate-risk group was identified, which consisted of patients less than 45 years of age with high-risk tumors and patients older than 45 years of age with low-risk tumors.

Dr Shaha, Shah, and Loree have been strong proponents of basing thyroid cancer therapy on risk group analysis and patterns of failure. They have contributed to a large body of literature, which has shown that patients in the high-risk group do poorly and have advocated aggressive treatment with total thyroidectomy, postoperative radioiodine therapy, and TSH suppressive doses of thyroid hormone. They have advanced the management of thyroid cancer, especially for patients at low risk for recurrence and mortality. They have helped to clarify the diverse biological behavior of differentiated thyroid cancer based on prognostic factors including: age greater than 45 years, size greater than 4 cm, aggressive histologic variants, extrathyroidal extension of disease, and distant metastases.

The authors have been proponents for treatment of patients at low risk for recurrence and mortality with thyroid lobectomy and isthmusectomy, which is a recognized therapeutic alternative supported by the National Comprehensive Cancer Network Guidelines. The American Thyroid Association recently recognized the importance of risk group stratification for predicting local and regional recurrence in patients with differentiated thyroid cancer and stratified risk of recurrence into low-, intermediate-, and high-risk groups.

In their seminal paper, 39% of patients were in the low-risk group, and they had a 13% recurrence rate, a 2% rate of distant metastases and mortality rate of 1% compared to 22% of patients in the high-risk group who had a recurrence rate of 50%, a 34% rate of distant metastases and a mortality rate of 33%. With only 2% of patients in the low-risk group developing distant metastases, the authors questioned the necessity for total thyroidectomy, the routine use of radioiodine, and lifelong TSH suppressive doses of thyroid hormone. They have been among the leading proponents for conservative therapy for patients with differentiated thyroid cancer in the low-risk group.

SECOND PRIMARY MALIGNANCIES IN
THYROID CANCER PATIENTS

Carole Rubino, Florent de Vathaire, Massimo E Dottorini, et al.

The late health effects associated with radioiodine (^{131}I) given as treatment for thyroid cancer are difficult to assess since the number of thyroid cancer patients treated at each center is limited. The risk of second primary malignancies (SPMs) was evaluated in a European cohort of thyroid cancer patients. A common database was obtained by pooling the 2-year survivors of the three major Swedish, Italian, and French cohorts of papillary and follicular thyroid cancer patients. A time-dependent analysis using external comparison was performed. The study concerned 6841 thyroid cancer patients, diagnosed during the period 1934–1995, at a mean age of 44 years. In all, 17% were treated with external radiotherapy and 62% received ^{131}I. In total, 576 patients were diagnosed with a SPM. Compared to the general population of each of the three countries, an overall significantly increased risk of SPM of 27% (95% CI: 15–40) was seen in the European cohort. An increased risk of both solid tumors and leukemias was found with increasing cumulative activity of 131 I administered, with an excess absolute risk of 14.4 solid cancers and of 0.8 leukemias per GBq of ^{131}I and 10^5 person-years of follow-up. A relationship was found between ^{131}I administration and occurrence of bone and soft tissue, colorectal, and salivary gland cancers. These results strongly highlight the necessity to delineate the indications of ^{131}I treatment in thyroid cancer patients in order to restrict its use to patients in whom clinical benefits are expected.

Rubino C, de Vathaire F, Dottorini ME, et al. Second primary malignancies in thyroid cancer patients. Br J Cancer. 2003;89;1638-1644.

Commentary by: *Jeremy L Freeman*

This is a seminal article in the field of thyroid oncology. For many years, the kneejerk response to patients with well-differentiated thyroid cancer was to automatically administer RAI. This was done with no regard to outcome measurement or toxicity of RAI. This article shows, in a statistically valid fashion, that there is an increased incidence of second primary malignancies when increasing doses of RAI are administered to patients with well-differentiated thyroid cancer. This is the largest cohort of patients in whom this has been reported.

This study is a mid-level type of study with respect to validity. The Rubino group made the thyroid oncology community more sensitive to the fact that there are indeed consequences to the administration of radioactive iodine, a fact that was largely unknown or ignored up until this study. This then triggered a number of studies as well as guideline policies by various interest groups to create evidence basis for indications for administration of radioactive iodine. Many of these guidelines/studies have now indicated that radioactive iodine is largely unnecessary in low-risk, well-differentiated thyroid cancer. This evidence-based approach is beginning to save the various health care systems money as well as mitigating against complications of administration of radioactive iodine.

All in all, this is an important study that has opened our eyes to the long-term consequences of radioactive iodine and has reduced cost and complications in patients because of responsible evaluation of a treatment modality's efficacy and consequence.

AN OBSERVATIONAL TRIAL FOR PAPILLARY THYROID MICROCARCINOMA IN JAPANESE PATIENTS

Yasuhiro Ito, Akira Miyauchi, Hiroyuki Inoue, et al.

Background: The recent development and spread of ultrasonography and ultrasonography-guided fine needle aspiration biopsy (FNAB) has facilitated the detection of small papillary microcarcinomas of the thyroid measuring 1 cm or less (PMC). The marked difference in prevalence between clinical thyroid carcinoma and PMC detected on mass screening prompted us to observe PMC unless the lesion shows unfavorable features, such as location adjacent to the trachea or on the dorsal surface of the thyroid possibly invading the recurrent laryngeal nerve, clinically apparent nodal metastasis, or high-grade malignancy on FNAB findings. In the present study we report comparison of the outcomes of 340 patients with PMC who underwent observation and the prognosis of 1,055 patients who underwent immediate surgery without observation.

Methods: Between 1993 and 2004, 340 patients underwent observation and 1,055 underwent surgical treatment without observation. These 1,395 patients were enrolled in the present study. Observation periods ranged from 18 months to 187 months (average 74 months).

Results: The proportions of patients whose PMC showed enlargement by 3 mm or more were 6.4 and 15.9% on 5-year and 10-year follow-up, respectively. Novel nodal metastasis was detected in 1.4% at 5 years and 3.4% at 10 years. There were no factors related to patient background or clinical features linked to either tumor enlargement or the novel appearance of nodal metastasis. After observation 109 of the 340 patients underwent surgical treatment for various reasons, and none of those patients showed carcinoma recurrence. In patients who underwent immediate surgical treatment, clinically apparent lateral node metastasis (N1b) and male gender were recognized as independent prognostic factors of disease-free survival.

Conclusions: Papillary microcarcinomas that are not associated with unfavorable features can be candidates for observation regardless of patient background and clinical features. If there are subsequent signs of progression, such as tumor enlargement and novel nodal metastasis it would not be too late to perform surgical treatment. Even though the primary tumor is small, careful surgical treatment including therapeutic modified neck dissection is necessary for N1b PMC patients.

Ito Y, Miyauchi A, Inoue H, et al. An observational trial for papillary thyroid microcarcinoma in Japanese patients. World J Surg. 2010;34:28-35.

Commentary by: *R Michael Tuttle, Ashok R Shaha*

The dramatic rise in the diagnosis of papillary microcarcinoma (PMC) over the last 50 years has resulted in an increasing proportion of thyroid surgeries being done for very small thyroid cancers. In the 1960s, only 5% of thyroid surgery was being done for MPC; this increased to 22% by the 1990s, and is now approaching 50% of thyroid surgeries at some centers. Until recently, such cancers were usually undetected subclinical disease, but high-resolution imaging and aggressive use of fine needle aspiration has resulted in an epidemic of these small tumors. Since autopsy studies demonstrate

PMC in 10–25% of adults dying of unrelated causes, it is likely that over 18 million adults in the USA harbor clinically undetected thyroid cancer, of which only 500,000 cases have been diagnosed and treated. Unless we change our approach to this disease, papillary cancer will continue to be one of the fastest growing malignancies worldwide for many more years.

These data force us to critically evaluate the benefit of treating (or even the benefit of identifying/diagnosing) PMC. While some thyroid cancers grow, invade, develop metastases, and result in death, many thyroid cancers pursue a much less indolent course, which more closely resembles a chronic disease rather than a life-threatening malignancy. Increasingly, oncology is coming to understand that the identification and treatment of small cancers with low-malignant potential is not required, and may even result in more harm than good. As a result, active surveillance has become a viable treatment option for properly selected patients with prostate cancer and low-grade lymphomas.

Therefore, the challenge we face is to be able to identify those thyroid cancers that are likely to progress and metastasize so that appropriate therapy can be applied, with excellent outcomes. Additionally, since salvage therapy is likely to be very effective in a slow growing disease, we must also identify time points in the progression of thyroid cancer that enable us to achieve the optimal risk/benefit treatment ratio.

It is in this context, that in 1993, Dr Akira Miyauchi and Dr Yasuhiro Ito and colleagues began to offer active surveillance as a treatment option for carefully selected PMC. Far ahead of their time in terms of thinking about the risk/benefit of aggressively treating small intrathyroidal cancers, these experts from Kuma Hospital in Kobe, Japan have provided us with a wealth of clinical experience and published data that is currently being used to justify clinical trials of observation of intrathyroidal PTC in the United States. In 1995, Dr Iwao Sugitani from Tokyo also began to offer active surveillance to PMC patients. As a result, we now have two large series of PMC patients carefully followed, with excellent clinical outcomes, at two major centers in Japan.

By excluding PMC patients with regional lymph node metastases, distant metastases, evidence of recurrent laryngeal nerve or tracheal invasion or tumors adjacent to the nerve or trachea, and patients whose cytopathology suggested a high-grade malignancy, they identified a carefully selected cohort of PMC patients who are excellent candidates for observation rather than immediate therapy. The primary follow-up consisted of physical examination and neck ultrasound on a yearly basis. Thyroid hormone suppressive therapy was not routinely employed. Surgical intervention was offered in the few patients who had disease progression manifest by either a 3 mm increase in the size of the primary tumor or identification of local or distant metastases.

In 2003, the authors published their first report of the outcome of 162 patients with PMC, showing that 70% of the tumors did not change from their initial size and that novel lymph node metastasis appeared in only 1.2% of the patients during the follow-up period, which was on average 47 months (18–113 months). They subsequently published a review article in 2007 in which they demonstrated that only 6.7% of the tumors showed enlargement by 3 mm or more during the 5-year period. Between 1993 and 2004, 340 patients underwent observation compared to 1,055 who underwent surgical treatment without observation. They enrolled these 1,395 patients in the present study. Here, the observational period ranged between 18 to 187 months (average 74 months). The summary of their results showed that the proportion of patients whose PMC showed enlargement by 3 mm or more were 6.4% at 5 years and 15.9% at 10 years. Nodal metastasis was detected in 1.4% at 5 years and 3.4% at 10 years.

In 2013, Dr Ito and colleagues once again updated their clinical outcomes in their PMC observation cohort. They now have 1,235 patients whose cancers have been observed with ultrasounds once or twice a year for at least 18 months; their average duration of observation is 5 years, with some patients having been observed for as long as 19 years. Among those observed for 10 years, only 8% grew by 3 mm or more, and only 3.8% developed nodal metastases. No patient has developed distant metastases or has died, and among the 191 patients having surgery after a period of observation, only 1 patient had recurrent disease in remnant thyroid tissue after a partial thyroidectomy (and the recurrence is being observed). These data suggested that PMC in young patients may be more likely to progress than PMC in older patients. The authors suggest that "most low-risk papillary microcarcinoma lacking aggressive features are harmless, and immediate surgery for all of them is definitely an overtreatment".

In a separate cohort of 230 Japanese MPC patients, Sugitani and colleagues reported very similar findings, demonstrating an increase in size of the primary tumor of 3 mm or more in only 7% and newly identified lymph node metastases in only 1% during a mean of 5 years of observation.

Both the Ito and Sugitani series provide compelling evidence that properly selected patients with MPC can safely avoid immediate thyroid surgery and be followed with an active surveillance management approach. During an observation period of 5–10 years, an increase in size of the primary tumor can be expected in approximately 5–10% of patients, with 2–4% developing clinically identifiable lymph node metastases. Importantly, appropriate therapy at the time of disease progression is associated with excellent clinical outcomes, suggesting that a "delay in treatment" is not associated with any clinically meaningful harm in the few patients who demonstrate disease progression while under observation. These compelling data led the thyroid cancer disease management team at Memorial

Sloan-Kettering Cancer Center to begin offering active surveillance as a clinical viable option to immediate surgical resection in properly selected PMC patients starting in around 2010 (preliminary data on 70 PMC patients followed with observation presented at the American Thyroid Association Annual Meeting, Puerto Rico, 2013). Furthermore, our group and others are trying to identify a molecular signature of disease progression that could be used to identify the small subset of PMCs that are destined to become clinically significant thyroid cancer. To date, no specific molecular profile can accurately predict disease progression in PMC.

Since there appears to be little benefit to the routine early detection and treatment of PMC, we must critically re-evaluate our current management paradigms to ensure that we are not causing more harm than good in our aggressive attempts to identify very small volume thyroid cancer. While widespread acceptance of an active surveillance management approach will require additional studies with longer follow-up, the currently available data does allow clinicians to discuss the option of observation rather than immediate surgery in properly selected PMC patients.

Chapter 13

Salivary Glands

SALIVARY GLAND TUMORS IN THE PAROTID GLAND, SUBMANDIBULAR GLAND, AND THE PALATE REGION

Carl-Magnus Eneroth

The relative incidence of the different types of salivary gland tumors and their prognoses has been shown to vary with the location in a study of 2,867 patients with tumors in the parotid gland, submandibular gland, and the palate region. After histologic re-examination and reclassification, 2,513 of the 2,867 tumors were classified as salivary gland tumors. The incidence of salivary gland tumors was strikingly high in the parotid gland, i.e. about twelve times more common in the parotid gland than in the submandibular gland. In all sites there was a striking predominance of pleomorphic adenoma, which altogether comprised 74% of the salivary gland tumors in the present series; the second largest group, mucoepidermoid carcinoma, only comprised 5%. The incidence of malignant salivary gland tumors was twice as high in the submandibular gland than in the parotid gland, but it was highest in the palate region. The prognosis for a given type of malignant tumor was most favorable when the primary tumor was located in the palate region, less favorable when it was in the parotid gland, and least favorable in the submandibular gland.

Eneroth CM. Salivary gland tumors in the parotid gland, submandibular gland, and the palate region, Cancer. 1971:27:6;1415–1418.

Commentary by: *Vincent van der Poorten*

Immediately following publication, the manuscript "Salivary gland tumors in the parotid gland, submandibular gland, and the palate region" in *Cancer (27;6:*1415-1418) by Carl-Magnus Eneroth became a landmark paper for everyone dealing with the extremely interesting but very complex field of salivary gland tumors. Proof of this is that this work until now has been referenced by more than 300 research groups dealing with salivary gland oncology. Dr Eneroth was an otolaryngologist—head and neck surgeon affiliated to the Department of Otolaryngology and the Institute of Tumor Pathology at the world famous Karolinska Sjukhuset in Stockholm, Sweden; a clinician with a strong interest in histopathology. This is reflected in many of his publications throughout his career. The manuscript was received for publication on New Year's Eve (December 31, 1970) after years of work, including presentations at the Royal Society of Medicine in the United Kingdom and at the XVIIth congress of the Scandinavian Oto-Laryngological Society in Helsingør, Denmark (June 27–30, 1969). *Carl-Magnus Eneroth kept on updating and* expanding the patient series, resulting in this landmark publication in June 1971 in a leading cancer journal. Eneroth published 69 papers on salivary gland tumors between 1961 and 1978 on histopathological and cytomorphologic features of salivary gland tumors, microspectrophotometric DNA analysis correlating nuclear DNA content to malignancy in, e.g. acinic cell carcinoma, fine needle aspiration cytology in the diagnosis of salivary gland tumors, and the effect of radiation on salivary function.

A meaningful comment on this landmark paper demands some historical context. The first detailed histological description of a salivary gland tumor type with characteristic structures was published by Billroth in 1859 who gave an extremely precise account of the histological and clinical features of 12 parotid tumors. He observed a complex structure of epithelial and mesenchymal components and denoted them as myxomas due to the predominance of the mesenchymal component. In 1874, Minssen introduced the term "mixed tumour", and in the same year Billroth reported a tumor type, which he called cylindroma; this term is still commonly used as a synonym for adenoid cystic carcinoma. In 1910, Albrecht and Arzt described the papillary cystadenoma lymphomatosum—nowadays called Whartin's tumor. Up until the mid-1940s, classifications of salivary gland tumors were based on these definitions, but many tumor types were diffusely defined and served as a collection bin for rarer tumors with uncertain histological features, e.g., frequently no difference was made between adenoma, cylindroma, and mixed tumor. Histological definition and corresponding clinical behavior remained ill-defined.

During the 1940s, an increase in surgery of parotid tumors followed improvements in surgical technique related to better knowledge of the facial nerve anatomy. This event went hand in hand with increasingly centralized tumor therapy so that larger operative series could be analyzed and specific histological structures were classified as separate tumor types. Especially in the United States during the years 1945–54, several tumor types were differentiated from earlier diffuse conceptions, and on this basis, Frank Foote and Edgar Frazell of Memorial Sloan-Kettering Cancer Center in New York presented the first solid classification of parotid tumors that was more differentiated than any previous one. Up until Dr Eneroth's work preceding his 1971 study, this classification had not become widely adopted outside the USA. It had not been possible to verify its clinical value because studied series were too small, too heterogeneously treated, or insufficiently analyzed. Several of the tumor types in Foote and

Frazell's classification, such as mucoepidermoid carcinoma and acinic cell carcinoma, remained assigned to various collective groups of tumors, or if they were considered independent, the concept of "semi-malignancy" still persisted.

Eneroth set out to eliminate this state of confusion. His goal was to definitively assign benign or malignant properties to the histologically well-delimited types of tumor in the proposed classification by Foote and Frazell, looking at the respective clinical behavior and long-term outcome of the specific tumor types. To that purpose he had at his disposal the patient series at Karolinska Sjukhuset and Radiumhemmet in Stockholm, where since 1909 the treatment of tumors—and thus also salivary gland tumors—in Sweden had been largely concentrated. As a result, an unprecedentedly large patient cohort had been registered and treated. Follow-up examinations of patients operated on for parotid tumors had been made at intervals of 3, 6, or 12 months for the rest of their lives. Sweden, being a small country with a relatively stationary population, only a few patients—less than 1%—had been lost to follow-up. A histological re-examination of all the material was possible since the whole paraffin-embedded material was preserved. Eneroth investigated the prognosis of the salivary gland tumors by studies of the rate of local recurrence, metastasis, mortality and determinate survival rate, the latter excluding indeterminate patients, i.e. the few lost to follow-up and those who died without signs of the tumor disease.

With the 1971 publication, CM Eneroth published the then largest single-center experience of this rare disease (2,867 patients treated in the Karolinska Sjukhuset and Radiumhemmet—Stockholm, 1919-1969). Eneroth recognized the importance of a population-based registry (two hospitals draining all salivary tumors in the south of Sweden), a long-term follow-up, and the importance of histological reclassification reflecting the high degree of pathological expertise needed to make an accurate typing and grading of tumors in this complicated area. This point has frequently been re-stressed and confirmed later. He also highlighted the at that time common mistake of mixing up squamous cell carcinoma of the palate and palatal minor salivary gland carcinoma; only 46% remained as true minor salivary gland tumors after his reclassification. The clinical parallelism that led to this confusion is still reflected in the application of the UICC/AJCC 'T' classification for oral SCC to MSGT of the oral cavity later on. His comments and observations further substantiated the move towards considering acinic cell en mucoepidermoid neoplasms as true malignant tumors. In the World Health Organization International Histological Classification of Tumours of 1972 (where Dr Eneroth was the representative of one of the main contributing centers), the definition was still "acinic cell tumour", and the proposition was only to use the term carcinoma if the tumor "happened to metastasize". In the same way the original term published by Thackray and Sobin in 1972 was "mucoepidermoid tumor", but based on the observations of Eneroth, these neoplasms would be called carcinoma later on. Eneroth divided the mucoepidermoid carcinoma group further into a highly differentiated (low grade) and poorly differentiated (high grade) subgroup as is still the most frequent subdivision used in many studies. Based on his long-term clinical behavior observations, he proposed the low-grade malignant variant of mucoepidermoid carcinoma and acinic cell carcinoma as the low-grade reference group for all salivary gland carcinomas.

The 1971 publication put forward many other observations that still today guide our clinical approach to a patient with a salivary gland lump. The notion "the smaller the gland the higher the malignancy rate" resulted from this series, where Eneroth noted that in the parotid gland, 1 of 6 tumors was malignant, in the submandibular gland 1 of 3 tumors was malignant, and half of the palate tumors were malignant. He gave the population-based estimate of about 4/5 tumors in the parotid (77%) and 1/2 tumors in the submandibular and minor salivary glands being pleomorphic adenomas, an observation that still today helps our clinical decision making ("rule of eighties" for parotid tumors). He suggested based on findings of univariate analysis, in an era when multivariate analysis was not widely used, that there was an effect of site on prognosis, patients with palatal tumors having a better disease-specific survival than patients having tumors at other sites. Eneroth explained this by correlating "duration of symptoms" to prognosis, the palatal tumors being the quickest to be noticed, thus having the best prognosis. Later, other authors using multivariate analysis identified this finding as "stage bias", with higher stage at presentation resulting in more difficult resection and worse prognosis. Stage at presentation differs among the sites, but corrected for stage, no more differences according to site could be retained. Important and very recognizable by clinicians today are the descriptions of different histological types preferably occurring in different sites: the observation that papillary adenolymphoma (Warthin), oncocytoma and acinic cell carcinoma occur almost exclusively in parotid, the observation that adenoid cystic carcinoma is the most frequent malignancy in submandibular and minor salivary gland tumors, and relating those findings to gland-specific differences is "normal histology".

Within the large mixed tumor group, Eneroth also delineated, on the basis of encapsulation, two distinct subgroups. About 98% are benign tumors, and about 2% are malignant tumors with infiltrative destructive growth (carcinoma ex pleomorphic adenoma). Before Eneroth's work, many pleomorphic adenoma features, such as high cellularity, predominance of epithelial component, cylindromatous structures and incomplete encapsulation, led to the use of the term "semi-malignancy" (in his own series about 50% of pleomorphic adenomas had been previously denoted semi-malignant on the basis of these criteria), which implied lifelong follow-up. Eneroth showed that 98% of these tumors could be uniformly considered benign, and lifelong follow-up as had been routinely performed, could be abandoned for these patients—this is still the basis of our current practice. His clinico-pathologic studies showed that Warthin's tumors are uniformly benign and that the notion of "recurrent Warthin's tumor" had to be ascribed to the multifocality and bilaterality of this tumor. His observation of adenoid cystic carcinoma disease-specific survival dropping from 73% at 5 years to 13% at 20 years is still the basis of our strong belief in the need of long-term follow-up of these patients.

It can be concluded that the work by CM Eneroth really brought substantial light to this previously dark area of head and neck oncology, and the evidence resulting from his huge efforts is still widely present in our current approach to patients with this disease.

SALIVARY NEOPLASMS: OVERVIEW OF A 35-YEAR EXPERIENCE WITH 2,807 PATIENTS

Ronald H Spiro

We have reviewed a 35-year experience with 2,807 patients treated for salivary tumors which arose in the parotid gland (1,695 patients; 70%), submandibular gland (235 patients; 8%), and seromucinous glands of the upper aerodigestive tract (607 patients; 22%). Pleomorphic adenomas comprised 45% of the total, most of which occurred in the parotid gland. The clinical findings and the distribution of patients according to the histology and the site of origin are summarized. Treatment was surgical and the resection was conservative when possible, depending upon the extent of the tumor. The impact of site, histology, grade, and tumor stage on the results is shown.

Spiro RH. Salivary neoplasms: overview of a 35-year experience with 2,807 patients. Head Neck Surg.1986;8:177-184.

Commentary by: *David W Eisele*

Neoplasms of the salivary glands represent a diverse group of uncommon benign and malignant tumors. Their management is a challenge due to their relative infrequency, their varied clinical behaviors, and their propensity to recur. The head and neck surgeon must understand the behavior of each tumor type in order to develop an appropriate treatment plan for a given patient.

In this publication, Dr Ronald Spiro reported a 35-year (1939–1973) experience of the Memorial Sloan-Kettering Head and Neck Service with a large series of patients with salivary gland neoplasms who had surgical treatment at their institution with at least a 10-year follow-up. Prior to this period of time, the management of salivary gland neoplasms lacked uniformity and included observation and primary radiation therapy. With more refined techniques of head and neck surgery, however, surgeons at Memorial Hospital and other major centers became leaders in the surgical management of salivary gland tumors. This report describes a surgical management approach in which the extent of surgery is tailored to the extent of tumor, and for parotid neoplasms, the facial nerve is preserved unless involved by the tumor. Neck dissections were usually done only for clinically apparent nodal metastases. This approach has stood the test of time and comports with contemporary treatment guidelines.

This report provides important information regarding the distribution of tumors for each type of gland, in particular, the proportion of malignant tumors that involve the parotid gland compared to the submandibular gland and the minor salivary glands, as well as the predominant tumor types for each gland. In addition, the presenting signs and symptoms are reported for benign and malignant tumors. The importance of clinical suspicion of a salivary gland neoplasm for any patient with a parotid or submandibular swelling or with a submucosal mass in the oral cavity or pharynx is emphasized.

Due to the relatively large numbers of cases and long follow-up period, this report provides important clinical outcome information regarding definitive surgery, as adjuvant radiation therapy was not yet routinely administered to patients with select malignant neoplasms. Significant survival differences are noted for low-grade malignant tumors, such as acinic cell carcinoma and mucoepidermoid carcinoma, compared to the high-grade neoplasms. Other prognostic factors are delineated and demonstrate the impact of tumor location and clinical stage on prognosis. Recommendations regarding adjuvant radiation therapy for select patients with adverse prognostic factors are described. The benefit of this adjuvant therapy would be the topic of subsequent reports from this institution.

In summary, this is a seminal report on a large group of patients with a diverse group of salivary gland tumors, in terms of location and type, managed surgically and with adequate follow-up. This article contributed significantly to our understanding of the behavior of and management principles for these neoplasms.

MALIGNANT TUMORS OF MAJOR SALIVARY GLAND ORIGIN
A Matched-Pair Analysis of the Role of Combined Surgery and Postoperative Radiotherapy

John G Armstrong, Louis B Harrison, Ronald H Spiro, et al.

Between 1966 and 1982, 46 patients with previously untreated malignant tumors of major salivary gland origin received combined surgery and postoperative radiotherapy. They were compared with 46 patients treated with surgery only between 1939 and 1965, who were matched according to prognostic criteria. Radiation doses ranged from 4,000 to 7,740 cGy (median, 5,664 cGy). The 5-year determinate survival rates for patients given combined therapy with stage I and II disease vs patients given surgery only was 81.9% vs 95.8%, while for stages III and IV it was 51.2% vs 9.5%, respectively. Local control for stage III and disease in patients given combined therapy vs patients given surgery only at 5 years was 51.3% vs 16.8%. For patients with nodal metastases, 5-year determinate survival for the combined-therapy group vs the surgery-only group was 48.9% vs 18.7%, and the corresponding local-regional control was 69.1% vs 40.2%. The results of this analysis suggest that postoperative radiotherapy significantly improves outcome for patients with stage III and IV disease and for patients with lymph node metastases.

Armstrong JG, Harrison LB, Spiro RH, et al. Malignant tumors of major salivary gland origin. A matched-pair analysis of the role of combined surgery and postoperative radiotherapy. Arch Otolaryngol Head Neck Surg. 1990;116:290-293.

Commentary by: *Jatin P Shah*

In the past, radiotherapy in general was felt to be ineffective in controlling tumors of salivary gland origin. However, radiotherapy had been employed on an empirical basis in patients undergoing surgery as adjuvant postoperative radiotherapy, particularly in patients who presented with advanced stage disease, cervical lymph node metastasis, or in whom ominous pathological features of the primary tumor were identified.

Although no randomized trial of adjuvant radiotherapy had been published in the past, Dr Armstrong and his colleagues attempted to define the role of adjuvant postoperative radiotherapy using the technique of matched pair analysis from historical controls to patients receiving postoperative radiotherapy. Their study included 155 patients with previously untreated major salivary gland tumors treated at Memorial Sloan-Kettering Cancer Center between 1966 and 1982. From this group, 46 patients were treated with combined surgery and postoperative radiotherapy. Matched pair controls were selected from a group of 319 patients treated between 1939 and 1965 at the same institution. A computerized search system was employed with the same prognostic factors as the patients receiving combined therapy to identify the matched controls. The median follow-up time for survivors was 5.8 years in the combined therapy group and 10.5 years in the control group. The 5-year survival rate was 68.9% in the combined therapy group compared to 55% in the control group. Similarly, local control was obtained in 73.4% of the combined therapy group vs 66.2% in the control group. The 5-year survival rate in patients with stage III and stage IV disease receiving combined therapy was 51% compared to 10% in the control group. Similarly, local control in the combined therapy group with stage III and stage IV disease was 51% vs 17% in the control group. On the other hand, the 5-year survival rate in patients with stage I and stage II disease was 82% for the combined therapy group vs 96% for the control group, a statistically insignificant difference. Similarly, local control in patients with stage I and stage II disease was 91% in the combined group vs 79% in the control group, again a statistically insignificant difference. On the other hand, patients with cervical lymph node metastases showed a significant positive impact of the combined therapy with a 49% 5-year survival rate compared to 19% in the control group.

This was the first such study comparing the value of adjunctive postoperative radiotherapy in patients with salivary gland cancer. This study clearly demonstrated the value of adjunctive postoperative radiation therapy in patients with stage III and stage IV disease with improved local control and 5-year survival. Similarly, it showed significant improvement in survival and regional control in patients with cervical lymph node metastases. The study also showed that there was little benefit of postoperative radiotherapy in stage I and II disease. The observations of this study clearly shifted paradigms in including radiotherapy as an integral component of the overall multidisciplinary treatment program for patients with advanced salivary gland cancers.

Chapter 14

Soft Tissue Tumors

HEAD AND NECK SOFT TISSUE SARCOMAS: A MULTIVARIATE ANALYSIS OF OUTCOMES

Brandon G Bentz, Bhuvanesh Singh, James Woodruff, et al.

Background: Soft tissue sarcomas of the head and neck represent a rare group of tumors of which a limited number of published individual- and institution-based experiences exist.

Methods: We performed an analysis of head and neck sarcoma patients identified from our institution between 1973 and 1999. Exclusion criteria included pediatric rhabdomyosarcomas, sarcomas of the neuromeningeal axis or non head and neck primary disease sites, and bone sarcomas. All cases underwent pathologic re-review before statistical analysis.

Results: After pathologic review, III head and neck sarcoma patients remained (mean age, 47 ± 20 years). The median duration of follow-up was 51 months; the actuarial 5-year relapse-free, disease-specific, and overall survivals were 55%, 52%, and 44%, respectively. Forty-six percent remained free of recurrence at the most recent follow-up, and the most common site of recurrence was local followed by distant sites. By multivariate analysis, size and grade significantly influenced relapse-free, disease-specific, and overall survivals, whereas margin status additionally influenced relapse-free survival. Subset analysis of the fibrosarcoma malignant fibrous histiocytoma and desmoid dermatofibrosarcoma protuberans histologies was undertaken.

Conclusions: Size > 5 cm and high-grade histology are considered poor prognostic indicators. Patients with either of these characteristics should be considered for adjuvant trials.

Bentz BG, Singh B, Woodruff J, et al. Head and neck soft tissue sarcomas: a multivariate analysis of outcomes. Ann Surg Oncol. 2004;11:619-628.

Commentary by: *Murray F Brennan*

Soft tissue sarcomas are unusual and uncommon lesions. In the Memorial Sloan-Kettering database of over 9,000 cases, less than 5% occurred in the head and neck. Given the complex histology with an excess of 50 different subtypes described, this makes comments on natural history, treatment, and outcome in the head and neck a difficult task. Wide variation in site within the head and neck adds further complexity, as does the fact that almost all histopathological subtypes are represented. The manuscript by Dr Bentz and colleagues was our first attempt to describe outcome for such lesions.

It is important to emphasize that this manuscript covers the period from 1973 to 1999. Despite this, the present study provides considerable information not available elsewhere. The most recent manuscripts are case reports or small institutional series.

Despite the rarity of the lesions in the head and neck, some inferences as to management can be developed based on the behavior of sarcomas in other sites. As with other sites, size and high-grade histology are poor prognostic indicators for local recurrence, disease-specific and overall survival. Margin positivity, as in other sites, is a factor in local recurrence but does not necessarily translate into disease-specific survival. It is always challenging to utilize percentage outcomes in relatively small subsets of patients. Nevertheless, in the manuscript described by Bentz et al. 111 patients were reviewed with a significant median follow-up of 51 months. As with other sites, death from disease was commonly associated with the development of metastatic disease. This was not seen in those subtypes, such as dermatofibrosarcoma protuberans and the desmoid tumor when metastatic disease is rare or non-existent, but advanced local disease can be associated with disease-specific survival as is seen in the retroperitoneum.

Utilization of nomograms, predictive tools for outcome, demonstrates the wide variation in potential outcome. For example, a 60-year-old male with a high grade 5–10 cm fibrosarcoma in the head and neck would be expected to have a 4-year mortality rate from sarcoma of 31%, whereas if that lesion occurred in the extremity, disease-specific death would be less than 15%. In similar fashion, if we examine malignant peripheral nerve sheath tumor (MPNST), a 60-year-old male with a high grade lesion 5–10 cm in size would have an 86% chance of dying of MPNST at 4 years, in comparison to 50% if that lesion occurred in the extremity.

An important issue for head and neck is the rare involvement of lymph nodes by sarcoma, with less than 3% of all sarcomas appearing in lymph nodes. This is an important observation, as with epithelial tumors of the head and neck, the majority will undergo lymph node dissection. Failure to understand the absence of lymph node metastasis in these lesions can result in significant unnecessary surgery or unnecessarily expanded radiation fields.

Despite the recommendations of the authors in 1999 for high-risk lesions (i.e. high grade, > 5 cm) to enter adjuvant systemic trials, such trials have been rare and with very limited proven success.

Chapter 15

Neurogenic Tumors and Paragangliomas

CAROTID BODY TUMOR (CHEMODECTOMA)
Clinicopathologic Analysis of Ninety Cases

William R Shamblin, William H ReMine, Sheldon G Sheps, et al.

The first excision of a carotid body tumor was performed by Riegner in 1880; the patient did not survive. In 1886, Maydl removed a carotid tumor; his patient survived but had hemiplegia and aphasia. In 1889, Albert first successfully excised a carotid body tumor without ligating the carotid vessels. The first successful removal of a carotid body tumor in the United States was reported by Scudder in 1903. Subsequently, more than 500 carotid body tumors have been reported in the literature.

Shamblin WR, ReMine WH, Sheps SG, et al. Carotid body tumor (chemodectoma). Clinicopathologic analysis of ninety cases. Am J Surg. 1971;122:732-739.

Commentary by: *Kerry D Olsen*

The paper on *Carotid Body Tumor (Chemodectoma): Clinical and Pathologic Analysis of 90 Cases* by Drs Shamblin, ReMine, Sheps, and Harrison was reported in the *American Journal of Surgery* in 1971. This paper demonstrates the Mayo Clinic approach to analyzing problems: utilizing the talents of a team of physicians, in this case, surgeons, an endocrinologist, and a pathologist. When the authors' paper was published, there was confusion regarding the behavior and treatment of carotid body tumors. The tumors were frequently misdiagnosed, and there was significant morbidity and mortality from surgical excision.

The article remains pertinent today as an excellent review of the anatomy of the carotid body, the physiology of chemodectomas, the microscopic appearance of these lesions, and the location of chemodectomas in the head and neck area. It also clarifies the terminology of chemodectoma, paraganglioma, and carotid body tumors.

Only 500 cases had been reported in the literature when the authors added the largest series of almost 100 cases. This gave new information as to the tumor's behavior, which has since shaped the treatment of this tumor. The authors showed that these tumors present at all ages, from 12 to 63, are more common in males, and generally present as an asymptomatic neck mass. They rarely are pulsatile and usually do not extend toward the hypopharynx or parapharynx. The authors did not know of the genetic predisposition of this tumor, but they did note that bilaterality was uncommon, and when it did occur, metachronous lesions were more common than synchronous ones.

These tumors were frequently misdiagnosed. An accurate preoperative diagnosis based on exam alone was very difficult. Their report showed the value of angiography in avoiding misdiagnosis. The authors report some of the earliest findings regarding the angiographic characteristics of these tumors. The tumors are highly vascular, have their blood supply from the external carotid artery, the arterial lumen of the carotid vessels does not appear to be compromised by even very large tumors; and they showed the classic lyra image of the internal and external carotid arteries displayed by a mass at the bifurcation of these vessels.

The authors sought to answer several questions important in understanding the behavior of these tumors. Their answers are still valuable today. The first question asked was, "Are these tumors benign or malignant?" At the time of this paper, it was felt that a large number of these tumors were malignant and, therefore, warranted an aggressive surgical approach. The authors concluded that malignancy is actually very rare. It occurs approximately 2% of the time. It is very difficult to determine malignancy by histologic appearance alone. They noted that one must find regional or distant metastasis to denote malignancy. It is first important to rule out synchronous or metachronous chemodectomas that occur in other locations as the microscopic appearance of metastases is similar to a benign lesion.

The second question asked was, "Do these tumors have endocrinologic function, i.e., are they secreting neoplasms?" They studied a subset of these tumors and concluded that none of these had secretory activity. Secretory activity from a carotid body tumor is very rare and corroborates our current understanding of these tumors.

They also wanted to know, "What is the history of untreated tumors?" The authors found that the duration of tumors prior to any treatment averaged 6 years. Some had a mass present for up to 47 years. They concluded that these tumors are slow-growing lesions and that death was rarely due to the neoplasm or metastasis. Even if large, the tumors did not compromise cerebral blood flow. Morbidity and mortality were generally due to iatrogenic injury to nerves and vessels and compromised cerebral blood flow. In many cases, they therefore recommended no treatment, as the risks of treatment did not outweigh the alternative of observation.

Another question asked was, "What therapy is beneficial?" Their patient series focused on surgical removal. They recommended a classification system based on operative risk that is still helpful today. Group 1 patients had tumors that were adjacent to the carotid vessels, in a classic location, and were at low risk for surgical injury. Group 2 patients had tumors that partially surrounded the carotid vessels, were much more adherent to the advential tissue, and had moderate surgical risk. And, finally, Group 3 patients had tumors that circumferentially involved the carotid bulb and bifurcation and were at high risk for vessel injury. They showed it could be impossible in these latter cases to separate the tumor from the vessel without getting into the lumen of the carotid artery.

They emphasized that any surgeon performing an operation on a carotid body tumor must have vascular surgical skills or work with a vascular surgeon. This approach would optimize safety of removal and reduce morbidity for the patient. Indeed, in an ideal situation, a head and neck surgeon today would work with a vascular surgeon. This team approach would lead to the greatest chance of avoiding nerve injury and optimizing care of the vessels.

The authors' final question was, "What is the treatment of choice?" They point out that no treatment may be best for some patients. This is clearly true today. They did not recommend surgical treatment for individuals with prior partial resection or for Group 3 tumors. In these cases, they felt the risks were too great. The tumor's slow growth and the advanced age of some patients warranted no treatment in many cases. They realized that patients did not die of these tumors—they died from surgery. They did show that if complete removal of the tumor is done, they will not recur. They also emphasized the importance of maintaining cerebral circulation with shunts or grafts, if necessary during excision. The role of radiation therapy was mentioned in cases in which one would not operate, but overall it was not recommended. They did not have availability of CT and MR scans or the use of embolization. The authors did, however, identify the need for a study that would tell them which patients could tolerate interruption of blood flow through the internal carotid artery. This led to our current balloon occlusion studies.

In summary, this paper provides important information about the behavior and approach to these tumors. It is clearly a landmark article. No one dies from a carotid body tumor. They die of iatrogenic causes, i.e. generally from surgery. The authors' impressions are still valid today. They recommended an individualized approach and, in some cases, observation. Surgical removal in the remaining patients can be safe and effective.

TRENDS IN NEUROVASCULAR COMPLICATIONS OF SURGICAL MANAGEMENT FOR CAROTID BODY AND CERVICAL PARAGANGLIOMAS: A FIFTY-YEAR EXPERIENCE WITH 153 TUMORS

John W Hallett, John D Nora, Larry H Hollier, et al.

Almost 75% of carotid body and cervical paragangliomas are adherent to or surround adjacent arteries and cranial nerves. Their resection can result in neurovascular injury, stroke, and excessive blood loss. To assess trends in neurovascular compli-cations, we reviewed 153 carotid body and cervical paragangliomas that were surgically managed between 1935 and 1985. Results of the past 10 years were comp-ared with two previous time periods: period I (1935 to 1965), when carotid artery reconstruction was uncommon at our institution, and period II (1966 to 1975), when methods of intraoperative electroencephalographic monitoring and carotid patch angioplasty were being developed. During the past 10 years (period III), surgical approach to these tumors has included intraoperative monitoring of cerebral blood flow, selective use of shunts, vein patch or graft reconstructions after extensive tumor resections, and mobilization of the parotid gland to facilitate adequate exposure of high tumors. Although tumor resection was attempted in 80% of patients in period I, surgical resection was complete in 98% during periods II and III. Three trends were observed: (1) The perioperative stroke rate has decreased dramatically from 23% in period I to 2.7% in period III (p = 0.007); (2) the perioperative mortality rate has been reduced from 6% in period I to no deaths in the past 10 years, but (3) the rate of postoperative cranial nerve dysfunction remains unchanged over 50 years (period I, 46%; period III, 40%). The median tumor size among patients with postoperative complications was significantly larger than those without complications (median size: 17 vs 7 cm³, p = 0.004). Forty-eight percent of cranial nerve problems were permanent. Our experience clearly demonstrates that nearly all carotid body and cervical chemodectomas can be completely resected with minimal risk of stroke or death. Future refinement of surgical technique for these difficult tumors must focus on methods to minimize cranial nerve dysfunction.

Hallett JW Jr, Nora JD, Hollier LH, et al. Trends in neurovascular complications of surgical management for carotid body and cervical paragangliomas: a fifty-year experience with 153 tumors. J Vasc Surg. 1988;7:284-291.

Commentary by: *John P Leonetti*

This 50-year review spanning the years 1935 to 1985 described the Mayo Clinic experience in the surgical management of 153 carotid body tumors or cervical paragangliomas treated at that institution. The patients were separated into three groups according to the time period in which the procedures were performed, with period one including the years 1935 to 1965, period two including the years 1966–1975, and period three including the years 1978 and 1985. The authors clearly state that in period one the tumor removal included carotid artery resection only, while in period two, intraoperative electroencephalography and carotid wall patch angioplasty were added. The period three patients underwent surgical resection with the addition of intraoperative cerebral blood flow monitoring, carotid artery shunting, carotid wall vein patching, or carotid resection with grafting, along with improved superior identification and protection of the internal carotid artery through the use of parotid gland mobilization.

The advantages of these newer techniques, which were developed and incorporated in the more recent time periods reviewed, are impressive and time tested. To begin, complete tumor resection was only attempted in 80% of those patients in group one; whereas complete tumor resection was achieved in all patients in groups two and three. Secondly, the stroke rate was significantly reduced from 23% in group one to only 2.2% in group three. More importantly, the overall mortality rate was reduced from 6% in group one to 0% in group three. The authors state that while the degree of tumor resections, stroke rate, and death were significantly reduced over time, the incidence and risk of lower cranial nerve deficits remained relatively unchanged, with group one patients experiencing these complications in 46% of the patients, and those in group three were noted to have lower cranial nerve deficits in 40% of the patients. In addition, 48% of these lower cranial nerve injuries were permanent. The authors concluded that carotid body tumor and cervical paraganglioma resection could be safely performed, and tumor resection could be complete as of 1985, but made the insightful recommendation that future efforts be made to reduce the risk and debilitating complications associated with lower cranial nerve deficits.

The number of patients reviewed in this series, as well as the impressive time span reviewed alone, make this a landmark publication. The advances in surgical technique are still utilized today to perform the complete and safe resection of these tumors. Improved preoperative imaging through the use of magnetic resonance angiography, intraoperative lower cranial never monitoring, and improved microscopic dissection have all contributed to the reduction in postoperative lower cranial nerve injury and the associated devastating postoperative complications with respect to speech, swallowing, and airway protection. As we surgeon-physicians strive to improve the methods for the safe and complete resection of these difficult tumors, we must refer to this landmark publication, which highlights improved exposure of the ICA above the tumor, maintenance of cerebral blood flow through shunting techniques, meticulous carotid patching or interposition grafting, and physiologic (not just anatomic) preservation of lower cranial nerves IX–XII.

Like most historical and well-respected contributions in our surgical literature, this manuscript should be studied as a foundation for future improvements in the management of patients with carotid body tumors and other cervical paragangliomas.

TUMORS AND SURGERY OF THE PARAPHARYNGEAL SPACE

Kerry D Olsen

The parapharyngeal space, an area of complex anatomic relationships, is involved in a wide variety of benign and malignant neoplasms. Because primary parapharyngeal space tumors are rare, it is difficult to obtain surgical experience in this region. This paper reviews the anatomy, presentation, evaluation, surgical approaches, and pathologic features and complications reported in managing patients with parapharyngeal space neoplasms.

Two surgical procedures have been used by the author to treat 44 tumors in the parapharyngeal space. The cervical-parotid approach was used in 35 patients, and the cervical-parotid approach with midline mandibulotomy was used in 9 patients. of the 44 tumors, 32 were benign lesions and 12 were malignant neoplasms. Forty tumors were primary parapharyngeal space tumors, and 4 cases represented isolated metastases to parapharyngeal nodes. Recurrent tumors accounted for 12 of the 44 cases. Discussion of the indications, surgical technique, and select points pertinent to using these two operative procedures is based on the operative experience gained from these 44 patients. The use of these two operations resulted in low morbidity and provided a safe, efficacious approach to the management of all parapharyngeal space neoplasms encountered.

Olsen KD. Tumors and surgery of the parapharyngeal space. Laryngoscope. 1994;104:1-28.

Commentary by: *Patrick J Gullane*

This paper from the Mayo Clinic, which was the candidate's thesis for his admission to the Triological Society, provides the most detailed overview of this highly complex space located bilaterally in the upper neck that contains numerous vital neurovascular structures. The author, Dr Kerry Olsen, is to be commended for the most complete and detailed review of this space currently published in the English literature, which has helped us to better understand the concepts of managing tumors that arise within or that invade this region.

Tumors involving this location are extremely rare, comprising less than 1% of all head and neck neoplasms. In this paper, a thorough knowledge of the surgical anatomy of the parapharyngeal space is addressed, which is fundamental to understanding the routes of passage of lesions to and from the space, awareness of the clinical presentation of parapharyngeal space tumors, an understanding of the variety of histological types, and the selection and interpretation of radiological investigations that has resulted in a much better understanding for the surgeon planning the most appropriate surgical approach to this area.

The author provides insight and detail into the various fascial planes that permit the spread of tumor and the differential diagnosis of the complexity of the contents, in addition to his recognition that 50% of the tumors in this location are of salivary gland origin and 20% neurogenic. His description of the investigational techniques, which have been replaced in a modern era with less invasive diagnostic tools, helped to minimize the complications associated with prior investigational techniques.

One cannot overstate the importance of this paper in the understanding of this space and the concepts around the surgical approaches previously described but not well understood.

The author's personal experience in the treatment of 44 tumors involving this space, which included the two standard approaches he advocates, i.e., cervical-parotid approach and cervical-parotid approach with midline mandibulotomy, has resulted in a dramatic reduction in the morbidity associated with surgery to this region. His work and experience has relegated the midline mandibulotomy approach to the resection of < 15% of tumors that involve this space. Those that require a mandibulotomy are mainly vascular neoplasms, malignant tumors, or those that have involved or invaded the skull base.

Olsen's thoughtful overview, detailed description of this challenging space, and the development of an algorithm for management of the neoplasms within this location has been transformative, and as a result, has enhanced the outcome and reduced the complications of patients undergoing surgery to the parapharyngeal space.

NORMAL LIFE EXPECTANCY FOR PARAGANGLIOMA
PATIENTS: A 50-YEAR-OLD COHORT REVISITED

Jeanette de Flines, Jeroen Jansen, Reinier Elders, et al.

The objective of this study was to assess the long-term survival of patients with a paraganglioma of the head and neck compared with the survival of the general Dutch population. This historic cohort study was conducted using nationwide historical data of paraganglioma patients. We retrieved a cohort of 86 patients diagnosed with a paraganglioma of the head and neck between 1945 and 1960 in the Netherlands. Dates of death were retrieved from the national bureau of genealogy. Survival after diagnosis was compared with age and sex adjusted survival in the general population, by means of Wilcoxon signed rank test and Kaplan-Meier actuarial survival curves. Although surgery had more complications in the studied era than today and the death of five patients with carotid body tumors caused immediate excess mortality, the survival of the followed cohort was not significantly reduced if compared with the general population. Paragangliomas of the head and neck do not reduce life expectancy.

de Flines J, Jansen J, Elders R, et al. Normal life expectancy for paraganglioma patients: a 50-year-old cohort revisited. Skull Base. 2011;6:385-388.

Commentary by: *Ian Ganly*

Paragangliomas arise from the paraganglia of the autonomic nervous system. In the head and neck, they most commonly occur in the carotid body (carotid body tumors) but also occur along the vagal nerve (glomus vagale) and temporal bone (glomus jugulare and glomus tympanicum tumors). They are slow growing and produce symptoms from cranial nerve involvement either from compression or infiltration. Options of treatment include surgical resection, radiation or observation, depending on patient and tumor-related factors. In general, elderly patients are treated with observation as these tumors typically grow very slowly at only 1 mm per year. However, in younger patients, treatment options are more involved due to the possible neurological sequelae, which can occur as complications of surgery. Some argue it is best to treat early either with surgery or radiation in the hope of preventing cranial nerve paralysis from tumor involvement. However, others argue for observation since any neurological loss of function is most likely to be of gradual onset, allowing compensatory mechanisms to develop. As such, patients who get paralysis may in fact have no symptoms at all due to this gradual onset of paralysis. This is an argument against surgical treatment. In addition, surgery may result in an acute paralysis of cranial nerves, particularly of cranial nerves 9–12. Acute paralysis of the vagus nerve will result in dysphagia, dysphonia and aspiration, which may necessitate vocal cord medialization procedures, nasogastric tube feeding, or insertion of a PEG in more long-term situations. Paralysis of cranial nerve 12 can result in ipsilateral paralysis of the tongue, again resulting in swallowing difficulties as well as speech impairment. Because of these neurological sequelae, surgical treatment of glomus vagale and glomus jugulare tumors has fallen out of favor due to the inevitable vagal nerve dysfunction produced. However, surgery is still the favored option in the treatment of carotid body tumors.

The long-term survival outcome of these patients has never been reported. This is mainly due to the rarity of these tumors, with few institutions having a large volume of such patients. However, it is also due to a lack of any reliable and prolonged follow-up information on these patients. The present study by de Flines is unique in that it reports the 50-year follow-up of a cohort of 86 patients from the Netherlands diagnosed from 1945–1960 with paragangliomas of the head and neck. In this study, patients were age and gender matched, stratified by year of birth using an online database of the Dutch Central Bureau of Statistics. Comparative analysis of survival was carried out using the Wilcoxon rank sum test. From their analysis, the authors report that there was no decreased life expectancy of patients with head and neck paragangliomas compared with the general population. This is the first ever report showing this type of information. However, the authors do report that quality of life can be reduced in these patients due to cranial nerve palsies of cranial nerves 7, 8, 9, 10, 11 and 12, as well as cerebrovascular injury during surgery. The authors conclude that the focus of management of paragangliomas should no longer be on cure of disease but rather quality of life.

This paper is significant because previously there had been great enthusiasm for the surgical resection of these tumors. With the knowledge that treatment does not impact survival such enthusiasm has now been dampened with the realization that surgery can inflict considerable morbidity with no apparent gain in outcome. Since the publication of this paper, many surgeons who previously carried out surgery for paragangliomas think more carefully about the benefits of surgical intervention balanced against the neurological risks as well as potential vascular risks with associated mortality. As such, there has been a change in paradigm of treatment. It is now much more common for patients with paragangliomas to be offered observation rather than surgery, thus avoiding the neurological and vascular morbidity of surgery.

Chapter 16

Reconstructive Surgery

A TWO-STAGE METHOD FOR PHARYNGOESOPHAGEAL RECONSTRUCTION WITH A PRIMARY PECTORAL SKIN FLAP

Vahram Y Bakamjian

Reconstruction of the pharynx and cervical esophagus following total laryngo-pharyngectomy for advanced cancer can be achieved more dependably with pedicled skin flaps than with free skin grafts. Methods based on Esser's principle of inlay grafting, such as those described by Negus, Edgerton, and Conley, using split-thickness skin dressed over a tubular or conical stent of one kind or another, have the merits of simplicity and immediate re-establishment of pharyngoesophageal continuity. With the natural tendency for considerable contracture to occur in split-thickness grafts, however, and the inordinately high incidence of poor "takes" in a critically mobile and contaminated region such as the pharynx, the goals of a primary, single-stage reconstruction are frequently defeated by the development of fistulas, severe strictures and occasionally a fulminating infection underneath the neck flaps.

Bakamjian VY. A two-stage method for pharyngoesophageal reconstruction with a primary pectoral skin flap. Plast Reconstr Surg.1965;36:173-184.

Commentary by: *Stephan Ariyan*

This landmark paper, published virtually a half century ago, reported some fundamental changes in concepts of reconstruction, which in turn led to significant research explaining the circulation of flaps, and ultimately the discovery and implementation of musculocutaneous, fasciocutaneous, and vascularized free flaps.

At the time shortly prior to the publication of this paper, MT Edgerton and others had proposed immediate reconstructions following resections of cancers of the head and neck region. This was contrary to the prevailing thought of waiting 2 or more years to make certain that there was no recurrence of the tumor before reconstructing the patient. Edgerton and others argued that it was incumbent upon surgeons to reconstruct the patients to bring them back to as normal a functional state and appearance as possible, and to do so as soon as possible. However, most of the techniques of reconstruction were either skin grafts or involved the use of tubed pedicled skin flaps that required several stages of surgical procedures for the completion of reconstruction.

Most notably, reconstructions following resection of the pharyngoeso-phageal region with skin grafts were often doomed to failure because of the high bacterial counts in the salivary flow overlying the constructed skin graft tubes. Furthermore, pharyngocutaneous fistulas were very common, and reliable flaps were in great need.

Bakamjian's paper illustrated 3 cases of reconstruction and reported on an additional 7 cases he had managed with a similar technique. In his paper, he named this flap the "pectoral skin flap", which was subsequently re-named the deltopectoral flap, and popularized by surgeons everywhere as the "Bakamjian flap" in honor of its inventor.

Interestingly, he noted in this paper that the first time he used this flap in a patient, he had based the flap laterally, on the deltoid area, elevating the skin obliquely across the chest over the pectoral region. However, he noted that in subsequent cases, he found it "...mechanically more convenient to base the flap medially over the perforating branches of the internal mammary vessels and to place its tip over the acromial or subacromial regions of the shoulder, depending on the availability of non-hairy skin in these areas".

He also pointed out that another advantage of basing it medially resulted in a tubed flap whose distal end was attached to the proximal end of the defect at the resected part of the oropharynx; this resulted in the opening of the reconstructed skin tube distally, allowing dependent drainage of salivary secretions down to the chest, below and away from the tracheostomy opening.

During the discussion portion of this paper, he pointed out that "...Many times...the need for such a flap, and definite specifications for it, become apparent more or less unexpectedly...." As such, there is no opportunity for delaying incisions to prepare a flap. And one of the distinct advantages of his reconstruction flap was that it required only one subsequent stage to complete the distal division and closure at 3–5 weeks after the initial operation. He went further in his discussion to point out that it "may seem foolhardy" to construct a flap of such length without prior delay. However, he pointed out that the success could be attributed to the location of the base of the flap overlying perforating branches of the internal mammary artery.

Within a few short years after the publication of this paper and the widespread recognition of the successful use of the deltopectoral flap, IA McGregor and IT Jackson studied this flap to determine why it survived to those lengths at all. They demonstrated that it was based on the very long intercostal perforating branches of the internal mammary vessels extending a long distance across the chest towards the deltoid region. They then introduced the concept differentiating between *random pattern* cutaneous flaps, which are nourished by communications of vessels in the dermal-subdermal plexus, and *axial pattern* cutaneous flaps, which are nourished by an anatomically recognized arterial and venous circulation following the long axis of this flap.

It was further noted that since there was a known axial blood supply along the undersurface of the length of the deltopectoral flap, the maximum viable length of the flap extended not only to the deltoid region but also over the surface of the deltoid muscle, which constituted the random portion extension of the distal end of the flap.

In fact, it was not long after the recognition of the axial circulation of this flap along the undersurface of the soft tissues, that one-stage recon-structions of the cheek and the floor of the mouth were performed by "de-epithelializing" that portion of the flap that ran along the undersurface of the neck skin. It was also found that flaps could be divided as early as 7–10 days. This flap continued for the next decade and a half to be the most important, reliable flap for head and neck reconstruction.

In the following two decades, further research identified various mus-culocutaneous flaps, osteocutaneous flaps, and microvascular free flaps that facilitated one-stage reconstructions of the head and neck region. Nevertheless, it is important to note that the observations of VY Bakamjian and his courage to use this flap to facilitate the healing of his patients, opened up new opportunities for research and the development of techniques of head and neck reconstruction that we use today.

SUPERIORITY OF THE DEEP CIRCUMFLEX ILIAC VESSELS AS THE SUPPLY FOR FREE GROIN FLAPS
Experimental Work

G Ian Taylor, Paul Townsend, Russell Corlett

The ability to transfer a free flap of groin skin and iliac bone to a distant site by microvascular techniques has considerable application to some of the difficult problems encountered in the repair of major jaw and leg defects. This paper traces the evolution of the free osteocutaneous groin flap from its initial design, based on the superficial circumflex iliac vessels, through its subsequent modification to use the deep circumflex iliac vessels as the pedicle.

Taylor GI, Townsend P, Corlett R. Superiority of the deep circumflex iliac vessels as the supply for free groin flaps: experimental work. Plast Reconstr Surg. 1979;64:595-604.

Commentary by: *Mark L Urken*

Although the earliest advances in microvascular surgery occurred prior to 1979 when this landmark article appeared in the literature, the importance of microvascular surgery in filling a genuine clinical need did not become widely accepted until Dr Taylor et al. introduced the deep circumflex iliac artery and vein as the major blood supply for use in the clinical transfer of the composite groin flap. The late 1970s and early 1980s represented the *perfect storm* in free flap surgery. Three major events occurred simultaneously:

1. The presence of a genuine clinical need in head and neck surgery for the long-standing clinical problem of deformity associated with segmental defects of the mandible leading to the Andy Gump deformity;
2. Technologic advances in the design of the microscope, the design of microsutures, the development of microsurgical instruments, and the introduction of endosteal implants for dental rehabilitation;
3. A rediscovery of the human body with respect to the vascular anatomy, leading surgeons to view the entire body as a potential source of vascularized tissue that could be transferred to the head and neck to reconstruct *postablative* defects that heretofore could not be restored.

In the 1960s and 1970s, the discipline of head and neck surgery was handicapped by the lack of available options to restore defects created by the removal of both benign and malignant tumors. Patients who underwent such deforming surgery were, more often than not, left with such severe functional and aesthetic challenges that they were forced to lead the rest of their lives as social recluses, unable to return to gainful employment or normal social interactions with friends and family. There was no clearer example of this than the patient who underwent a segmental resection of the mandible leading to the development of the aptly named *Andy Gump* deformity. Secondary reconstruction of the mandible was attempted using nonvascularized bone, but the unfavorable vascular bed created by radiation often led to failure. In addition, the exposure of nonvascularized bone to oral secretions led to infection and the spiraling downhill course that inevitably resulted in the removal of that bone. The recognition that primary reconstruction could only be accomplished with vascularized bone led to several creative attempts to transfer bone with its native blood supply left intact. Many options to solve this problem were attempted, such as the use of regional flaps to transfer segments of rib, sternum, and scapular spine. The limited vascular supply to the segment of transferred bone and the inability to contour that bone to simulate the shape of the missing mandible were insurmountable problems. The emergence of biocompatible hardware led to the use of bridging reconstruction plates to hold the remaining segments of the mandible in position. However, most of these options were fraught with complications and led to the common necessity to return to the operating room to manage those complications. Perhaps the most significant deficiency of these techniques, in addition to their lack of reliability, was the inability to restore functional dentition so that patients could return to normal mastication.

The decade of the 1970s and 1980s saw an explosion in technology that affected many aspects of head and neck reconstructive surgery. The advances in the microscope that were so important to otologic and neuro-surgical advances, along with the development of microsurgical instruments conducive to the performance of microvascular surgery, set the stage for the wide-scale emergence of the era of free tissue transfer that would revolutionize head and neck surgery and forever change the way we manage patients with head and neck and skull base tumors. Another very important technologic advance was the development of microsutures that could be mass-produced for the anastomosis of blood vessels that were as small in size as a millimeter in diameter. These technologic advances permitted free flaps to be transferred to the head and neck in experienced hands, with a rate of success that now approaches 99%. These confluent events led to the emerging recognition that microvascular techniques could be applied for transfer of tissue from distant sites in the body, no longer restricted by the arc of rotation of regional flaps. One of the final pieces in the puzzle to restore normal function following extensive ablative surgery of the oral cavity was the application of endosteal implants that could be placed directly into the transferred bone to serve as tooth root analogues that would permit anchorage of dental prostheses for functional dental rehabilitation.

The article by Ian Taylor and colleagues reflects the third major advance in microsurgery that involved the discovery of new donor sites that met the criteria for inclusion in the armamentarium of the head and neck micro-surgeon. There were three major criteria for a donor site to emerge as a valued site for head and neck reconstruction. First and foremost, that donor site had to have a composition of tissue that would fit the needs of the defect created in the head and neck. Secondly, it had to have a reliable vascular supply with vessels that were of adequate length and size for transfer to the head and neck. Thirdly, the removal of that flap from its native location in the body could not cause a secondary functional or aesthetic problem. In short, the flap had to be *expendable*. Skin is the most readily available organ in the body. However, the interruption of the skeletal structure in order to transfer bone requires that the remaining skeletal support will not be adversely affected. The iliac crest was the first of the three major donor sites for widespread use in reconstruction of the mandible. The other two donor sites, the scapula and fibula, would not emerge for several years following Taylor's landmark article that revolutionized the iliac crest donor site.

Prior to this article and the body of anatomic research that led up to it, the iliac crest flap was transferred on the superficial circumflex iliac artery and vein. Taylor et al. demonstrated the superiority of the deep circumflex iliac arterial and venous (DCIA/DCIV) vascular system in its supply of the iliac bone, the overlying skin and the internal oblique muscle. The reliability, diameter, and the length of this pedicle, clearly indicated the merits of these vessels. The rich vascularity of the bone was evident on cross sectional evaluation of the ilium, performed after dye injection studies, and set the stage for the use of the iliac composite flap for mandibular reconstruction. In addition, the authors described the anatomic variability of the perforators to the skin, as well as the limits of the cutaneous territory supplied by those perforators. This article also highlighted the anatomy of the ascending branch of the DCIA/DCIV and its axial supply to the internal oblique muscle. The importance of the latter was not immediately evident. However, the ability to harvest a second soft tissue flap, along with the traditional skin paddle, added tremendously to the versatility of this composite flap. One of the major drawbacks of the iliac osteocutaneous flap was the thickness of the overlying skin and its lack of suitability to replace the mucosal lining of the oral cavity. In addition, the anatomy of the cutaneous perforators did not permit the skin to be freely maneuvered relative to the bone, without putting the vascular supply at risk. Taylor et al. clearly defined the anatomy of the ascending branch in their detailed anatomic descriptions, and our group applied this composite flap of bone and the internal oblique muscle for oromandibular reconstruction. It was later adapted for use in 3-dimensional palatomaxillary reconstruction.

The anatomic detail delineated in this article by Taylor and colleagues represented the gold standard for future donor site descriptions. This landmark article clearly defined both the normal anatomy as well as the most common anatomic anomalies. In addition, it detailed the muscular anatomy surrounding the iliac bone and the optimal approach to safe harvest of this composite flap based on the DCIA/V. While the iliac crest donor site is no longer as popular for composite flap harvest as it was in the 1980s and early 1990s, its anatomic description led to widespread advances in micro-vascular surgery of the head and neck that paved the way for the application of the fibular, as well as the scapular donor sites, that would soon follow and emerge as the mainstays for use in mandibular and maxillary reconstruction. Ultimately, advances in microsurgical transfer of skin and muscle allowed the reconstruction of virtually any ablative defect in the head and neck and permitted surgeons to resect tumors that would otherwise not be considered for ablative surgery. These advances in reconstruction, which permitted advances in ablative surgery, have impacted the lives of countless patients who otherwise would not have been considered candidates for successful lifesaving surgical treatment.

THE *PECTORALIS MAJOR* MYOCUTANEOUS FLAP
A Versatile Flap for Reconstruction in the Head and Neck

Stephan Ariyan

The surgical treatment of advanced carcinomas of the head and neck area often requires extensive resections, necessitating large flaps for reconstruction. In recent years, there has been more acceptance of immediate repairs following the removal of these large cancers. As a result, patients are more willing to undergo these extensive resections to improve their chances of cure with the reasonable expectation that an immediate reconstruction will provide an adequate cosmetic result.

If the cancer has progressed beyond any hopes for cure, sometimes palliative surgery with repair may be offered to lessen the suffering.

Repairs in the head and neck area have been facilitated by the recent development of myocutaneous flaps. In this paper we present out experience with a newly developed pectoralis major myocutaneous flap.

Ariyan S. The pectoralis major myocutaneous flap: a versatile flap for reconstruction in the head and neck. Plast Reconstr Surg. 1979;63:73-81.

Commentary by: *Neal Futran*

Head and neck reconstruction is unique in the demand for fairly complex closures, requiring attention to coverage, support, and lining often in a 3-dimensional nature. The goals are not only functional (i.e. speech, swallowing, and respiration) but aesthetic as well. Pedicled myocutaneous flaps have been recognized as one of the most important reconstructive methods in major head and neck cancer surgery. The pectoralis major muscle has been applied to the reconstruction variety of chest wall defects since 1947, when Pickerel reported its use as a turnover flap. In 1968, Hueston and McConchie reported a case in which this muscle was used as a carrier for the overlying skin to repair an upper sternal defect. However, it was Ariyan's work in 1979 that showed that the flap could be raised as an axial myocutaneous flap based on the thoraco-acromial artery. He recognized the tremendous potential of the musculocutaneous unit based on the pectoralis major for the reconstruction of a large number of head and neck defects. This initial publication described four cases, two of which were raised as peninsula flaps; one as an island flap, and one as a double-paddle island flap.

This discovery was of paramount importance, because it allowed the possibility of obtaining a large amount of well-vascularized tissue to cover skin and/or mucosal defects from the neck up to and including the midface and skull base. Furthermore, the low morbidity to the donor site and the execution in a one-stage procedure resulted in more efficient and superior patient care. (Previously, these defects could only be restored with staged procedures, and ineffectively at that). The main reasons for this are the ease of its technical aspects, versatility, and proximity to the head and neck region. The major advantages of this flap, which distinguishes it from the three previously described major cutaneous flaps (deltopectoral, nape of neck and forehead) that were in use prior to the time of Ariyan's report, are the following: rich vascularity; large skin territory; ability to transfer without prior delay; improved arc of rotation; increased bulk; primary donor site closure; ease of harvest in the supine position; and ability to transfer two epithelial surfaces for inner and outer lining. Coverage is possible almost anywhere within the oral cavity and can be extended to reach the level of the lateral orbital rim if necessary. The muscle component is well vascularized and often enough to minimize fistula formation when used for intraoral defects, provide bulk for contour defects, or cover neck structures protecting the carotid artery, especially in patients who have undergone prior radiation therapy with or without chemotherapy.

This paper was a remarkable step in head and neck reconstruction and set the stage for it to be undoubtedly the most reliable and versatile type of flap for this purpose. It rapidly replaced many of the existing reconstructive methods and became the "workhorse" in head and neck reconstruction throughout the 1980s and 90s. As the cumulative experience in the use of this flap has increased, its limitations have been identified and modifications have been ascribed. A large series of cases were spawned from a variety of different medical centers and were reported as testimony to the reliability, versatility, and ease of harvesting this flap. Surgeons have incorporated a costochondral segment or a portion of the sternum for simultaneous mandibular reconstruction. The use of a double-paddle flap for through-and-through defects, with the skin islands either placed vertically above each other or side by side, also has been reported. Another method of obtaining two flaps from the same muscle, by splitting the skin and muscle vertically and basing one flap on the thoraco-acromial artery and one flap on the lateral thoracic artery, was advocated by Tobin. To avoid the bulkiness associated with the flap, the pectoralis major also has been used as a pure muscle flap with or without skin grafting.

Now 30 years later, with the use of microvascular free tissue transfer as the primary method for major head and neck reconstruction, the role of the pectoralis major flap is gradually fading in its use for immediate reconstruction. Despite this, the pectoralis major flap continues to play a useful role and is still the subject of many published papers. It may be considered to be the first reparative choice for patients disfigured by cancer or presenting with severe medical morbidities and can provide a reliable reconstructive option in patients with a vessel-depleted neck. The flap is especially useful in centers worldwide that have limited microvascular capabilities and resources. It is also commonly used in salvage for complications after tumor resection, particularly to obliterate dead space, achieve coverage of exposed vessels, and act as a barrier of salivary contamination. In all these situations, it is advisable to opt for a flap of this type, which in addition to reliability requires shorter operative time.

The pectoralis major flap is cemented in the armamentarium of the head and surgeon through Stephen Ariyan's vision and innovation, and will continue to be a vital tool in the restoration of form and function in our patients well into the future.

THE RADIAL FOREARM FLAP: A VERSATILE METHOD FOR INTRA-ORAL RECONSTRUCTION

David S Soutar, Luis R Scheker, Norman SB Tanner, et al.

Summary: The radial forearm flap is ideal for intra-oral reconstruction, offering thin, pliable predominantly hairless skin to replace oral mucosa. The vascularity of the area allows considerable variation in the design of this fasciocutaneous flap and offers the possibility of including bone as an osteocutaneous flap. Furthermore, the vascular anatomy of the flap simplifies the technical aspects of free tissue transfer. Based on ten clinical cases the design of the flap is described and its versatility in differing clinical situations is illustrated. The advantages of this method of intra-oral reconstruction are discussed and evaluated.

Soutar DS, Scheker LR, Tanner NSB, McGregor IA. The radial forearm flap: a versatile method for intra-oral reconstruction. Br J of Plast Surg.1983:36;1-8.

Commentary by: *Ralph Gilbert*

This paper from the Canniesburn Plastic Surgery Unit in Glascow, Scotland, by Soutar et al. represents the first description in the English literature of the use of the cutaneous and osteocutaneous forearm flap in oral cavity reconstruction. The concept of this flap was first described by Yang Guofan (Yonghe, Yuanjian, & Guofan, 1982) in China for neck resurfacing after burn injury. Building on Guofan's description, David Soutar and his colleagues conceptualized the use of the forearm flap in oral reconstruction.

In this paper, the anatomy of this flap is described along with a harvest technique including the potential harvest of the radius as an osteocutaneous transfer. Interestingly, in this original description, Soutar and colleagues conceptualized the potential of this being a flow-through flap with repair of the distal radial artery to the facial artery and the proximal vessel to the external carotid. They described the fact that in many patients the venae comitantes join the medial cubital vein, raising the possibility of harvesting this flap with two venous circulations via the venae and the cephalic vein. They described the concept of a subfascial harvest as a technique that has been replaced in the modern era by the suprafacial harvest to reduce donor site morbidity (Lutz, Wei, Chang, & Yang, 1999). They also described a number of flap designs, including the concept of a reverse flow flap.

One cannot overstate the importance of this paper in the rehabilitation of oral cavity patients. At the time of this description, the vast majority of patients were either undergoing reconstruction with the relatively bulky pectoralis major flap or not undergoing repair at all, with the direct suturing of the margins of the surgical defect to the mandible. From a patient's perspective, the introduction of the flap was transformative. Patients had thin pliable mobile reconstructions with the potential for defect volume matching and sensation. This certainly resulted in a dramatic improvement in oral cavity function for this group of patients.

The opportunity to transfer bone with the cutaneous island raised the possibility of primary mandibular or maxillary reconstruction. The length and volume of bone available was limited, with a maximum length of 10 cm, a vertical component of less than 1 cm, and the inability to reliably osteotomize the bone transfer. In addition, the donor site for bone transfer was problematic, with high rates of distal radial fracture, particularly in older patients (Swanson, Boyd, & Mulholland, 1990; Villaret & Futran, 2003). The introduction of the fibular transfer along with the scapular and iliac crest transfers has largely relegated this transfer to limited bone defects such as orbital or nasal reconstruction.

The forearm flap over the past two decades has been ubiquitous in head and neck reconstruction and remains the workhorse flap for oral reconstruction. The advantages of this flap continue to be its reliable anatomy, ease of harvest, and limited donor site morbidity. Its use has extended to small-volume skin defects, orbital reconstruction, (Chepeha et al., 2005) nasal reconstruction, and as a vascularized carrier for a variety of complex reconstructions, including the larynx and trachea.

Soutar's description of the flap for head and neck reconstruction has been transformative for head and neck reconstructive surgeons and the patients they serve and will likely remain as a workhorse flap for many decades to come.

FIBULA FREE FLAP: A NEW METHOD OF MANDIBLE RECONSTRUCTION

David A Hidalgo

The fibula was investigated as a donor site for freeflap mandible reconstruction. It has the advantages of consistent shape, ample length, distant location to allow a two-team approach, and low donor-site morbidity. It can be raised with a skin island for composite-tissue reconstruction.

Twelve segmental mandibular defects (average 13.5 cm) were reconstructed following resection for tumor, most commonly epidermoid carcinoma. Five defects consisted of bone alone, and four others had only a small amount of associated intraoral soft-tissue loss. Eleven patients underwent primary reconstructions. At least two osteotomies were performed on each graft, and miniplates were used for fixation in 11 patients. Six patients received postoperative radiation, and two patients received postoperative chemotherapy.

The flaps survived in all patients. All osteotomies healed primarily. The septocutaneous blood supply was generally not adequate to support a skin island for intraoral soft-tissue replacement. The aesthetic result of the reconstruction was excellent in most patients, particularly in "bone only" defects. There was no long-term donor-site morbidity.

Hidalgo DA. Fibula free flap: a new method of mandible reconstruction. Plast Reconstr Surg. 1989;84: 71-77.

Commentary by: *Joseph J Disa*

Volume 84, Issue Number 1 of the journal *Plastic and Reconstructive Surgery* was published in July of 1989. In that journal was the seminal article by David A Hidalgo, MD, plastic surgeon at Memorial Sloan-Kettering Cancer Center (MSKCC). Dr Hidalgo trained at New York University with William Shaw, MD, a pioneer in reconstructive microsurgery. Together with Dr Shaw's experience and Dr Hidalgo's ingenuity and artistry, they developed the beautifully illustrated text "Microsurgery in Trauma". While an attending surgeon at MSKCC, Dr Hidalgo brought head and neck reconstruction to a new level with the introduction of microvascular head and neck reconstruction. The existing paradigm of reconstruction with inadequate tissues, multiple procedures, and sub optimal results was supplanted with a new era of replacing like with like, restoring form and function, and limiting donor site morbidity. This paradigm shift is no better exemplified than the article under discussion "Fibula Free Flap: A New Method of Mandible Reconstruction".

The paper is an extended case report describing 12 patients who underwent mandible reconstruction with the fibula free flap. Eleven were immediate and one was delayed reconstruction. Epidermoid carcinoma was the typical disease state, and the average mandibular defect was 13.5 cm. All flaps survived in this series, although the fibula free flap skin island suffered a different fate. In 7 cases the skin island was not used. The other

5 cases used a skin island, but this was problematic. The skin island was deemed not viable in 3 cases and was excised intraoperatively. The other 2 cases had one complete skin island survival and one partial survival. Although some patients in whom the skin did not survive required a vestibuloplasty at a later date, the aesthetic results were considered excellent in most patients, particularly those requiring a "bone only" reconstruction. Additionally, there was no long-term donor site morbidity.

Perhaps the most challenging mandibular defects are those requiring anterior arch reconstruction. In this series, this represented 50% of the patients. The remaining were lateral or hemimandibular defects. Dr Hidalgo demonstrated through the use of preoperatively obtained X-ray templates that the fibula free flap can be osteotomized in multiple segments to match the contours of the native mandible. The segmental blood supply to the fibula based upon the peroneal vessels allow for multiple osteotomy segments while preserving blood supply to the bone.

To date, the fibula free flap is the gold standard in microvascular mandibular reconstruction. While the scapula, forearm, and iliac crest have a role, the fibula free flap is the most versatile, easy to harvest and allows for a two-team approach, and the fibula is long enough to reconstruct the vast majority of mandibular defects. There is no question that limitations exist, including mobility of the skin island, bone thickness in some situations, and the potential for problems in patients with peripheral vascular disease; however, the fibula free flap remains the most ideal donor site for this indication. A major focus for Dr Hidalgo was subsequently published in *Plastic and Reconstructive Surgery* in the "Aesthetic Improvements in Mandible Reconstruction" article. This was the emphasis on precise graft shaping that yielded superior aesthetic results. The templates, fibula anatomy, and the use of miniplates all facilitated the segmental construction of the graft that could produce an exact duplicate of the specimen shape.

Since Dr Hidalgo's original work, there have been some modifications and improvements. Knowledge of the septocutaneous perforator anatomy has made design and survival of the skin island the norm, not the exception. Tourniquet insufflation pressure does not need to be 450 mm Hg, as described in the original article, to have an avascular environment for flap harvested. Enhanced knowledge of the anatomy of the peroneal vascular system allows for the safe dissection of the pedicle under tourniquet control. Experience has also taught us that 2 weeks of intermaxillary, fixation as described in the original description, can be replaced with a much shorter duration of fixation and early mobilization.

One final, brilliant concept from the original paper merits comment: the use of the mandibular condyle as an autologous bone graft. Dr Hidalgo conceptualized and successfully executed the use of the native condyle (if disease-free) as an autologous bone graft rigidly fixed the end of the fibula flap to reconstruct the temporal mandibular joint. This technique currently remains an attractive alternative over other methods of joint reconstruction.

"Fibula Free Flap: A New Method of Mandible Reconstruction" is a must read for any student of head and neck surgery. The technique is useful for both benign and malignant conditions. It is highly reliable, and in the vast majority of situations, is the preferred method of mandible reconstruction. Dr Hidalgo is to be congratulated for his ingenuity.

A CLASSIFICATION SYSTEM AND ALGORITHM FOR RECONSTRUCTION OF MAXILLECTOMY AND MIDFACIAL DEFECTS

Peter G Cordeiro, Eric Santamaria

Maxillectomy defects become more complex when critical structures such as the orbit, globe, and cranial base are resected, and reconstruction with distant tissues becomes essential. This study reviews all maxillectomy defects reconstructed immediately using pedicled and free flaps to establish (1) a classification system and (2) an algorithm for reconstruction of these complex problems.

Over a 5-year period, 60 flaps were used to reconstruct defects classified as the following: type I, limited maxillectomy (n = 7); type II, subtotal maxillectomy (n = 10); type IIIa, total maxillectomy with preservation of the orbital contents (n = 13); type IIIb, total maxillectomy with orbital exenteration (n = 18); and type IV, orbitomaxillectomy (n = 10). Free flaps (45 rectus abdominis and 10 radial forearm) were used in 55 patients (91.7 percent), and the temporalis muscle was transposed in five elderly patients who were not free-flap candidates. Vascularized (radial forearm osteocutaneous) bone flaps were used in four of the 60 patients (6.7 percent) and nonvascularized bone grafts in 17 (28.3 percent). Simultaneous reconstruction of the oral commissure using an Estandler procedure was performed in 10 patients with maxillectomy and through-and-through soft-tissue defects.

Free-flap survival was 100 percent, with re-exploration in five of 55 patients (9.1 percent) and partial-flap necrosis in one patient. Seven of the 60 patients (11.7 percent) had systemic complications, and four died within 30 days of hospitalization. Fifty patients had more than 6 months of follow-up with a mean time of 27.7 (± 15.6) months. Postoperative radiotherapy was administered in 32 of these patients (64.0 percent). Chewing and speech functions were assessed in 36 patients with type II, IIIa, and IIIb defects. A prosthetic denture was fixed in 15 of 36 patients (41.7 percent). Return to an unrestricted diet was seen in 16 patients (44.4 percent), a soft diet in 17 (47.2 percent), and a liquid diet in three (8.3 percent). Speech was assessed as normal in 14 of 36 patients (38.9 percent), near normal in 15 (41.7 percent), intelligible in six (16.7 percent), and unintelligible in one patient (2.8 percent). Globe and periorbital soft-tissue position was assessed in 14 patients with type I and IIIa defects. There were no cases of enophthalmos, and one patient had a mild vertical dystopia. Ectropion was observed in 10 of 14 patients (71.4 percent). Oral competence was considered good in all 10 patients with excision/reconstruction of the oral commissure; however, two patients (20 percent) developed microstomia after receiving radiotherapy. Aesthetic results were evaluated at least 6 months after reconstruction in 50 patients. They were good to excellent in 29 patients (58 percent) for whom cheek skin and lip were not resected, and poor to fair (42 percent) when the external skin or orbital contents were excised. Secondary procedures were required in 16 of 50 patients (32.0 percent).

Free-tissue transfer provides the most effective and reliable form of immediate reconstruction for complex maxillectomy defects. The rectus abdominis and radial forearm flaps in combination with immediate bone grafting or as osteocutaneous flaps reliably provide the best aesthetic and functional results. An algorithm based on the type of maxillary resection can be followed to determine the best approach to reconstruction.

Cordeiro PG, Santamaria E. A classification system and algorithm for reconstruction of maxillectomy and midfacial defects. Plast Reconstr Surg. 2000;105:2331-2346.

Commentary by: *Mark K Wax*

This article by Drs Cordeiro and Santamaria describes a functional reconstruction of maxillectomy defects based on an easily communicated classification system. The authors used their experience, garnered from patients reconstructed at Memorial Sloan-Kettering Cancer Center, and describe an excellent algorithm to be considered for these defects. Going beyond this, the authors examined the long-term functional and aesthetic results in their patients. The authors took reconstructive surgery of these maxillectomy defects to the next level by defining an algorithm for reconstruction and techniques to optimize functional rehabilitation as well as cosmetic outcomes.

The authors look at a series of 60 patients with maxillectomy defects that were immediately reconstructed over a 5-year period. All patients had vascularized free tissue transfer. While most patients had squamous cell carcinoma (60%), there was the usual mix of other sarcomas and rarer type tumors. At Memorial Sloan-Kettering Cancer Center, maxillectomy defects were classically described in one of four ways. The authors utilized and modified this system so that functional reconstruction with composite free tissue transfer could be applied to optimize the rehabilitative potential. Type I defects include resection of one or two walls of the maxilla but preservation of the palate. Type II defects include resection of the maxillary arch, the palate, and the anterior and lateral walls with preservation of the orbital floors. Type III defects involve the classic total maxillectomy with: (a) orbital preservation or (b) orbital exenteration. Type IV defects involve a classic total maxillectomy, except the palate is preserved. The authors use a variety of free tissue transfer donor sites, demonstrating the versatility of free tissue transfer by allowing for multiple composite tissues to reconstruct the specific tissue defect that was created. Bony reconstruction was performed in 35% of patients, and 10 patients had reconstruction of the upper lip.

The authors performed an extensive functional and aesthetic evaluation of the patients at 6 months following surgery. Patients that had Type I defects did well in terms of aesthetic results. Patients with palatal resection were able to obtain normal or near normal speech in greater than 80% of the patient population. When evaluating patients as to dietary intake, greater than 90% of patients were able to eat either a soft or regular diet. No patient required a feeding tube, and almost 40% of patients could be dentally rehabilitated with a prosthesis. Fourteen patients were evaluated following resection of the orbital floor with reservation of the orbital contents. All of these patients maintained their preoperative vision without the need for eye patching. Ectropion developed in 71% of patients.

Oral competence was achieved in all patients who underwent resection and reconstruction of either the oral commissure or upper lip. Fifty-eight percent of patients had good or excellent aesthetic results. The larger the surgical procedure, the larger the surface area of skin that was affected, the poorer the aesthetic outcome. The authors noted that while increasing volume of resection leads to decreasing aesthetic outcomes, overall functional and rehabilitative outcomes are excellent in the majority of patients.

The maxilla bears a close relationship with many critical anatomic structures. The close proximity of the orbit, oral cavity, nasal cavity, and skin and lips of the mid face makes treatment of maxillary cancer potentially very debilitating from a functional and cosmetic perspective. Prior to free tissue transfer, reconstruction depended mainly on prosthetic rehabilitation. While in expert hands acceptable outcomes were available, not everyone could expect to be rehabilitated. Surgical reconstruction of defects of the maxillary complex and adjacent structures was very difficult. The tremendous value of this manuscript was that it built upon the ability of surgeons to use composite free tissue transfer to reconstruct composite tissue defects. By examining both the tissue volume as well as the type of tissues that were excised, the authors were able to develop an algorithm that allowed one to determine which tissue would provide the best replacement. Furthermore, by classifying the defects as to which adjacent structures, orbital or oral cavity, were impacted by the surgical resection, the reconstructive surgeon could determine the best tissue for reconstruction. What makes this manuscript unique is the foundation for rehabilitation that the authors laid down. Through the superb use of photo documentation and artistic drawings the authors were able to convey a large range of maxillary defects and classify them into four categories based on a paradigm of reconstruction, with the goal being rehabilitation and cosmetic optimization. Having done this, the authors then went on to analyze their results from a functional and cosmetic perspective. This laid the groundwork for other reconstructive surgeons to develop a paradigm for reconstruction. The authors, by analyzing their results, also demonstrated the benefits of free tissue transfer in this patient population. The morbidity of free tissue transfer, while minimal in this institution, had not been entirely well accepted by the general reconstructive population. By being able to demonstrate and analyze their functional outcomes the authors established free tissue transfer as a viable and better alternative to prosthetic rehabilitation.

In summary, this landmark work by Drs Cordeiro and Santamaria described a reconstructive paradigm for a potentially devastating functional defect. Their graphic depiction of outcomes and analyses of the multiple functions of the maxillofacial complex determined that functional rehabilitation of these defects was possible in the majority of patients. The authors brought forward a standard by which other reconstructive surgeons could compare their outcomes.

HAVE WE FOUND AN IDEAL SOFT-TISSUE FLAP?
AN EXPERIENCE WITH 672 ANTEROLATERAL THIGH FLAPS

Fu-chan Wei, Vivek Jain, Naci Celik, et al.

The free anterolateral thigh flap is becoming one of the most preferred options for soft-tissue reconstruction. Between June of 1996 and August of 2000, 672 anterolateral thigh flaps were used in 660 patients at Chang Gung Memorial Hospital. Four hundred eighty-four anterolateral thigh flaps were used for head and neck region reconstruction in 475 patients, 58 flaps were used for upper extremity reconstruction in 58 patients, 121 flaps were used for lower extremity reconstruction in 119 patients, and nine flaps were used for trunk reconstruction in nine patients. Of the 672 flaps used in total, a majority (439) were musculocutaneous perforator flaps. Sixty-five were septocutaneous vessel flaps. Of these 504 flaps, 350 were fasciocutaneous and 154 were cutaneous flaps. Of the remaining 168 flaps, 95 were musculocutaneous flaps, 63 were chimeric flaps, and the remaining ten were composite musculocutaneous perforator flaps with the tensor fasciae latec. Total flap failure occurred in 12 patients (1.79 percent of the flaps) and partial failure occurred in 17 patients (2.53 percent of the flaps). Of the 12 flaps that failed completely, five were reconstructed with second anterolateral thigh flaps, four with pedicled flaps, one with a free radial forearm flap, one with skin grafting, and one with primary closure. Of the 17 flaps that failed partially, three were reconstructed with anterolateral thigh flaps, one with free radial forearm flap, five with pedicled flaps, and eight with primary suture, skin grafting, and conservative methods.

In this large series, a consistent anatomy of the main pedicle of the anterolateral thigh flap was observed. In cutaneous and fasciocutaneous flaps, the skin vessels (musculocutaneous perforators or septocutaneous vessels) were found and followed until they reached the main pedicle, regardless of the anatomic position. There were only six cases in this series in which no skin vessels were identified during the harvesting of cutaneous or fasciocutaneous anterolateral thigh flaps. In 87.1 percent of the cutaneous or fasciocutaneous flaps, the skin vessels were found to be musculocutaneous perforators; in 12.9 percent, they were found as septocutaneous vessels. The anterolateral thigh flap is a reliable flap that supplies a large area of skin. This flap can be harvested irrespective of whether the skin vessels are septocutaneous or musculocutaneous. It is a versatile soft-tissue flap in which thickness and volume can be adjusted for the extent of the defect, and it can replace most soft-tissue free flaps in most clinical situations.

Wei FC, Jain V, Celik N, et al. Have we found an ideal soft-tissue flap? An experience with 672 anterolateral thigh flaps. Plast Reconstr Surg. 2002;109:2219-2226.

Commentary by: *Peter G Cordeiro*

The paper "Have We Found an Ideal Soft-Tissue Flap? An Experience with 672 Anterolateral Thigh Flaps" by Fu-chan Wei et al. is a review of Dr Wei's initial experience with the anterolateral thigh flap, which was used for a variety of reconstructive problems, between June 1996 and August 2000. He describes his experience with 672 free flaps, of which 484 were used in the head and neck. The anterolateral thigh flap was originally described by Song, but was popularized by Dr Wei and his colleagues who used this flap extensively at the Chang Gung Memorial Hospital. In the past decade, the flap has become much more utilized on a worldwide basis, not just in Asia, but also in Europe and the United States. The paper is significant because it defines the utility of the flap as well as documents the reliability of the blood supply, which has always been in question. The flap was originally described as a fasciocutaneous perforator flap but, as ascertained by Wei, can also be elevated as a fasciocutaneous flap with septocutaneous perforators, musculocutaneous perforators, or as a musculocutaneous flap with a segment of the vastus lateralis, or as a chimeric flap with other muscles such as the rectus femoris or tensor fascia lata. Although this is an excellent soft tissue flap that is useful for a variety of different purposes, I do not think that it (or any other flap) can ever be labeled the "ideal soft tissue flap" as suggested by the article. It is, however, an extremely useful flap for a variety of different purposes.

In head and neck reconstruction, as a general principle one should first establish the requirements of the defect and then select the flap. Defects can be small, medium, or large with regard to volume requirement and also small, medium, or large based on the surface area requirement. I most commonly use two to three soft tissue flaps; the selection process is based on the combination of surface area to volume requirement as well as other features that might be provided by the flap. Thus, a defect that requires a small volume flap with small to moderate amounts of surface area would be best reconstructed with a radial forearm fasciocutaneous flap, while a very large volume defect with extensive surface area requiring multiple skin islands would be best served by a rectus abdominis myocutaneous flap. Defects that fall between these two extremes are reconstructed best by the anterolateral thigh flap, specifically a defect that requires a moderate volume and a moderate to large surface area type flap. My own bias in this scenario would be to use a gracilis myocutaneous flap or a parascapular flap depending on the quality of skin that is required as well as the volume of the defect; however, the anterolateral thigh flap is excellent in this scenario, because it does provide both the skin and the volume required by these types of defects.

Other benefits of this flap, as outlined by Wei, are a fairly long pedicle, which is useful in head and neck reconstruction and the ability to use muscle in combination with the flap, which will provide volume as well as excellent blood supply. The options provided by the myocutaneous ALT flap include the vastus lateralis muscle, the rectus femoris or even the tensor fasciae lata. The flap also can provide excellent fascia, if necessary. As described by Wei, the flap can also be thinned and elevated in the suprafascial level to provide a thinner more pliable flap. In many surgeons' hands, however, this is less reliable, and the potential for necrosis increases. In this scenario, I think there are some shortcomings to use of the ALT. My own perspective is that if needed for reconstruction of the tongue or resurfacing of mucosa, this flap, unless thinned to the extreme, can be too stiff or too bulky. The Asian patient population that Dr Wei works with might perhaps be more suited to use of this donor site. In North American Caucasians, the ALT flap can be quite bulky and stiff. One of the other relative disadvantages of this flap is that a fair amount of surgical experience is needed to reliably raise a well-vascularized flap, particularly because, as Wei points out, a majority of these flaps are derived from musculocutaneous perforators, which can be difficult to dissect and decrease the reliability of the blood supply.

Thus, there is no question that the ALT is an excellent adjunct to the armamentarium of the reconstructive plastic surgeon. There is also no question that this paper has contributed significantly to our literature and to reconstruction in the head and neck since it added one more reliable "multi-faceted flap". However, I would not label this the ideal soft tissue flap since it is ideal for certain applications but not others. As with any type of reconstruction in the head and neck, the selection of the flap should be based on the requirements of the defect.

Chapter 17

Radiation Oncology

THE PLACE OF RADIOTHERAPY IN THE MANAGEMENT OF THE SQUAMOUS CELL CARCINOMA OF THE SUPRAGLOTTIC LARYNX

Gilbert H Fletcher, Richard H Jesse, Robert D Lindberg, et al.

The supraglottic larynx is composed of the epiglottis, the aryepiglottic folds, false cords, and arytenoids. The epiglottis itself is divided into supra and infrahyoid epiglottis. The squamous cell carcinomas originating on these various anatomic structures differ with respect to local extensions and regional lymph node metastases; therefore, their management must be planned accordingly.

The three modalities of treatment are surgical resection alone, irradiation alone, or a combination of both. As a rule, in our institution, the combined treatment includes surgical resection and postoperative irradiation.

The purpose of this paper is to analyze the results obtained by these three modalities and to draw guidelines for the treatment of patients with cancer of the supraglottic larynx.

Fletcher GH, Jesse RH, Lindberg RD, et al. The place of radiotherapy in the management of the squamous cell carcinoma of the supraglottic larynx. Am J Roentgenol Radium Ther Nucl Med. 1970;108: 19-26.

Commentary by: *Jacques Bernier*

This contribution, published in 1970 in the *American Journal of Roentgenology*, is one of the strongest symbols of the prominent role played by Gilbert H Fletcher and the MD Anderson Cancer Center (MDACC) in the management of head and neck cancers. This article counted indeed among the very first reports, which, by assessing on such a large scale the place of radiotherapy in the management of supraglottic larynx carcinoma, pioneered a number of treatment policies for tumors arising from this anatomical entity. More than 40 years after the publication of this paper, we can only admire the rigorous methodologies used by the authors to record, analyze, and report the results of the treatments they had given. Likewise the way they derived, from their clinical observations, a significant number of treatment policies— still fully valid, and almost half a century later—deserves all of our respect.

What strikes the reader at first is the impressive number of patients entered in this study at a time when many radio-oncologists, both in the US and in Europe, had just completed their learning curve after the advent of mega-voltage radiotherapy, and hardly succeeded in gathering homogeneous cohorts of patients, especially when presenting with head and neck carcinoma.

To report on 267 patients, with only the supraglottic larynx as an analysis site, enabled the authors to identify distinct policies of treatment according to the various larynx subsites, such as supra- and infra-hyoid epiglottis, aryepiglottic fold, false cord, and arytenoids.

Beyond the advantages drawn from this large population sample, the ability shown by Fletcher and his team to elicit what were already robust conclusions, also resulted from the judicious evaluation they had made throughout the 50s and 60s of the clinical situations justifying postoperative radiotherapy (PORT), namely the tumor and/or lymph node volume, positive surgical margins, and extracapsular spread in the neck.

One of the numerous merits of GH Fletcher and his team were to demonstrate that PORT policies, thanks to their significant impact on residual malignant microfoci, had to be privileged in high-risk situations, such as the presence of advanced tumor stages (T3-4 lesions) or for subsites in which it is difficult to secure surgical margins (i.e. aryepiglottic folds). Likewise, the well-recognized value in our current practice of PORT in patients with lymph node metastases was strongly influenced by the publication of this report, which had yielded a drastic increase in nodal failures from 38% up to 71%, when PORT had been omitted.

This MDACC contribution was among the first ones that made a clear distinction, in terms of both natural history and response to treatment, between tumors arising in the aryepiglottic fold and false cord. Indeed, the often infiltrative pattern presented by the former ones and their lymphophilic pattern—even at early stages—implied, according to the authors, to favor for this subsite, the delivery of postoperative radiotherapy, more often than in patients with false cord carcinoma.

The article by Fletcher and colleagues also emphasizes their outstanding role in pioneering head and neck cancer radiotherapy: first, through the optimization of irradiation doses and volumes in the framework of conventionally fractionated radiotherapy; second, by throwing the bases of what we call nowadays "conformal radiotherapy", by implementing the "unequal loading, 3:2 or 2:1" concept through parallel opposed fields for laterally sided lesions, and underlining the advantages offered by the application of booster doses at the end of the treatment; and third, via the subtle use of irradiation combining different beam qualities. Being myself a trainee in Gilbert H Fletcher's department a few years after the publication of this article, I was very impressed by the wonderful coordination existing among the physicians and radiographers operating at the Cobalt-60 and Betatron (Allis-Chalmers and Siemens) units, especially when mixing with great expertise photon and electron beams, and ensuring a perfect match between upper-neck (lateral) and lower-neck (anterior) fields.

Another interesting message of this article relates to the prerequisite for radiotherapy efficacy, namely the pre-therapeutic work-up. Although the power of resolution from X-ray examinations was not, by definition, comparable to that offered by the imaging tools available nowadays, the conjunction of very careful clinical examinations and the high expertise in reviewing roentgenographic findings, which the authors clearly underline in this contribution, paved the way for developing these "combined" clinical skills among the next generations of physicians dealing with head and neck cancer.

As mentioned before, another critical point of this article is the rigorous methodologies used by Fletcher and his team in recording and reporting their results, specifically with regard to the way to present treatment outcomes following definitive radiotherapy or PORT, both in terms of efficacy results and complications. In regard to efficacy, the presentation of the tables, ranging from patients statistics to local-regional recurrence and metastasis rates, and stratified by tumor and nodal site and size, and treatment types (postsurgical versus postirradiation failures), is as an utmost perfect example of stratification and methodology to validate a given treatment approach. In this, GH Fletcher is a precursor if we consider the modern ways to present efficacy results following head and neck local treatment.

Last but not least, this paper offers some strong clues on the dose-control relationships: beyond their ability to draw the first dose-response curve for T2 and T3 lesions of the supraglottic larynx cancer, Fletcher and his colleagues also emphasized the interactions existing between the irradiation doses and overall treatment time to control supraglottic larynx carcinomas. The clear benefit these patients could draw from accelerating the treatment was indeed shown when the authors reported on optimal doses to control these tumors stages, with 6,100 rads in 5 weeks, 6,500 rads in 6 weeks, and 6,850 rads in 7 weeks, respectively. The time-dose factor would become, throughout the next decades, one of the major algorithms used in clinical radiobiology, especially to treat head and neck cancers. It is nowadays part of the design of any prospective trial investing in treatment intensity-related issues in this patient population.

Interestingly enough, this article also established firmer correlations between dose-volume parameters and complications, for instance for both laryngeal edema and necrosis. In addition, Fletcher had clearly identified the deleterious impact of smoking habits, since he showed that "Patients in whom persistent edema developed almost *universally* persisted in smoking cigarettes"... The authors of very recent and influential papers on persistence of smoking during treatment and its impact on outcome could not agree more.

Last but not least, by integrating a section entitled "Preservation of larynx function" into this contribution, the authors not only paved the way for all efforts put forth in that direction during the last 4 decades, they had also made a clear distinction, as far back as the 60s, between the concepts of organ and function preservation!

For all these reasons, this visionary paper by Fletcher and his colleagues is undoubtedly, to us radio-oncologists, a milestone in the literature of head and neck radiotherapy.

A RADIATION THERAPY ONCOLOGY GROUP (RTOG) PHASE III RANDOMIZED STUDY TO COMPARE HYPERFRACTIONATION AND TWO VARIANTS OF ACCELERATED FRACTIONATION TO STANDARD FRACTIONATION RADIOTHERAPY FOR HEAD AND NECK SQUAMOUS CELL CARCINOMAS: FIRST REPORT OF RTOG 9003

Karen K Fu, Thomas F Pajak, Andy Trotti, et al.

Purpose: The optimal fractionation schedule for radiotherapy of head and neck cancer has been controversial. The objective of this randomized trial was to test the efficacy of hyperfractionation and two types of accelerated fractionation individually against standard fractionation.

Methods and Materials: Patients with locally advanced head and neck cancer were randomly assigned to receive radiotherapy delivered with: (1) standard fractionation at 2 Gy/fraction/day, 5 days/week, to 70 Gy/35 fractions/7 weeks: (2) hyperfractionation at 1.2 Gy/fraction, twice daily, 5 day/week, to 81.6 Gy/68 fractions/7 weeks; (3) accelerated fractionation with split at 1.6 Gy/fraction, twice daily, 5 days/ week, to 67.2 Gy/42 fractions/6 weeks including a 2-week rest after 38.4 Gy; or (4) accelerated fractionation with concomitant boost at 1.8 Gy/fraction/day, 5 days/week and 1.5 Gy/fraction/day to a boost field as a second daily treatment for the last 12 treatment days to 72 Gy/42 fractions/6 weeks. Of the 1113 patients entered, 1073 patients were analyzable for outcome. The median follow-up was 23 months for all analyzable patients and 41.2 months for patients alive.

Results: Patients treated with hyperfractionation and accelerated fractionation with concomitant boost had significantly better local-regional control (p = 0.045 and p = 0.50 respectively) than those treated with standard fractionation. There was also a trend toward improved disease-free survival (p = 0.067 and p = 0.054 respectively) although the difference in overall survival was not significant. Patients treated with accelerated fractionation with split had similar outcome to those treated with standard fractionation. All three altered fractionation groups had significantly greater acute side effects compared to standard fractionation. However, there was no significant increase of late effects.

Conclusions: Hyperfractionation and accelerated fractionation with concomitant boost are more efficacious than standard fractionation for locally advanced head and neck cancer. Acute but not late effects are also increased.

Fu KK, Pajak TF, Trotti A, et al. A Radiation Therapy Oncology Group (RTOG) phase III randomized study to compare hyperfractionation and two variants of accelerated fractionation to standard fractionation radiotherapy for head and neck squamous cell carcinomas: first report of RTOG 9003. Int J Radiat Oncol Biol Phys. 2000;48:7-16.

Commentary by: *Louis B Harrison*

This article from Fu et al. represents a landmark contribution to the head and neck cancer literature. It is the largest randomized trial that evaluates the role of various radiation therapy fractionation schedules. Eligible patients included individuals aged 18 years or older, with a Karnofsky performance

score greater than 60, with previously untreated stages III or IV squamous cell carcinomas of the oral cavity, oropharynx, supraglottic larynx, base of tongue, or hypopharynx. For the base of the tongue and hypopharynx, patients with stage II disease were eligible. All patients were free of distant metastasis. The patients were randomized to one of four treatment schedules:

1. Standard fractionation at 2 Gy per fraction 5 days a week to 70 Gy in 35 fractions in 7 weeks.
2. Hyperfractionation at 1.2 Gy per fraction, twice daily, 6 hours apart, 5 days a week to 81.6 Gy in 68 fractions over 7 weeks.
3. Accelerated fractionation with split at 1.6 Gy per fraction, twice daily, 6 hours apart, 5 days a week to 67.2 Gy in 42 fractions over 6 weeks including a 2-week split after 38.4 Gy.
4. Accelerated fractionation with concomitant boost at 1.8 Gy per fraction 5 days a week to the large field plus 1.5 Gy per fraction as a p.m. concomitant boost given 6 hours after treatment of the large field for the last 12 treatments to a total of 72 Gy in 42 fractions over 6 weeks.

This trial accrued 1,113 patients, of which 1,073 patients were evaluable and formed the basis of the outcome analysis. This is a very large series, and will probably be the largest fractionation trial ever conducted in head and neck cancer. Patients were treated using older techniques that were pertinent to the era of therapy. Most patients were treated using linear accelerators or cobalt machines, and most patients were treated using lateral opposed fields, anterior and lateral wedge fields, or other field arrangements that are today considered outdated.

The median follow-up was approximately 41 months for surviving patients. This trial showed a statistically significant improved local-regional control at 2 years for patients receiving either hyperfractionation (schedule 2) or accelerated fractionation with concomitant boost (schedule 4). The trend toward improved disease-free survival also was noted for these two fractionation schedules. There was a higher rate of acute toxicity with the hyperfractionation or accelerated fractionation programs, but late toxicity (toxicity occurring from 6 to 24 months) was not increased. Overall survival was the same for all four arms. This clinical trial validated that local-regional control could be enhanced by manipulating the radiation therapy fractionation schedule.

When analyzed by the rationale of the study, this clinical trial demonstrates that local-regional control is increased with either an increase in total dose (hyperfractionation arm) or by shortening the overall treatment time (accelerated fractionation with concomitant boost). Both of these approaches led to improved local-regional control, with a trend towards improved disease-free survival. It is not a surprise that the improved local-regional control did not change overall survival. Changes in local treatment rarely affect the risk of distant metastasis, and this trial is certainly no different.

When put into context, the results of this trial must be explained in the context of current head and neck cancer management. Nowadays, patients with stages III and IV disease would be treated with a concomitant chemotherapy-radiotherapy program. Given that concomitant chemotherapy/radiotherapy has become a standard of care, radiotherapy alone is rarely used for this patient population. In the era of concomitant chemotherapy-radiotherapy, hyperfractionation or accelerated fractionation programs are not as commonly used. In addition, current radiation therapy techniques call for intensity-modulated radiation therapy (IMRT), to be a standard of care for most of these patients. In the same way, in the IMRT era, concomitant boost techniques or hyperfractionation techniques have not been commonly used. Thus, we do not know whether these manipulations in radiation therapy fractionation would have an impact when IMRT is utilized, or in the concomitant chemotherapy era. However, for patients who are being treated by radiation therapy alone, the results of this trial remain valid.

The largest percentage of patients in this study represented oropharynx as the primary site—approximately 60% of the patients in each arm. This study was done prior to the HPV era, so we do not know what percentage of patients might have had HPV-related malignancies. While it is hard to predict the impact that this may have had on the outcome, it is certainly worthy of notation.

As expected, acute toxicity was the most common limiting factor in the hyperfractionation and accelerated fractionation arms. This is enhanced, nowadays, with the use of concomitant chemotherapy. Many radiation therapy technical modifications as well as pharmacologic modifications are being studied to reduce acute toxicity and improve patient comfort.

In summary, this landmark paper is one of the most important local-regional therapy trials ever to be performed in head and neck cancer. The results of this trial still have relevance to modern thinking, although the results are not currently being applied in most centers. The fact that shorter treatment times and higher radiation therapy doses led to improved local-regional control should be considered in developing new studies. Also, in the HPV era, where treatment de-intensification is being considered, these findings should also be remembered. While treatment de-intensification is being studied for more favorable HPV-positive patients, treatment intensification may be considered for less favorable HPV-negative patients. The findings of this study could have relevance in developing clinical trials for these subsets. The findings should also be considered in de-intensification programs that rely on radiation alone.

It is unlikely that a clinical trial of this size will ever be performed again, in which the main topic is a manipulation in local treatment. The authors are to be congratulated for this historical study and landmark achievement.

RANDOMIZED TRIAL ADDRESSING RISK FEATURES AND TIME FACTORS OF SURGERY PLUS RADIOTHERAPY IN ADVANCED HEAD AND NECK CANCER

K Kian Ang, Andy Trotti, Barry W Brown, et al.

Purpose: A multi-institutional, prospective, randomized trial was undertaken in patients with advanced head and neck squamous cell carcinoma to address (1) the validity of using pathologic risk features, established from a previous study, to determine the need for, and dose of, postoperative radiotherapy (PORT); (2) the impact of accelerating PORT using a concomitant boost schedule; and (3) the importance of the overall combined treatment duration on the treatment outcome.

Methods and Materials: Of 288 consecutive patients with advanced disease registered preoperatively, 213 fulfilled the trial criteria and went on to receive therapy predicated on a set of pathologic risk features: no PORT for the low-risk group (n = 31); 57.6 Gy during 6.5 weeks for the intermediate-risk group (n = 31); and, by random assignment, 63 Gy during 5 weeks (n = 76) or 7 weeks (n = 75) for the high-risk group. Patients were irradiated with standard techniques appropriate to the site of disease and likely areas of spread. The study endpoints were locoregional control (LRC), survival, and morbidity.

Results: Patients with low or intermediate risks had significantly higher LRC and survival rates than those with high-risk features (p = 0.003 and p = 0.0001, respectively), despite receiving no PORT or lower dose PORT, respectively. For high-risk patients, a trend toward higher LRC and survival rates was noted when PORT was delivered in 5 rather than 7 weeks. A prolonged interval between surgery and PORT in the 7-week schedule was associated with significantly lower LRC (p = 0.03) and survival (p = 0.01) rates. Consequently, the cumulative duration of combined therapy had a significant impact on the LRC (p = 0.005) and survival (p = 0.03) rates. A 2-week reduction in the PORT duration by using the concomitant boost technique did not increase the late treatment toxicity.

Conclusions: This Phase III trial established the power of risk assessment using pathologic features in determining the need for, and dose of, PORT in patients with advanced head-and-neck squamous cell cancer in a prospective, multi-institutional setting. It also revealed the impact of the overall treatment time in the combination of surgery and PORT on the outcome in high-risk patients and showed that PORT acceleration without a reduction in dose by a concomitant boost regimen did not increase the late complication rate. These findings emphasize the importance of co-ordinated interdisciplinary care in the delivery of combined surgery and RT.

Ang KK, Trotti A, Brown BW, et al. Randomized trial addressing risk features and time factors of surgery plus radiotherapy in advanced head-and-neck cancer. Int J Radiat Oncol Biol Phys. 2001;51:571-578.

Commentary by: *June Corry*

The terms "total treatment package" and "overall treatment time" have long been part of the head and neck vernacular—these terms were derived from work relating to this study. The article provides long-term outcome data of a trial of risk-adjusted postoperative radiotherapy (PORT) dose, confirming the preliminary results first reported in 1993. The aims of the study were to (1) prospectively validate using clusters of pathological risk factors to assign PORT, (2) assess whether shortening the radiotherapy duration but not dose would counter accelerated repopulation, and (3) assess the impact of the total duration of treatment on patient outcomes.

Like all good research, this study built upon previous work. Starting with the work of Rod Withers et al. back in 1988, we know that during a course of radiotherapy, the initial reduction in tumor cell growth was followed, at around the 4-week mark, by accelerated regrowth or repopulation of clonogenic cancer cells. An important intellectual connection was subsequently made by realizing that accelerated repopulation could occur following any treatment modality that resulted in a reduction in the head and neck cancer cell population, not only that occurring during radiotherapy but also after surgery. Supportive information for this concept came from retrospective analyses of clinical results showing poorer outcomes when commencement of PORT was delayed > 6 weeks. Hence evolved the concept of connecting the day of surgery to the day of completion of PORT to describe an "overall treatment time" that could be potentially important in optimizing loco-regional control (LRC).

The schema for this trial was that all patients treated with curative surgical intent were registered, and then those eligible for PORT were allocated to intermediate- or high-risk groups. The intermediate group received 57.6 Gy in 32 fractions (1.8 Gy per fraction) over 6 ½ weeks. The high-risk group were randomized to either conventional radiotherapy (CF), 63 Gy in 35 fractions over 7 weeks or accelerated radiotherapy (AF), 63Gy in 35 fractions over 5 weeks. The intermediate group had only 1 risk factor (other than ECE), and the high-risk group had ECE or at least 2 or more of other pathological risk factors (oral cavity primary site, surgical margins < 5 mm, > 1 positive node, > 1 positive nodal group, largest node > 3 cm).

The results of this study prospectively validated the use of pathological risk factors to differentiate the need for and the dose of PORT. Patients with no adverse pathological features did not need PORT as their 5-year LRC, and overall survival (OS) rates with surgery alone were 90% and 83%, respectively. The intermediate risk group, receiving intermediate dose PORT, had a similarly good LRC rate (94%), and a 66% OS rate. In contrast, the high-risk group had an LRC of only 68% and OS of 42%, despite receiving higher dose PORT.

This study established prospectively the impact of the overall treatment time on LRC and OS. High-risk patients with < 11 weeks of overall treatment time had significantly better LRC and OS compared to those with 11–13 and > 13 weeks of overall treatment time. The LRC rate in the < 11 week group was more than double that of the > 13 week group. The randomized component of the study—between CF or AF PORT in the high-risk group—showed a trend for improved LRC and OS in the AF group. The importance of overall treatment time was further supported by the fact that patients with > 13 weeks of overall treatment time who received CF PORT had a significantly poorer LRC and OS compared to the AF group. So shortening the overall treatment time by 1 week could be seen to compensate for the delay in commencement of PORT. Another way to shorten overall treatment time by 1 week is to increase the fraction size from 1.8 Gy to 2 Gy. This has the added advantage of decreasing the number of fractions, i.e., less machine time (resources) required, and it is the current standard practice in many radiation therapy centers.

This prospective information regarding the importance of overall treatment time on patient outcomes has become widely used around the world by radiation therapy departments with significant waiting times. This study contributes to an evidenced-based method for the development of a priority system for all patients requiring radiotherapy. In our department, high-risk postoperative head and neck patients are allocated the highest priority regarding commencement date of PORT.

With coordinated care, the majority of patients should be able to commence PORT treatment within 4 weeks of surgery, and hence, an overall treatment time of < 11 weeks is readily achievable. This study emphasized the importance of coordinated care from the head and neck team (surgeons, radiation oncologists, dieticians, nurses, speech pathologists, and dentists) to enable the patient to be ready to commence PORT within 4 weeks of surgery. This "coordinated care" was a forerunner to the current multidisciplinary care model in most head and neck cancer departments.

The increased rate of confluent (Grade 3) mucositis was, not surprisingly, significantly higher in the patients receiving 63 Gy compared to 57.6 Gy, but this study quantified that increase (36% versus 16%). This information is another building block of knowledge that can be incorporated into subsequent, quite different studies. For example, there are various current studies aiming to reduce the acute and late treatment toxicity in good prognosis patients, such as those with HPV-positive oropharyngeal cancer. With this in mind the ECOG 1308 study is using similar doses (54 Gy in 27 fractions over 5.5 weeks) to the postoperative intermediate dose of this study in HPV-positive patients who have had a complete response to induction chemotherapy.

This current study also demonstrated the poor outcomes of high-risk patients treated *optimally* with surgery and PORT (24% LR failure) and suggested the need for more intensive treatment in this group. This work has subsequently been completed by cooperative study groups (RTOG and EORTC). Those studies showed that the outcomes for patients with ECE and/or positive surgical margins could be improved by adding concurrent chemotherapy to PORT.

The overall message is the value of clinical research in improving patient outcomes. Each block of information scientifically obtained and shared within the international and interdisciplinary head and neck communities builds a bigger and clearer picture of how we can optimize patient care.

INTENSITY-MODULATED RADIOTHERAPY IN THE TREATMENT OF NASOPHARYNGEAL CARCINOMA: AN UPDATE OF THE UCSF EXPERIENCE

Nancy Y Lee, Ping Xia, Jeanne M Quivey, et al.

Purpose: To update our experience with intensity-modulated radiotherapy (IMRT) in the treatment of nasopharyngeal carcinoma (NPC).

Methods and Materials: Between April 1995 and October 2000, 67 patients underwent IMRT for NPC at the University of California-San Francisco (UCSF). There were 20 females and 47 males, with a mean age of 49 (range 17–82). The disease was Stage I in 8 (12%), Stage II in 12 (18%), Stage III in 22 (33%), and Stage IV in 25 (37%). IMRT was delivered using three different techniques: (1) manually cut partial transmission blocks, (2) computer-controlled auto-sequencing segmental multileaf collimator (SMLC), and (3) sequential tomotherapy using a dynamic multivane intensity modulating collimator (MIMiC). Fifty patients received concomitant cisplatinum and adjuvant cisplatinum and 5-FU chemotherapy according to the Intergroup 0099 trial. Twenty-six patients had fractionated high-dose-rate intracavitary brachytherapy boost and 1 patient had gamma knife radiosurgery boost after external beam radiotherapy.

The prescribed dose was 65–70 Gy to the gross tumor volume (GTV) and positive neck nodes, 60 Gy to the clinical target volume (CTV), 50-60 Gy to the clinically negative neck, and 5-7 Gy in 2 fractions for the intracavitary brachytherapy boost. Acute and late normal tissue effects were graded according to the Radiation Therapy Oncology Group (RTOG) radiation morbidity scoring criteria. The local progression-free, local-regional progression-free, distant metastasis-free rates, and the overall survival were calculated using the Kaplan-Meier method.

Results: With a median follow-up of 31 months (range 7 to 72 months), there has been one local recurrence at the primary site. One patient failed in the neck. Seventeen patients developed distant metastases; 5 of these patients have died. The 4-year estimates of local progression-free, local-regional progression-free, and distant metastases-free rates were 97%, 98%, and 66% respectively. The 4-year estimate of overall survival was 88%. The worst acute toxicity documented was as follows: Grade 1 or 2 in 51 patients, Grade 3 in 15 patients, and Grade 4 in 1 patient. The worst late toxicity was Grade 1 in 20 patients, Grade 2 in 15 patients, Grade 3 in 7 patients, and Grade 4 in 1 patient. At 3 months after IMRT, 64% of the patients had Grade 2, 28% had Grade 1, and 8% had Grade 0 xerostomia. Xerostomia decreased with time. At 24 months, only one of the 41 evaluable patients had Grade 2, 32% had Grade 1 and 66% had Grade 0 or no xerostomia. Analysis of the dose-volume histograms (DVHs) showed that the average maximum, mean, and minimum dose delivered were 79.3 Gy, 74.5 Gy, and 49.4 Gy to the GTV, and 78.9 Gy, 68.7 Gy, and 36.8 Gy to the CTV. An average of only 3% of the GTV and 3% of the CTV received less than 95% of the prescribed dose.

Conclusion: Excellent local-regional control for NPC was achieved with IMRT. IMRT provided excellent tumor target coverage and allowed the delivery of a high dose to the target with significant sparing of the salivary glands and other nearby critical normal tissues.

Lee N, Xia P, Quivey JM, et al. Intensity-modulated radiotherapy in the treatment of nasopharyngeal carcinoma: an update of the UCSF experience. Int J Radiat Oncol Biol Phys. 2002;53:12-22.

Commentary by: *Brian O'Sullivan*

The paper by Lee et al. "Intensity-modulated radiotherapy in the treatment of nasopharyngeal carcinoma: an update of the UCSF experience" changed radiotherapy practice for nasopharyngeal cancer (NPC) significantly, globally, and through a process that might be considered unusual in today's medicine.

In contemporary medicine, we are taught to adopt changes in practice based on robust data and experience, generally considered to require randomized controlled trials, preferably supported by results of confirmatory trials. It is useful to also have properly conducted systematic studies that integrate experience from the randomized trials in the form of individual patient-based meta-analyses. Indeed, some critical academics might argue that these are the only acceptable standards and that other forms of evidence are not relevant, could be misleading, and certainly should not influence worldwide practice for a generation of physicians; even more importantly, the patients of those physicians should not be exposed to the potential risks and costs associated with certain medical innovations in the absence of Level 1 evidence. It is interesting to reflect on these principles as we look back at this landmark paper under discussion and published more than a decade ago by our colleagues at the University of California, San Francisco.

So what can we say about an understated updated experience from an individual center on just 67 patients with NPC treated in the 1990s without a control group and who were not enrolled in a clinical trial? Undoubtedly, for the reasons mentioned already, some might have felt it should not be regarded seriously, or would claim that the experience should at least have been subjected to validation in a randomized trial. And in principle they would be right, and most of us would generally embrace that standard; however, in the case of Nancy Lee's report of IMRT for NPC, time has shown that they would also have been wrong.

Possibly only those who actually treat NPC truly appreciated the impact of the 2001 paper published on the maturing results of a treatment applied to NPC by Karen Fu and her colleagues in the prior decade. Such a treatment had already been used in other head and neck cancers, especially by investigators at the University of Michigan, and with results indicating the ability to spare many patients from the morbidity of permanent and irreversible xerostomia. But NPC is not a common disease in Michigan, and no reports emanated about its treatment with IMRT from those investigators. Instead, an accident of geography yielded a population in large need of a treatment that improved outcome in terms of tumor control and amelioration of normal tissue toxicity. And medicine overall, head and neck oncology in particular, and especially our patients, have been rewarded by the disciplined innovation and careful application of radiation oncology principles to a new radiotherapy modality by clinical investigators in San Francisco. Thus, Asian people residing in proximity to San Francisco and who understandably suffered from NPC in greater numbers than the remainder of the North American population became the subjects and beneficiaries of IMRT for this disease, which led to this remarkable practice-changing report.

In previous eras, radiation therapy alone had shown efficacy in local control for early-stage nasopharyngeal carcinoma, but the available radiotherapy techniques had been associated with loco-regional recurrence rates as high as 50%. For example, even large experienced centers exemplified by the Hong Kong study reported by Anne Lee and her colleagues, provided a local control rate of only 61% in 5,037 patients treated over a 10-year period. Several factors might have contributed to these low reported local control rates, but inadequate dose to the primary site and treatment of more advanced stage disease are the likely culprits. At the same time, Carlos Perez and colleagues at Washington University observed that increasing doses of radiation resulted in nasopharynx tumor control in 80% of patients receiving 66–70 Gy and 100% of those receiving over 70 Gy in the T1, T2, and T3 tumors. However, the tumor control rate did not rise above 55% even for doses over 70 Gy in T4 lesions, illustrating the problem of larger, more complex tumors being more difficult to treat without risk of damage to critical structures. And while Palazzi and colleagues in Milan reported a 5-year local control rate of 84% with conventional radiotherapy in 2004, it was at the cost of significantly higher adverse effects, making the continuation if this approach untenable if an alternative radiotherapy strategy was available. It also underlined the ethical problems of performing randomized trials of IMRT in the more advanced settings of NPC. Such patients are faced with the dual hazard in a control arm of potential underdosage of tumor to avoid vulnerable normal anatomy or alternatively maintaining the control rate but accepting toxicity that could be extreme and indeed unacceptable (e.g., visual loss due to the proximity of the optic apparatus).

When Nancy Lee and her colleagues at UCSF reported a loco-regional control approaching 100% using IMRT, the landscape of the treatment of NPC changed forever. The paper was an update of an equally dramatic prior report but with additional patients and longer follow-up. Only one local failure was seen, a patient with T4N1 disease who was not a candidate for concurrent chemotherapy due to underlying medical conditions. The report also provides detailed technical and toxicity information concerning the delivery and outcome of IMRT and emphasizes the need for chemotherapy in locally advanced disease.

The change to using IMRT was understandably slow in some jurisdictions, likely related to the rarity of the disease in those areas and the need to implement a technological laden nascent treatment approach. But the change has still been unyielding and occurred quickly in other jurisdictions and now represents the contemporary standard for the treatment of NPC. Unfortunately, it likely remains beyond reach in some areas of the developing world where NPC has its greatest incidence and remains a challenge for those countries and their governments. Nonetheless, the UCSF paper set the bar for a modern standard that exceeds 90% local control in a disease in which this was so difficult to achieve previously. Once a clear advantage in favor of IMRT for NPC was generally accepted in the radiation oncology community, clinical equipoise was no longer considered present, and IMRT came to be considered as the standard of care in jurisdictions where it could be provided.

And how did such a small study achieve this impact, and was the reported effect correct and reproducible, the true test of the value and impact of a new treatment? In fact, publications in the intervening years have recapitulated the result in numerous institutions, and clinical trials have also addressed specific issues. The RTOG confirmed that it can be applied with the same success across numerous institutions in a single-arm phase II study, two groups in Hong Kong have independently reported randomized trials in early-stage NPC and showed improvement in xerostomia and/or quality of life in the IMRT arm, and a recent large randomized phase III trial from China addressing all stages of NPC is positive, thereby confirming the overall principles of toxicity and efficacy originally reported from UCSF.

In finalizing this commentary about this unusual, powerful, and pivotal report on a small cohort of patients, it is worth considering it again in the context of our views about evidence-based medicine. As noted earlier, we regard the robust randomized trial and accompanying meta-analysis as the gold standard in providing level 1 evidence appropriate to change practice. However, forgotten in this principled philosophy is a third element in the nature of evidence that might also be suitable but is less common, certainly rarely emphasized, but was described in the original outline of the principles of evidence-based medicine by Sackett and colleagues. Specifically, they also included the situation when a specific result can be considered the equivalent of level 1 evidence when there is complete elimination of an adverse event and there is no plausible reason to suspect inferior efficacy; in such very rare situations a randomized study is not required to support the assertion of benefit. This has happened from time to time in medicine. Penicillin is one example. So too, seems IMRT in the case of NPC. For this, we must congratulate Nancy Lee, Karen Fu, and their colleagues at UCSF for changing the practice of head and neck oncology so directly and specifically with one small pivotal report, and so meaningfully for countless generations of our patients.

HYPERFRACTIONATED OR ACCELERATED RADIOTHERAPY IN HEAD AND NECK CANCER: A META-ANALYSIS

Jean Bourhis, Jens Overgaard, Hélène Audry, et al.

Background: Several trials have studied the role of unconventional fractionated radiotherapy in head and neck squamous cell carcinoma, but the effect of such treatment on survival is not clear. The aim of this meta-analysis was to assess whether this type of radiotherapy could improve survival.

Methods: Randomized trials comparing conventional radiotherapy with hyper-fractionated or accelerated radiotherapy, or both, in patients with non-metastatic HNSCC were identified and updated individual patient data were obtained. Overall survival was the main endpoint. Trials were grouped in three pre-specified categories: hyperfractionated, accelerated, and accelerated with total dose reduction.

Findings: 15 trials with 6,515 patients were included. The median follow-up was 6 years. Tumors sites were mostly oropharynx and larynx; 5,221 (74%) patients had stage III-IV disease (International Union Against Cancer, 1987). There was a significant survival benefit with altered fractionated radiotherapy, corresponding to an absolute benefit of 3.4% at 5 years (hazard ratio 0.92, 95% CI 0.86–0.97; p = 0.003). The benefit was significantly higher with hyperfractionated radiotherapy (8% at 5 years) than with accelerated radiotherapy (2% with accelerated fractionation without total dose reduction and 1.7% with total dose reduction at 5 years, p = 0.02). There was a benefit on locoregional control in favor of altered fractionation versus conventional radiotherapy (6.4% at 5 years; p < 0.0001), which was particularly efficient in reducing local failure, whereas the benefit on nodal control was less pronounced. The benefit was significantly higher in the youngest patients [hazard ratio 0.78 (0.65–0.94) for under 50-year olds, 0.95 (0.83–1.09) for 51–60-year olds, 0.92 (0.81–1.06) for 61–70-year olds, and 1.08 (0.89–1.30) for over 70-year olds; test for trends p = 0.007].

Interpretation: Altered fractionated radiotherapy improves survival in patients with head and neck squamous cell carcinoma. Comparison of the different types of altered radiotherapy suggests that hyperfractionation has the greatest benefit.

Bourhis J, Overgaard J, Audry H, et al.; Meta-Analysis of Radiotherapy in Carcinoma of Head and Neck (MARCH) Collaborative Group. Hyperfractionated or accelerated radiotherapy in head and neck cancer: a meta-analysis. Lancet. 2006;368:843-854.

Commentary by: *David M Brizel*

Standard fractionation radiotherapy (RT) for head and neck cancer (HNC) typically consists of once daily 2 Gy fractions to total doses of 66–70 Gy. Local-regional control and overall survival range from 70% to 90% for early stage (I and II) disease. This approach is far less effective for locally advanced stage III and IV disease. Overall, locoregional control and survival range from 10% to 40% in this setting.

Both tumor and patient host-related factors limit the effectiveness of conventionally fractionated RT in the treatment of locally advanced head and neck cancer. RT is given on a fractionated daily basis in order to take advantage of important radiobiologic principles including re-oxygenation of hypoxic cells and redistribution of cells into more sensitive phases of the cell cycle. One tradeoff to the benefits of daily fractionation is prolongation of the total treatment time. Squamous cell head and neck cancers have rapid potential cellular doubling times of 3–5 days. It has been estimated that 0.5–0.6 Gy of a typical 2 Gy fraction of radiation is used to compensate for tumor repopulation that has taken place in the day elapsed since a previous fraction. Consequently, the probability of eradicating a tumor with any given cumulative total dose of irradiation is dependent not just on the magnitude of that cumulative dose but also the total time in which that dose is delivered, shorter total times being expected to succeed more often than longer times.

Accelerated fractionation (AF) is the strategy designed to address tumor repopulation. The total treatment time is shortened via the use of multiple daily fractions, which are either the same size as conventional once daily fractions or slightly smaller, e.g. 1.6–2.0 Gy. The shortening of the overall treatment time will increase the severity of acute side effects such as mucositis. A decrease in the total dose delivered becomes necessary to prevent acute toxicity from escalating to intolerable levels as total treatment times become very short (< 6 weeks).

Hyperfractionation (HF) represents a different strategy for improving the therapeutic index. HF also uses multiple daily fractions, but they are considerably smaller (1.1–1.2 Gy) than those utilized in accelerated regimens. Hyperfractionated regimens are designed to overcome therapeutic resistance by increasing the total cumulative dose delivered compared to conventional once daily fractionation without increasing the risk of long-term late toxicity. Long-term complications are largely a function of the size of the dose per fraction, with smaller fractions being less toxic.

Retrospective evaluations of single-institution programs of both AF and HF that were published in the 1970s and 1980s suggested that both of these approaches might be superior to conventional once daily fractionation in locally advanced non-metastatic disease settings. Subsequently, prospective randomized trials of AF and/or HF were conducted to test these hypotheses. The results of these first studies were published in the early 1990s. These studies all suggested that there were improvements in locoregional control and perhaps survival.

The meta-analysis of fractionation study (MARCH) by Bourhis et al. provides extensive insight into the effect that HF and AF have on survival. It represents the second of three landmark publications that have significantly influenced the management of head and neck cancer. The findings are very robust because of the vigorous methodology employed by the investigators. The analysis plan was developed prospectively, and the protocol itself was published in the Cochrane Library. A steering committee comprised of an internationally prominent group of head and neck oncologists was constituted at the outset. They prospectively identified three distinct fractionation strategies by which to classify trials that were comparing altered fractionation against standard fractionation. The first of these was HF, which examined the effect of an increased total dose given in the same total treatment time relative to conventional fractionation. The second group of studies, AF, measured the effect of a reduction in the total treatment time without any reduction in the total dose delivered. The third group of trials used AF to decrease the total treatment time but also reduced the total dose delivered. Additional inclusion criteria were that trials had to use radiotherapy as the primary treatment modality with curative intent, use fraction sizes ≤ 2.5 Gy in the control arm, and deliver the equivalent of 66–70 Gy in 2 Gy fractions. Postoperative radiotherapy trials and studies that included concurrent chemotherapy were excluded. Trials performed from 1969–1999 were eligible.

Several aspects of this meta-analysis make its findings particularly powerful. Many meta-analyses only evaluate trials that have been published in the peer-reviewed literature. The MARCH Group also identified unpublished trials and those reported in abstract format only and incorporated them into their database. This approach helps to overcome the effect of publication bias, which often leads to the non-publication of negative trials, and it provides a more realistic picture of the effectiveness of the therapeutic interventions under investigation. Furthermore, the investigators contacted the principal investigators from the individual trials and subsequently obtained updated individual patient data from each trial for their analysis. This strategy provides the most up-to-date results of the trials being evaluated, quite often more contemporary than that contained in the original publications themselves.

The steering committee initially identified 26 potentially eligible trials but excluded 9 of them: three were postoperative trials, two used unconventional fractionation schemes in the control arm, one had a biased randomization scheme, and three utilized hypofractionated irradiation in the investigational arm. The remaining 15 trials, with a total of 6,515 patients and a median follow-up of 6 years (range 4–10 years), constituted the population for this meta-analysis.

The MARCH study showed that altered fractionation resulted in an 8% reduction in the risk of death compared with standard fractionation, which translated into an absolute improvement in survival of 3.4% at 5 years. The survival benefit resulted primarily from an improvement in local control, with a lesser but still significant improvement in regional disease control. Distant recurrence was not affected by the fractionation strategy. HF and AF without dose reduction were equally effective in the improvement of local control, but HF led to an 8% absolute improvement in survival compared to 2.2% for AF without dose reduction. AF with total dose reduction did not significantly improve survival.

The superior survival of HF compared to AF without dose reduction must be interpreted cautiously given that local control was the same with the two regimens. The AF studies had a higher proportion of patients with early stage disease and larynx cancer than the HF trials, which may explain part of the discrepancy. Survival tends to be very good in both of these settings even with improvements in local control because of the availability of effective salvage options when failure does occur.

Concurrent chemoradiation constitutes the current non-surgical standard of care for locally advanced HNC. Most of the trials that comprise the MARCH study were conducted in an era when RT alone was the standard of care. They were also performed in an era of non-conformal radiotherapy prior to the widespread adoption of intensity-modulated radiotherapy (IMRT). These two facts must also be kept in mind as one interprets the findings of MARCH.

A higher incidence of non-cancer related deaths was observed in the trials that used AF without dose reduction compared to the trials that used HF. Concurrent chemoradiation is known to cause both more acute and late morbidity than conventional RT alone. RTOG 9003 showed that AF without dose reduction has more late morbidity than HF. Recently, the accelerated RT alone control arm of GORTEC 9902 demonstrated increased acute and late morbidity compared with standard fractionation chemoradiation. Since HF is designed to maintain parity vis a vis conventional fractionation with respect to late toxicity and AF is not, it is reasonable to expect that excessive morbidity from AF may negate much of the improvement in efficacy when non-conformal techniques are used.

RTOG 0129 and GORTEC 9902 both compared standard fractionation chemoradiation against chemoradiation that used AF without dose reduction. Both studies showed that AF did not add any benefit in this setting. The finding in MARCH that conventional fractionation is inferior to altered fractionation therefore cannot be applied to the concurrent chemoradiation arena. The *de facto* radiotherapeutic dose escalation derived from concurrent chemotherapy as originally reported in 2007 by Kasibhatla may exceed that which is achievable from modification of fractionation.

IMRT is more time and labor expensive and more costly than 3-D conformal or 2-D non-conformal RT. The cost of delivering hyperfractionated IMRT is 75–100% more than for non-IMRT techniques. It is also more logistically challenging for patients. IMRT allows for much more precise delineation of both tumor/target volumes and normal organs with improved ability to spare critical structures including the mandible, major salivary glands, and pharyngeal constrictor muscles. This ability should help to make AF without dose reduction a more attractive strategy for RT alone than the MARCH study would otherwise suggest.

Chapter 18

Medical Oncology

THE USE OF THE NITROGEN MUSTARDS IN THE PALLIATIVE TREATMENT OF CARCINOMA
With Particular Reference to Bronchogenic Carcinoma

David A Karnofsky, Walter H Abelmann, Lloyd F Craver, et al.

The therapeutic value of the nitrogen mustards in the palliative treatment of Hodgkin's disease, lymphosarcoma, leukemia, and allied disorders has been established by numerous publications in the past two years. Other types of cancer have been treated much less extensively with the nitrogen mustards, largely because the results, in the occasional cases reported, have not been impressive. In the course of our study of the effects of the nitrogen mustards on various types of neoplastic disease, we obtained a remarkable temporary remission in a patient with an anaplastic carcinoma of the lung. This observation prompted the more extensive trial of the nitrogen mustards in primary lung carcinoma, and our results form the basis for this report. Our therapeutic experiences with several other types of cancer are also briefly described in order to compare them with the lung-tumor group.

Karnofsky DA, Abelmann WH, Craver LF, et al. The use of nitrogen mustards in the palliative treatment of carcinoma. Cancer. 1948;1:634-656.

Commentary by: *Matthew G Fury*

Karnofsky, Abelmann, Craver, and Burchenal described the first extensive experience with nitrogen mustards in the treatment of advanced solid tumors in 1948. Table 1 presents the baseline performance status scores of the subjects in the study population. In this study population, the reported baseline performance scores ranged from 20 ("Very sick; hospitalization necessary; active supportive treatment necessary") to 70 ("Cares for self. Unable to carry on normal activity or do active work").

The study population included 35 patients with inoperable lung cancer. The average age was 57 years. Pathologic confirmation was obtained in all cases. Thirteen cases were described as anaplastic bronchogenic carcinoma, including 6 of the oat-cell type. The dose of nitrogen mustard (HN2) given usually was 0.1 mg/kg daily for 4 days, although different dosing schemes were used for some patients. The most important toxic effect of the treatment was deemed to be hematopoietic injury. The therapeutic principle was "...to give the maximum amount of HN2 that will not produce serious

Table 1: Performance Status		
Definition	*%*	*Criteria*
Able to carry on normal activity and to work. No special care is needed	100	Normal; no complaints; no evidence of disease
	90	Able to carry on normal activity; minor signs or symptoms of disease
	80	Normal activity with effort; some signs or symptoms of disease
Unable to work. Able to live at home, care for most personal needs. A varying amount of assistance is needed	70	Cares for self. Unable to carry on normal activity or to do active work
	60	Requires occasional assistance, but is able to care for most of his needs
	50	Requires considerable assistance and frequent medical care
Unable to care for self. Requires equivalent of institutional or hospital care. Disease may be progressing rapidly	40	Disabled; requires special care and assistance
	30	Severely disabled; hospitalization is indicated although death not imminent
	20	Very sick; hospitalization necessary; active supportive treatment necessary
	10	Moribund; fatal processes progressing rapidly
	0	Dead

toxic complications". Using broadly defined efficacy criteria that included symptomatic improvement, 74% of the lung cancer patients "showed some immediate, favorable response". Radiographic response to treatment also was evaluated with X-rays. The average survival of this group of patients was 3 months, ranging from 2 months to 8 months.

The manuscript also describes a separate population of 18 patients with advanced solid tumors other than lung cancer, including 5 patients with genitourinary malignancies and 2 men with squamous cell carcinoma of the base of the tongue that had been previously irradiated. The two head and neck cancer patients did not respond to therapy and had a rapid downhill course. However, evidence of brief clinical improvement was observed against genitourinary malignancies (3 patients), neurogenic cancers (2 patients), and gastrointestinal and gynecological malignancies (1 each).

Table 1 of this manuscript went on to become one of the most widely used instruments in oncology clinical research. It became known as the Karnofsky Performance Status (KPS), and helped establish uniform criteria for describing the fitness of cancer patients in a research study. Use of the KPS provided early insight into the fundamental oncologic principle that cancer patients with lower fitness are less likely to derive any benefit from exposure to chemotherapy compared with patients with higher KPS scores.

Prior to this manuscript, the clinical efficacy of nitrogen mustards against certain hematologic malignancies had been well established, but there was limited experience using this type of treatment for patients with solid tumors. The concept of dose-limiting bone marrow toxicity guided the development of many of the subsequent chemotherapy agents that are in use today. The manuscript provided proof-of-principle that systemic chemotherapy can achieve a palliative benefit in some patients with advanced solid tumors. Karnofsky and colleagues also helped establish standards for the systematic evaluation of chemotherapy agents, such as the description of baseline characteristics of the study population, pathologic confirmation of each case, detailed explanation of the administration of therapeutic regimen, description of treatment-related toxicities, and the use of defined criteria to assess efficacy. Although the conventions for evaluating new chemotherapy agents have become increasingly formalized over the years—and the technological impacts of high resolution radiologic imaging and of cellular and molecular biology have transformed the field of medical oncology entirely—much of the basic framework for collecting and reporting clinical data in this landmark study still is evident in contemporary oncology research.

A PHASE III RANDOMIZED STUDY COMPARING CISPLATIN AND FLUOROURACIL AS SINGLE AGENTS AND IN COMBINATION FOR ADVANCED SQUAMOUS CELL CARCINOMA OF THE HEAD AND NECK

Charlotte Jacobs, Gary Lyman, Enrique Velez-Garcia, et al.

Purpose: To determine whether combination chemotherapy is superior to single agents for recurrent/metastatic head and neck cancer, we compared the efficacy and toxicity of cisplatin (CP) and fluorouracil (5-FU), alone and in combination in a phase III trial.

Patients and Methods: Two hundred forty-nine patients with recurrent head and neck cancer were randomized to one of three treatment: CP (100 mg/m²) and 5-FU (1 g/m² × 4), CP, or 5-FU every 3 weeks.

Results: The overall response rate to the combination (32%) was superior to that of CP (17%) or 5-FU (13%) (p = .035). Response was associated with good performance status (PS) but not with primary site, site of recurrence, histology, prior irradiation, or relative dose intensity. Median time to progression was less than 2.5 months, and there was no significant difference in median survival (5.7 months) among the groups. By multivariate analysis, patients with better PS and poorly differentiated tumors had superior survival. Hematologic toxicity and alopecia were worse in the combination arm.

Conclusion: Although the response rate to the combination of CP plus 5-FU was superior to that achieved with single agents, survival did not improve.

Jacobs C, Lyman G, Velez-Garcia E, et al. A phase III randomized study comparing cisplatin and fluorouracil as single agents and in combination for advanced squamous cell carcinoma of the head and neck. J Clin Oncol.1992;10;257-263.

Commentary by: *Merril S Kies*

While head and neck cancer doctors know that powerful local treatment strategies with surgery and radiotherapy have traditional and secure roles in the management of this diverse group of diseases, there has long been a huge need for complementary systemic treatments. Patients often present with advanced regional tumors and have significant risk of recurrence after primary surgery or radiotherapy. Indeed, some patients present with distant metastases, and subgroups of patients with nasopharyngeal cancer or bulky cervical nodal metastases at diagnosis may have a 25–40% risk of developing distant disease despite effective local treatment. These patients have long been candidates for drug therapy. And so much excitement was generated with the early observations of tumor responses to cytotoxic drugs such as methotrexate, fluorouracil, and cisplatin. The capacity for substantial tumor responses was first observed in patients with distant metastases, but found to be more profound when chemotherapy was administered as an induction regimen to patients with regionally advanced disease but no previous therapy.

Questions quickly arose as to how best to administer these cytotoxic principles—should there be sequential therapies and drug combinations? Could chemotherapy be administered as an effective adjunct to surgery or radiotherapy for organ preservation, or even to improve local and regional disease control?

In the 1970s, as medical oncology was approaching adolescence, Muhyi Al-Sarraf and colleagues demonstrated the high activity and promise of the cisplatin and infusional fluorouracil combination, and in the setting of recurrent or distant metastatic disease, the regimen was widely used. However, there were important ancillary questions: was toxicity excessive? Did a tumor response lead to advancing survival? Could scientific data be generated that would give direction to clinical practice, which we now refer to as the practice of evidence-based medicine? And how were cancer doctors to ask questions in a practical way that honored the need of patients for best available treatment while providing critical outcomes data to ultimately advance clinical care? Charlotte Jacobs and her associates showed us a way.

This early paper by Jacobs C, Lyman G, Velez-Garcia, et al. addressed some of these clinically and critically important questions in a prospective and definitive manner. In a multicenter protocol, 243 patients with recurrent or advanced squamous cancer of the head and neck, not amenable to curative salvage local therapy, were randomized to receive cisplatin and 5-fluorouracil or either of these agents as a single compound. The results of the trial were disappointing, as the tumor response rates were modest and there was no demonstration of a tumor control or survival advantage for the combination despite the predictable increase in toxicity. Still, the impact of this paper was as a notable contribution to our understanding of the actual efficacy of the available systemic options at that time and how to start to test the hypotheses. This study provided tangible data. We needed to know where we were with this new clinical science, and of a practical and reliable research strategy for the identification of potentially effective novel therapies. This study demonstrated a workable clinical trial platform that would influence future investigators and contribute to present efforts to practice evidence based medicine. The fundamental approach of the investigators for this report has been a continuing model, affecting the design of numerous studies, among them the EXTREME trial reported by Jan Vermorken, which demonstrated in a similarly prospective controlled trial the statistically significant response and survival value of adding cetuximab to the cisplatin-fluorouracil combination.

CHEMOTHERAPY ADDED TO LOCOREGIONAL TREATMENT FOR HEAD AND NECK SQUAMOUS-CELL CARCINOMA: THREE META-ANALYSES OF UPDATED INDIVIDUAL DATA

Pignon JP, Bourhis J, Domenge C, et al.

Background: Despite more than 70 randomized trials, the effect of chemotherapy on non-metastatic head and neck squamous-cell carcinoma remains uncertain. We did three meta-analyses of the impact of survival on chemotherapy added to locoregional treatment.

Methods: We updated data on all patients in randomized trials between 1965 and 1993. We included patients with carcinoma of the oropharynx, oral cavity, larynx, or hypopharynx.

Findings: The main meta-analysis of 63 trials (10,741 patients) of locoregional treatment with or without chemotherapy yielded a pooled hazard ratio of death of 0.90 (95% CI 0.85–0.94, p < 0.0001), corresponding to an absolute survival benefit of 4% at 2 and 5 years in favor of chemotherapy. There was no significant benefit associated with adjuvant or neoadjuvant chemotherapy. Chemotherapy given concomitantly to radiotherapy gave significant benefits, but heterogeneity of the results prohibit firm conclusions. Meta-analysis of six trials (861 patients) comparing neoadjuvant chemotherapy plus radiotherapy with concomitant or alternating radiochemotherapy yielded a hazard ratio of 0.91 (0.79–1.06) in favor of concomitant or alternating radiochemotherapy. Three larynx-preservation trials (602 patients) compared radical surgery plus radiotherapy with neoadjuvant chemotherapy plus radiotherapy in responders or radical surgery and radiotherapy in non-responders. The hazard ratio of death in the chemotherapy arm as compared with the control arm was 1.19 (0.97–1.46).

Interpretation: Because the main meta-analysis showed only a small significant survival benefit in favor of chemotherapy, the routine use of chemotherapy is debatable. For larynx preservation, the non-significant negative effect of chemo-therapy in the organ-preservation strategy indicates that this procedure must remain investigational.

Pignon JP, Bourhis J, Domenge C, et al. Chemotherapy added to locoregional treatment for head and neck squamous-cell carcinoma: three meta-analyses of updated individual data. MACH-NC Collaborative Group. Meta-Analysis of Chemotherapy on Head and Neck Cancer. Lancet. 2000;355:949-955.

Commentary by: *Jennifer Grandis*

Head and neck squamous cell carcinoma (HNSCC) has historically been treated by primary surgical extirpation followed by adjuvant radiation. The role of chemotherapy has long been debated, and the paucity of appro-priately powered, randomized clinical trials has limited any definitive determination of the relative contribution of systemic chemotherapeutic agents in this disease. To address this gap in knowledge, these authors performed three meta-analyses of all published randomized trials of patients with carcinomas of the oral cavity, pharynx, and larynx. Published in the high-impact scientific journal, *The Lancet*, in 2002, this study summarized the cumulative experience and defined the role of chemotherapy in HNSCC.

The primary meta-analysis focused on 10,741 HNSCC patients enrolled on 63 clinical trials studying locoregional treatment with or without chemotherapy. In these trials, the addition of chemotherapy to radiation as definitive treatment (concomitant chemoradiation) was associated with an absolute survival benefit of 4% at 2 and 5 years. Notably, there was no benefit of chemotherapy when administered in the neoadjuvant or adjuvant setting. The three clinical trials that focused on larynx preservation (total of 602 patients) compared surgery and radiation to neoadjuvant chemotherapy plus radiotherapy in responders or surgery and radiation in non-responders. In these studies, the increased hazard ratio of death in the chemotherapy arm compared with the control arm (1–19; 0.97–1.46) underscored the risks of systemic delivery of cytotoxic agents in this setting. Overall, the authors concluded that there was only a small, but statistically significant, survival benefit with the addition of chemotherapy for locoregional HNSCC.

The strengths of this study included the rigorous methodology employed by the co-authors and attempts to harmonize patient and treatment characteristics across diverse populations. However, meta-analyses are associated with several limitations, including an inability to investigate mechanisms, numerous cases of missing or incomplete data, and a sole reliance on published data without access to primary results. In addition, the authors chose to focus on overall survival rather than any disease-specific survival assessment. While this approach is understandable in the setting of a large-scale meta-analysis, the cause of death is unknown in most cases and the impact of treatment on disease remains elusive. Since the publication of this manuscript, the oncology community has embraced disease-specific endpoints as more likely reflecting the impact of a specific therapeutic intervention.

This study was published prior to several important developments in our understanding of the biology and treatment of head and neck cancer. In the next decade, combined chemoradiation (generally platinum but often taxanes), in which the addition of chemotherapy was understood as radiosensitizing, would replace primary surgical resection for the treatment of many cancers of the pharynx and larynx due to the probably equivalent survival outcomes and improved preservation of key anatomic structures (including the tongue and larynx) with non-operative therapy. The epidermal growth factor receptor (EGFR) was recognized as a prognostic biomarker and therapeutic target, leading to the FDA approval of the monoclonal antibody cetuximab in 2006, in combination with radiation for locally advanced HNSCC. The emergence of the human papilloma virus (HPV) as a primary causative agent in pharyngeal cancer is now widely appreciated in

North America, and the distinct prognosis and clinical characteristics of this virally induced HNSCC suggests that treatments specific for HPV-HNSCC are warranted.

Finally, in this genomic era of medicine, we are now beginning to appreciate the genetic heterogeneity of human HNSCC. The explosion of molecular targeting agents as cancer treatments coupled with the emerging information from large-scale human HNSCC whole exome sequencing studies underscores our need to incorporate personalized medicine approaches based on our understanding of the biology of each patient's tumor. Chemotherapeutic agents that selectively target dividing cells are clearly associated with dose-limiting toxicities. While these agents likely have a role in the treatment of locoregional HNSCC, ongoing and future studies that assess predictive biomarkers will allow us to determine the role of chemotherapy for biologically distinct subsets of this malignancy.

PHASE III RANDOMIZED TRIAL OF CISPLATIN PLUS PLACEBO COMPARED WITH CISPLATIN PLUS CETUXIMAB IN METASTATIC/RECURRENT HEAD AND NECK CANCER: AN EASTERN CO-OPERATIVE ONCOLOGY GROUP STUDY

Barbara Burtness, Meredith A Goldwasser, William Flood, et al.

Purpose: Therapy of recurrent/metastatic squamous cell carcinoma of the head and neck results in median progression-free survival (PFS) of 2 months. These cancers are rich in epidermal growth factor receptor (EGFR). We wished to determine whether the addition of cetuximab, which inhibits activation of EGFR, would improve PFS.

Patients and Methods: Patients with recurrent/metastatic squamous cell carcinoma of the head and neck were randomly assigned to receive cisplatin every 4 weeks, with weekly cetuximab (arm A) or placebo (arm B). Tumor tissue was assayed for EGFR expression by immunohistochemistry. The primary endpoint was PFS. Secondary endpoints of interest were response rate, toxicity, overall survival, and correlation of EGFR with clinical endpoints.

Results: There were 117 analyzable patients enrolled. Median PFS was 2.7 months for arm B and 4.2 months for arm A. The hazard ratio for progression of arm A to arm B was 0.78 (95% CI, 0.54 to 1.12). Median overall survival was 8.0 months for arm B and 9.2 months for arm A (p – 21). The hazard ratio for survival by skin toxicity in cetuximab-treated patients was 0.42 (95% CI, 0.21 to 0.86). Objective response rate was 26% for arm A and 10% for arm B (p – .03). Enhancement of response was greater for patients with EGFR staining present in less than 80% of cells.

Conclusion: Addition of cetuximab to cisplatin significantly improves response rate. There was a survival advantage for the development of rash. Progression-free and overall survival were not significantly improved by the addition of cetuximab in this study.

Burtness B, Goldwasser M, Flood W, et al. Phase III randomized trial of cisplatin plus placebo compared with cisplatin plus cetuximab in metastatic/recurrent head and neck cancer: an Eastern Co-operative Oncology Group study. J Clin Oncol. 2005;23:8646-8654.

Commentary by: *Marshall R Posner*

In 2005, Barbara Burtness and her colleagues published the first randomized phase III clinical trial testing cetuximab plus another agent in recurrent and metastatic head and neck cancer in the *Journal of Clinical Oncology*. The study compared cetuximab plus platinum to cisplatin alone for recurrent and metastatic squamous cell cancer of the head and neck. While the trial did not achieve a positive outcome in its primary endpoint, improved survival in the experimental arm, it did demonstrate in multiple secondary endpoints the value of cetuximab as a treatment for patients with recurrent and metastatic head and neck cancer. This study heralded the dawn of molecularly targeted, EGFR-directed therapy in head and neck cancer, and the positive outcomes and trends identified by the study supported further investigations. Since the publication of this trial in 2005, the value of cetuximab in the treatment of neck cancers has been demonstrated definitively by the EORTC-managed Extreme Trial, which proved a significant response, progression-free survival and survival advantage in recurrent and metastatic squamous cell cancer of the head and neck with combination therapy that included cetuximab compared to treatment without cetuximab. Several other trials of EGFR-directed monoclonal antibodies in recurrent and metastatic squamous cancer of the head and neck have now been studied in phase III trials and have also shown advantages compared to chemotherapy alone.

The ECOG trial was small, ambitious, and relatively underpowered. Only 117 randomized patients were entered, and a modification late in the trial allowed 13 patients who progressed on the control arm to receive cetuximab after progression. Despite being underpowered for survival and allowing crossover, which also diminished the power to observe a significant difference in survival, Burtness and her colleagues demonstrated the safety and feasibility of performing a randomized trial, reported compelling data in several important endpoints that were ultimately assessed in the Extreme Trial, and defined the toxicity of cetuximab in combination with cisplatin. One of the most important positive outcomes in the ECOG trial was a difference in response rates. A significant difference in response rate between the placebo arm (10%) and cetuximab arm (26%) was reported. By achieving a higher response rate in recurrent disease, the combination was shown to have substantial efficacy and potential. There are also a number of other subtle findings in the study that were not fully addressed in the discussion because of the careful and conservative nature of the presentation by ECOG. Notably, although the median survival was not increased significantly, the 2-year survival for patients on the cetuximab arm (16%) was substantially higher than that seen on the control arm (9%), further supporting the positive impact of this agent. This finding suggests that there are some patients who derive long-lasting benefit from cetuximab therapy. Progression-free survival also showed a trend towards improvement, although not significantly so.

Dr Burtness and her colleagues pursued translational studies in this trial and demonstrated the counterintuitive fact that high tumor EGFR expression was associated with a lower response rate compared to moderate and low EGFR expression. While the data are limited because of the small number of patients with informative samples, this work has provided guidance for the extremely difficult task of investigating biomarkers suitable for predicting cetuximab response. Finally, the careful attention and reporting of the nuances of treatment and management were critically important in the design and logistics of future trials and set the stage for the eventual successful evaluation of this agent as part of combination regimens for treatment of patients with advanced recurrent and metastatic cancer. Ultimately, this work provided the basis for the design of the Extreme Trial, which led to the approval of combination therapy with cetuximab in Europe and has guided modern standard therapy in North America.

As a result of the ECOG Team efforts and the works of others as a result of this paper, cetuximab has become a standard, useful therapy for patients with recurrent and metastatic squamous cell cancer of the head and neck.

RADIOTHERAPY PLUS CETUXIMAB FOR SQUAMOUS-CELL CARCINOMA OF THE HEAD AND NECK

James A Bonner, Paul M Harari, Jordi Giralt, et al.

Background: We conducted a multinational, randomized study to compare radiotherapy alone with radiotherapy plus cetuximab, a monoclonal antibody against the epidermal growth factor receptor, in the treatment of locoregionally advanced squamous-cell carcinoma of the head and neck.

Methods: Patients with locoregionally advanced head and neck cancer were randomly assigned to treatment with high-dose radiotherapy alone (213 patients) or high-dose radiotherapy plus weekly cetuximab (211 patients) at an initial dose of 400 mg per square meter of body-surface area, followed by 250 mg per square meter weekly for the duration of radiotherapy. The primary end point was the duration of control of locoregional disease; secondary end points were overall survival, progression-free survival, the response rate, and safety.

Results: The median duration of locoregional control was 24.4 months among patients treated with cetuximab plus radiotherapy and 14.9 months among those given radiotherapy alone (hazard ratio for locoregional progression or death, 0.68; p = 0.005). With a median follow-up of 54.0 months, the median duration of overall survival was 49.0 months among patients treated with combined therapy and 29.3 months among those treated with radiotherapy alone (hazard ratio for death, 0.74; p = 0.03). Radiotherapy plus cetuximab significantly prolonged progression-free survival (hazard ratio for disease progression or death, 0.70; p = 0.006). With the exception of acneiform rash and infusion reactions, the incidence of grade 3 or greater toxic effects, including mucositis, did not differ significantly between the two groups.

Conclusions: Treatment of locoregionally advanced head and neck cancer with concomitant high-dose radiotherapy plus cetuximab improves locoregional control and reduces mortality without increasing the common toxic effects associated with radiotherapy to the head and neck.

Bonner JA, Harari PM, Giralt J, et al. Radiotherapy plus cetuximab for squamous-cell carcinoma of the head and neck. N Engl J Med. 2006;354:567-78.

Commentary by: *Jatin P Shah*

The increased effectiveness of combining chemotherapy with radiotherapy in organ preservation and overall tumor control of squamous cell carcinomas of the head and neck sparked interest in extending that philosophy to other primary sites. However, the high-grade acute toxicity and long-term sequelae of cytotoxic drugs given concurrently or sequentially with radiotherapy dampened the enthusiasm to intensify the concurrent chemoradiotherapy treatment programs. Clearly, there was the need to identify combinations of other drugs with radiotherapy to reduce toxicity while maintaining oncologic efficacy. Cetuximab, a IgG1 monoclonal antibody against the ligand-binding domain of EGFR, had been shown to enhance the cytotoxic effects of radiation therapy in squamous cell carcinoma.

This study attempted to demonstrate the increased therapeutic index combining cetuximab with radiotherapy compared to radiotherapy alone in a randomized fashion.

This is the report of a multi-center randomized trial comparing high-dose radiotherapy alone to high-dose radiotherapy plus cetuximab. A total of 424 patients from 73 centers in the United States and 14 from other countries were accrued on the trial. The duration of local-regional control was significantly longer in patients on the treatment arm compared to the radiotherapy alone arm. The median duration of locoregional control in the study arm was 24.4 months compared to 14.9 months with radiation alone. Overall, adding cetuximab to radiotherapy resulted in a 32% reduction in the risk of locoregional progression. Similarly, the median survival time on the study arm was 49 months compared to 29.3 months with radiotherapy alone. Thus, there was a 26% reduction in the risk of death. Median progression-free survival in the study arm was 17.1 months compared to 12.4 months with radiotherapy alone. However, the cumulative rates of incidence of distant metastases at 1 and 2 years were similar in the two groups.

This trial demonstrated a significantly increased duration of locoregional control of disease and survival among patients with locoregionally advanced head and neck cancer. Thus, cetuximab plus radiotherapy was observed to be superior to radiotherapy alone in increasing both the duration of locoregional disease control and survival in locoregionally advanced head and neck cancer. One criticism of this study, however, is that this randomized trial compared radiotherapy alone vs radiotherapy plus cetuximab. It would have been highly desirable if a direct comparison was made between cetuximab with radiotherapy compared to cisplatinum with radiotherapy. Such a trial would have given an answer to many unanswered questions regarding the role of EGFR inhibitors and its comparison to cytotoxic drugs such as cisplatinum. Nevertheless, this is the first trial which demonstrated the efficacy and utility of EGFR inhibitors given concomitantly with radiotherapy. A major paradigm shift has occurred as a result of this study with reference to the utility of this drug in those patients who are either not candidates for or unable to tolerate cisplatinum concurrently with radiotherapy for locoregionally advanced head and neck cancer.

CISPLATIN AND FLUOROURACIL ALONE OR WITH DOCETAXEL IN HEAD AND NECK CANCER

Marshall R Posner, Diane M Hershock, Cesar R Blajman, et al.

Background: A randomized phase 3 trial of the treatment of squamous-cell carcinoma of the head and neck compared induction chemotherapy with docetaxel plus cisplatin and fluorouracil (TPF) with cisplatin and fluorouracil (PF), followed by chemoradiotherapy.

Methods: We randomly assigned 501 patients (all of whom had stage III or IV disease with no distant metastases and tumors considered to be unresectable or were candidates for organ preservation) to receive either TPF or PF induction chemotherapy, followed by chemoradiotherapy with weekly carboplatin therapy and radiotherapy for 5 days per week. The primary end point was overall survival.

Results: With a minimum of 2 years of follow-up (≥ 3 years for 69% of patients), significantly more patients survived in the TPF group than in the PF group (hazard ratio for death, 0.70; p = 0.006). Estimates of overall survival at 3 years were 62% in the TPF group and 48% in the PF group; the median overall survival was 71 months and 30 months, respectively (p = 0.006). There was better locoregional control in the TPF group than in the PF group (p = 0.04), but the incidence of distant metastases in the two groups did not differ significantly (p = 0.14). Rates of neutropenia and febrile neutropenia were higher in the TPF group; chemotherapy was more frequently delayed because of hematologic adverse events in the PF group.

Conclusions: Patients with squamous-cell carcinoma of the head and neck who received docetaxel plus cisplatin and fluorouracil induction chemotherapy plus chemoradiotherapy had a significantly longer survival than did patients who received cisplatin and fluorouracil induction chemotherapy plus chemoradiotherapy.

Posner MR, Hershock DM, Blajman CR, et al. Cisplatin and fluorouracil alone or with docetaxel in head and neck cancer. N Engl J Med. 2007;357:1705-1715.

Commentary by: *Matthew G Fury*

This 2007 TAX 324 manuscript by Posner and colleagues established TPF (Taxotere, Cisplatin, 5-Fluorouracil) as superior induction chemotherapy compared with PF. This manuscript was published in the same issue of the *New England Journal of Medicine* with the similar TAX 323 study. Taken together, the TAX 323 and TAX 324 studies established TPF as the regimen of choice for fit patients with head and neck cancer deemed to be appropriate candidates for induction chemotherapy.

PF was studied as an induction chemotherapy regimen in the 1980s. For patients with bulky locally and/or regionally advanced HNSCC, the strategy of induction chemotherapy prior to definitive radiation therapy (RT) had several theoretical advantages. Induction chemotherapy allows for early systemic therapy of microscopic disease, which might decrease the risk of the subsequent development of gross distant metastatic disease. Induction chemotherapy can also decrease the size of the primary tumor and involved lymph nodes, thereby facilitating delivery of subsequent definitive RT with concurrent low-dose weekly chemotherapy. Weekly chemotherapy usually is better tolerated than the high dose q3 week cisplatin regimen that is typically administered concurrently with RT for patients who have not received induction chemotherapy. For patients with resectable oral cavity tumors, induction PF was described as a strategy to reduce the number of patients who require mandibulectomy.

However, many head and neck oncologists raised significant concerns about the role of induction chemotherapy in head and neck cancer. One concern was that, after induction chemotherapy, patients might not be compliant with subsequent RT, which is the curative backbone of the treatment plan. Another concern was that early systemic therapy might engender tumor resistance, thereby compromising local control with subsequent definitive RT.

The role of induction chemotherapy remained relatively limited in the treatment of HNSCC until the discovery of taxane chemotherapy and the development of the TPF regimen. The taxanes, paclitaxel (Taxol®) and docetaxel (Taxotere®), provided a major advance in the systemic treatment of HNSCC. Investigators evaluated the addition of taxanes to induction PF. Two phase I studies demonstrated the feasibility of docetaxel + PF, or "TPF". A unique feature of these phase I studies was that the maximum-tolerated dose (MTD) was deemed to be that dose at which 3 of 6 patients experienced the same dose-limiting toxicity (DLT). In phase I studies for patients with incurable disease, MTD is defined as the dose level at which no more than 1 of 6 patients experience any DLT. The definition of DLT in the phase I TPF studies reflects a consideration that, for patients being treated with curative intent, a relatively aggressive regimen is often needed. The relatively high bar for defining MTD in the phase I TPF studies underscores that TPF was developed to be an aggressive chemotherapy regimen for previously untreated patients with potentially curable disease.

TAX 324 was a randomized phase III clinical trial that compared TPF versus PF as induction chemotherapy for patients with stage III or IV disease without distant metastases. After 3 cycles of induction TPF or PF, patients from both groups then received the same definitive RT with concurrent low-dose weekly carboplatin. Five hundred one patients were randomized. Median age was approximately 56 years, more than 80% of the patients were men, and the most common primary site was oropharynx. PF was administered as cisplatin 100 mg/m^2 on day 1 and 5-fluorouracil 1000 mg/m^2/day as a continuous infusion for 5 days of a 21-day cycle. TPF was administered as docetaxel 75 mg/m^2 on day 1, cisplatin 100 mg/m^2 on day 1, and 5-fluorouracil 1000 mg/m^2/day as a continuous infusion for 4 days of a 21-day cycle.

The most common grade 3 or 4 adverse event was neutropenia, occurring in 83% of the TPF patients and 56% of the PF patients. Febrile neutropenia occurred in 12% of the TPF patients. Grade 3 or 4 mucositis occurred somewhat more frequently in the PF group than in the TPF group (27% versus 21%), probably due to the higher 5-fluorouracil dose in the PF regimen.

Survival outcomes significantly favored the TPF group compared to the PF group; median overall survival was 71 versus 30 months, respectively, and median progression-free survival was 36 versus 13 months, respectively. The overall response to induction chemotherapy was 72% in the TPF group and 64% in the PF group (p = 0.07). Locoregional failure was significantly less common in the TPF group than in the PF group (30% versus 38%), but there was not a significant difference in the incidence of distant metastases between the two groups.

The TAX 323 study featured a similar design, but with some differences in the chemotherapy regimen doses. Another difference was that in TAX 323, patients received radiation therapy alone after induction chemotherapy. TAX 323 was restricted to patients with unresectable disease. TAX 323 again showed superior efficacy outcomes for TPF versus PF, although the survival times were shorter, likely reflecting the inclusion of only patients with unresectable disease.

TAX 324 and TAX 323 established TPF as the induction chemotherapy regimen of choice and reignited the debate about the appropriate role of induction chemotherapy in the management of locally and/or regionally advanced HNSCC. Three randomized studies were launched to compare primary chemoradiation versus induction TPF followed by chemoradiation. The PARADIGM and DeCIDE studies, as reported at the 2012 Annual Meeting of the American Society of Clinical Oncology, both failed to demonstrate improved overall survival with the induction chemotherapy approach. Both studies may have been statistically underpowered. Paccagnella and colleagues have conducted a larger randomized study of TPF followed by chemoradiation versus primary chemoradiation, and the pending results of that study may provide further guidance regarding the use of TPF.

TAX 324 demonstrated that the addition of docetaxel to induction PF leads to improved survival, compared to PF, when administered as part of a sequential therapy program that includes subsequent definitive radiation therapy. The remarkable finding was that the addition of a mere 3 cycles of docetaxel improved overall survival. This highlights the chemosensitive nature of newly diagnosed HNSCC, and motivates the search for new classes of drugs to combat this cancer. While the optimal role of induction chemotherapy in the management of locally and/or regionally advanced HNSCC remains unresolved, the development of TPF provided a new, more effective option for clinical situations in which the treating physician feels that induction chemotherapy is warranted.

PLATINUM-BASED CHEMOTHERAPY PLUS CETUXIMAB IN HEAD AND NECK CANCER

Jan B Vermorken, Ricard Mesia, Fernando Rivera, et al.

Background: Cetuximab is effective in platinum-resistant recurrent or metastatic squamous-cell carcinoma of the head and neck. We investigated the efficacy of cetuximab plus platinum-based chemotherapy as first-line treatment in patients with recurrent or metastatic squamous-cell carcinoma of the head and neck.

Methods: We randomly assigned 220 of 442 eligible patients with untreated recurrent or metastatic squamous-cell carcinoma of the head and neck to receive cisplatin (at a dose of 100 mg per square meter of body-surface area on day 1) or carboplatin (at an area under the curve of 5 mg per milliliter per minute, as a 1-hour intravenous infusion on day 1) plus fluorouracil (at a dose of 1000 mg per square meter per day for 4 days) every 3 weeks for a maximum of 6 cycles and 222 patients to receive the same chemotherapy plus cetuximab (at a dose of 400 mg per square meter initially, as a 2-hour intravenous infusion, then 250 mg per square meter, as a 1-hour intravenous infusion per week) for a maximum of 6 cycles. Patients with stable disease who received chemotherapy plus cetuximab continued to receive cetuximab until disease progression or unacceptable toxic effects, whichever occurred first.

Results: Adding cetuximab to platinum-based chemotherapy with fluorouracil (platinum-fluorouracil) significantly prolonged the median overall survival from 7.4 months in the chemotherapy-alone group to 10.1 months in the group that received chemotherapy plus cetuximab (hazard ratio for death, 0.80; 95% confidence interval, 0.64 to 0.99; p = 0.04). The addition of cetuximab prolonged the median progression, 0.54; p < 0.001) and increased the response rate from 20% to 36% (p < 0.001). The most common grade 3 or 4 adverse events in the chemotherapy-alone and cetuximab groups were anemia (19% and 13%, respectively), neutropenia (23% and 22%), and thrombocytopenia (11% in both groups). Sepsis occurred in 9 patients in the cetuximab group and in 1 patient in the chemotherapy-alone group (p = 0.02). Of 219 patients receiving cetuximab, 9% had grade 3 skin reactions and 3% had grade 3 or 4 infusion-related reactions. There were no cetuximab-related deaths.

Conclusions: As compared with platinum-based chemotherapy plus fluorouracil alone, cetuximab plus platinum-fluorouracil chemotherapy improved overall survival when given as first-line treatment in patients with recurrent or metastatic squamous-cell carcinoma of the head and neck.

Vermorken JB, Mesia R, Rivera F, et al. Platinum-based chemotherapy plus cetuximab in head and neck cancer. N Engl J Med. 2008;359:1116-1127.

Commentary by: *David G Pfister*

The management of patients with recurrent and/or metastatic squamous cell cancer of the upper aerodigestive tract (SCHNC) is challenging. Long-term disease control and cure can be obtained in selected patients with disease amenable to local therapies. But for those patients without a feasible surgical or radiation option, chemotherapy has been the principle treatment modality used. While there are many drugs with activity—methotrexate, cisplatin, carboplatin, 5-fluorouracil, paclitaxel, docetaxel, and cetuximab being among the most commonly used—the efficacy of these single agents is disappointing in this disease setting. The minority of patients will have a major response; cures are anecdotal, so treatment is given with palliative intent; and median survivals in studies are consistently less than 1 year.

Combinations of these drugs, such as cisplatin/5-fluorouracil, may increase the response rate at the expense of more toxicity, but response durations remain limited to a few months on average, and historically, randomized trials have failed to convincingly demonstrate an improvement in overall survival compared to therapy with single agents. The availability of taxane combinations changed the observed side effect profiles but did not lead to overall survival improvement.

With this as background, the above paper reported by Vermorken and colleagues is particularly important. In this clinical study (the so-called "EXTREME" trial), the treatment of patients with recurrent and/or metastatic SCHNC with a platinum doublet plus the anti-epidermal growth factor receptor antibody cetuximab improved overall survival compared to treatment with a platinum doublet alone. In addition, the paper highlights the utility of targeted therapy in SCHNC.

The epidermal growth factor receptor (EGFR) has been of great interest as a therapeutic target in SCHNC, as it is commonly overexpressed in these tumors and associated with a poor prognosis. Cetuximab is a IgG1 monoclonal antibody that blocks relevant ligand binding to the receptor and is the best studied of this class of agent in SCHNC. The drug demonstrates synergy with cisplatin when combined in a murine model. When used in patients with recurrent and/or metastatic SCHNC, an estimated 13% of patients will have a major response. A randomized trial of cisplatin versus cisplatin plus cetuximab in this population led to a significant improvement in response (10% versus 26%, $p = 0.09$). There was not a clear improvement in the primary endpoint of median progression-free survival (2.7 months versus 4.2 months, $p = 0.09$) nor in overall survival (8.0 months versus 9.2 months, $p = 0.21$), but the sample size (N = 123) to address false negative concerns was relatively modest for comparisons of this nature.

In the EXTREME trial, 442 eligible patients with untreated recurrent and/or metastatic SCHNC were randomized to a platinum doublet (cisplatin or carboplatin plus 5-fluorouracil) with or without cetuximab for a maximum of six cycles. At that point, patients treated with the triplet who had stable disease or better continued on single-agent cetuximab maintenance until there was progression of disease or toxicity that precluded further treatment. Both median overall (7.4 months versus 10.1 months, $p = 0.04$) and progression-free (3.3 months versus 5.6 months, $p < 0.001$) survivals were superior on the cetuximab-containing arm. Sepsis, hypomagnesemia, and skin reactions were all more common with the addition of cetuximab ($p = 0.02$, 0.05, and

0.001, respectively). The initial United States Food and Drug Administration (FDA) approved labeling for cetuximab in patients with recurrent and/or metastatic SCHNC was for use in platinum-refractory disease as a single agent; the results of the EXTREME trial led to a further expansion of this indication.

Although cetuximab appeared synergistic with cisplatin in a murine model, the therapeutic benefit of cetuximab in recurrent and/or metastatic SCHNC may be predominantly additive. In patients with SCHNC refractory to cisplatin-based therapy, the response rate is similar whether cetuximab is then given alone or combined with cisplatin-based treatment. In another study, patients with SCHNC who had progressed through platinum-based therapy and cetuximab each given alone demonstrated no responses when platinum-based therapy and cetuximab were then combined. Given these data, a question not answered by the EXTREME trial becomes apparent, i.e., would sequential administration of a platinum doublet alone followed by cetuximab alone at progression yield similar survival results to treatment with the cetuximab containing triplet followed by cetuximab maintenance reported in the Vermorken et al. study?

A biomarker to predict response to cetuximab-based therapy in SCHNC remains elusive, and is an important area of ongoing research. The development of a skin rash to EGFR-targeted agents is associated with improved outcome, but this is a marker that only becomes known after the commencement of treatment. In a correlative study done in conjunction with the EXTREME trial, tumor EGFR copy number was not predictive of efficacy on the cetuximab arm.

IMPROVED SURVIVAL OF PATIENTS WITH HUMAN PAPILLOMAVIRUS-POSITIVE HEAD AND NECK SQUAMOUS CELL CARCINOMA IN A PROSPECTIVE CLINICAL TRIAL

Carole Fakhry, William H Westra, Sigui Li, et al.

Background: The improved prognosis for patients with human papillomavirus (HPV)-positive head and neck squamous cell carcinoma (HNSCC) relative to HPV-negative HNSCC observed in retrospective analyses remains to be confirmed in a prospective clinical trial.

Methods: We prospectively evaluated the association of tumor HPV status with therapeutic response and survival among 96 patients with stage III or IV HNSCC of the oropharynx or larynx who participated in an Eastern Cooperative Oncology Group (ECOG) phase II trial and who received two cycles of induction chemotherapy with intravenous paclitaxel and carboplatin followed by concomitant weekly intravenous paclitaxel and standard fractionation radiation therapy. The presence or absence of HPV oncogenic types in tumors was determined by multiplex polymerase chain reaction (PCR) and in situ hybridization. Two-year overall and progression-free survival for HPV-positive and HPV-negative patient were estimated by Kaplan-Meier analysis. The relative hazard of mortality and progression for HPV-positive vs HPV-negative patients after adjustment for age, ECOG performance status, stage, and other covariables was estimated by use of a multivariable Cox proportional hazards model. All statistical tests were two-sided.

Results: Genomic DNA of oncogenic HPV types 16, 33, or 35 was located within tumor cell nuclei of 40% [95% confidence interval (CI) = 30% to 50%] of patients with HNSCC of the oropharynx or larynx by in situ hybridization and PCR. Compared with patients with HPV-negative tumors, patients with HPV-positive tumors had higher response rates after induction chemotherapy (82% vs 55%, difference = 27%, 95% CI = 9.3% to 44.7%, p = .01) and after chemoradiation treatment (84% vs 57%, difference = 27%, 95% CI = 9.7% to 44.3%, p = .007). After a median follow-up of 39.1 months, patients with HPV-positive tumors had improved overall survival [2-year overall survival = 95% (95% CI = 87% to 100%) vs 62% (95% CI = 49% to 74%), difference = 33%, 95% CI = 18.6% to 47.4%, p = .005, log-rank test] and, after adjustment for age, tumor stage, ECOG performance status, lower risks of progression [hazard ratio (HR) = 0.27, 95% CI = 0.10 to 0.75], and death from any cause (HR = 0.36, 95% CI = 0.15 to 0.85) than those with HPV-negative tumors.

Conclusion: For patients with HNSCC of the oropharynx, tumor HPV status is strongly associated with therapeutic response and survival.

Fakhry C, Westra WH, Li S, et al. Improved survival of patients with human papillomavirus–positive head and neck squamous cell carcinoma in a prospective clinical trial. J Natl Cancer Inst. 2008;100: 261-269.

Commentary by: *Erich M Sturgis*

This article reports the first prospective clinical trial to show that oropharyngeal cancers positive for human papillomavirus (HPV) were associated with better overall and progression-free survival than HPV-negative cancers. The authors represented the Eastern Cooperative Oncology Group (ECOG). Drs Fakhry, Westra, Forastiere, and Gillison were from Johns Hopkins

Medical Institutions; Drs Li, Cmelak, Ridge, and Pinto were from the Dana-Farber Cancer Institute, Vanderbilt University, Fox Chase Cancer Center, and Stanford University, respectively. While numerous case series from single institutions as well as meta-analyses had previously indicated an improved prognosis for patients with HPV-positive versus HPV-negative head and neck cancer, this was the first prospective clinical trial with a homogeneous patient set undergoing the same standardized treatment approach to confirm the better prognosis associated with HPV-positive cancer. Also notable is that this correlative biomarker study was included as part of the original clinical trial plan.

Patients eligible for the ECOG 2399 organ preservation phase II trial were those with stage III or IV (specifically, T2N1-3M0 or T3-4N0-3M0) laryngeal or oropharyngeal squamous cell carcinoma. Patients with unresectable disease were not eligible. The treatment schema was two cycles of induction chemotherapy (paclitaxel and carboplatin) followed by concurrent paclitaxel and 70 Gy of radiation. As noted in the original report of the results from ECOG 2399, 105 patients were enrolled: 36 with laryngeal cancer and 69 with oropharyngeal cancer. The 2-year overall survival rate was 63% for those with laryngeal cancer and 83% for those with oropharyngeal cancer, and the organ preservation rate was 74% for the larynx and 84% for the oropharynx. As part of the original protocol, patients consented to a biomarker study of HPV positivity of patients' formalin-fixed and paraffin-embedded specimens from biopsy of the primary tumor. Specimens from 96 patients (91% of trial participants) were available for HPV analysis.

The researchers were blinded to all clinical data until the HPV analysis was completed and the results were reported to ECOG. All histopathologic slides were reviewed by a single study pathologist who confirmed the presence of tumor and assigned a pathologic grade and degree of basaloid features. HPV status (positive vs negative) was determined by HPV16 *in situ* hybridization for detection of oncogenic HPV16 DNA in tumor cell nuclei, and HPV status was confirmed by polymerase chain reaction (PCR) on DNA extracted from the tumor. A multiplex PCR assay was used to screen for 37 oncogenic HPV types, and for tumors that were PCR positive for HPV other than HPV16, *in situ* hybridization was used to confirm nuclear localization of the HPV DNA. HPV positivity was graded (1+ to 3+) according to the number of focal hybridization signals per nucleus. In addition, HPV16 viral load was estimated using real-time quantitative PCR. Finally, p16 immunohistochemistry was performed, and the results were recorded as positive (strong and diffuse nuclear and cytoplasmic staining, a marker of HPV-driven oropharyngeal malignancy) or negative (absence of staining or weak staining).

Overall, 38 (40%) of 96 tumors were HPV positive, and 58 (60%) of 96 tumors were HPV negative. All of the HPV-positive tumors were oropharyngeal tumors. Of the 62 oropharyngeal tumors, 38 (61%) were HPV positive, and 24 (39%) were HPV negative. Of the 38 HPV-positive tumors, 36 were attributed to HPV16 by HPV *in situ* hybridization and confirmatory PCR analysis, while 1 was attributed to HPV33 and 1 was attributed to HPV35 by HPV PCR analysis and confirmatory HPV33 or HPV35 *in situ* hybridization. HPV positivity was scored as 1+ for 11 tumors, 2+ for 7 tumors, and 3+ for 20 tumors. The median HPV16 viral copy number per cell by real-time PCR was estimated to be 0, 0.3, 2.4, and 17.6 for tumors graded as 0, 1+, 2+, and 3+ by *in situ* hybridization, respectively. Finally, all 36 of the HPV-positive tumors with sufficient material for p16 immunohistochemistry were positive for p16, while 28% of the HPV-negative tumors (the number of such tumors tested was not reported) were positive for p16.

Compared to patients with HPV-negative tumors, patients with HPV-positive tumors were younger and more likely to be male, white, never smokers, have an ECOG performance status of 0, and have a less than 20 pack-year history of smoking, though these differences were not all significant. Compared to HPV-negative tumors, HPV-positive tumors were more likely to be poorly differentiated, basaloid, of a lower T category, of a higher N category, and stage IV; though again, these differences were not all significant. Unfortunately, the authors did not provide a complete comparison of these demographic and clinical characteristics between patients with HPV-positive and HPV-negative tumors restricted to patients with oropharyngeal cancer. However, patients with HPV-positive oropharyngeal cancer were significantly more likely than patients with HPV-negative oropharyngeal cancer to be white, have an ECOG performance status of 0, and have a less than 20 pack-year history of smoking.

Because patients with either laryngeal or oropharyngeal cancer were eligible for and enrolled in the ECOG 2399 trial, much of the presentation of outcomes compares all patients with HPV-positive tumors to all patients with HPV-negative tumors, even though no laryngeal tumor was HPV positive and the most relevant comparisons are those between patients with HPV-positive and HPV-negative oropharyngeal cancer. Overall, the rate of response to induction chemotherapy was higher for HPV-positive tumors (82%) than HPV-negative tumors (55%, P = 0.01; 58% for HPV-negative oropharyngeal cancers and 53% for HPV-negative laryngeal cancers). Median follow-up time was 39.1 months (minimum 20.1 months).

In analyses limited to patients with oropharyngeal tumors, on Kaplan-Meier analysis, the overall survival and progression-free survival rates were both better for patients with HPV-positive than those with HPV-negative tumors (P = 0.004 and P = 0.05, respectively). The 2-year overall survival rate and progression-free survival rate for patients with HPV-positive oropharyngeal cancer were 95% and 86%, respectively. Local/regional recurrence occurred in only 2 patients with HPV-positive and 8 patients with HPV-negative oropharyngeal cancer, while distant metastases occurred in 3 patients with HPV-positive but only 1 patient with HPV-negative oropharyngeal cancer. Only 7 of 38 patients with HPV-positive oropharyngeal cancer versus 12 of 24 patients with HPV-negative oropharyngeal cancer died.

In multivariate analysis including patients with laryngeal cancer, those with HPV-positive tumors had significantly lower risks of death and progression than those with HPV-negative tumors after adjustment for age, performance status, and stage (hazard ratios = 0.36 and 0.27, respectively). Because no patient with laryngeal cancer had an HPV-positive tumor, there was no method for adjusting for tumor site (oropharynx vs larynx). In multivariate analysis limited to patients with oropharyngeal cancer, the effect of HPV status on overall or progression-free survival was not significant, most likely because of sample size and limited power. However, among patients with oropharyngeal tumors, on univariate analysis, having an HPV-positive tumor was associated with a 71% lower risk for death ($p = 0.01$) and a 68% lower risk for progression ($p = 0.04$), and on multivariate analysis, having an HPV-positive tumor was associated with a 61% lower risk for death ($p = 0.06$) and a 62% lower risk for progression ($p = 0.09$).

Despite the shortcomings of limited sample size and the inclusion of patients with laryngeal cancer in much of the analysis, this landmark work firmly established HPV as a critically important prognostic factor for patients with oropharyngeal cancer. This work laid the foundation for critical advances in the field, including the following:

1. Several phase III trials from Europe, North America, and Australia have confirmed the major prognostic significance of HPV in patients with oropharyngeal cancer treated with chemotherapy and radiation.
2. A multicenter phase II clinical trial (ECOG 1308) restricted to patients with HPV-positive oropharyngeal cancer has completed enrolment. This trial is exploring the possibility of reduced-dose radiotherapy for HPV-positive oropharyngeal cancers after complete response to induction chemotherapy.
3. A multicenter phase III clinical trial (Radiation Therapy Oncology Group 1016) restricted to patients with HPV-positive oropharyngeal cancer will soon complete enrolment. This trial is comparing survival and toxic effect profiles between patients treated with concurrent cetuximab and radiation and those treated with concurrent cisplatin and radiation.
4. Two multicenter phase II clinical trials will evaluate the role of transoral surgery in deintensifying therapy for HPV-positive oropharyngeal cancer (ECOG 3311) and in intensifying therapy for HPV-negative oropharyngeal cancer (Radiation Therapy Oncology Group 1221).

FACTORS ASSOCIATED WITH SEVERE LATE TOXICITY AFTER CONCURRENT CHEMORADIATION FOR LOCALLY ADVANCED HEAD AND NECK CANCER: AN RTOG ANALYSIS

Mitchell Machtay, Jennifer Moughan, Andrew Trotti, et al.

Purpose: Concurrent chemoradiotherapy (CCRT) for squamous cell carcinoma of the head and neck (SCCHN) increases both local tumor control and toxicity. This study evaluates clinical factors that are associated with and might predict severe late toxicity after CCRT.

Methods: Patients were analyzed from a subset of three previously reported Radiation Therapy Oncology Group (RTOG) trials of CCRT for locally advanced SCCHN (RTOG 91-11, 97-03, and 99-14). Severe late toxicity was defined in this secondary analysis as chronic grade 3 to 4 pharyngeal/laryngeal toxicity (RTOG/European Organization for the Research and Treatment of Cancer late toxicity scoring system) and/or requirement for a feeding tube ≥ 2 years after registration and/or potential treatment-related death (e.g. pneumonia) within 3 years. Case-control analysis was performed, with a multivariable logistic regression model that included pretreatment and treatment potential factors.

Results: A total of 230 patients were assessable for this analysis: 99 patients with severe late toxicities and 131 controls; thus, 43% of assessable patients had a severe late toxicity. On multivariable analysis, significant variables correlated with the development of severe late toxicity were older age (odds ratio 1.05 per year; p = .001); advanced T stage (odds ratio, 3.07; p = .0036); larynx/hypopharynx primary site (odds ratio, 4.17; p = .0041); and neck dissection after CRT (odds ratio, 2.39; p = .018).

Conclusion: Severe late toxicity after CCRT is common. Older age, advanced T-stage, and larynx/hypopharynx primary site were strong independent risk factors. Neck dissection after CCRT was associated with an increased risk of these complications.

Machtay M, Moughan J, Trotti A, et al. Factors associated with severe late toxicity after concurrent chemoradiation for locally advanced head and neck cancer: an RTOG analysis. J Clini Oncol. 2008;26:3582-3589.

Commentary by: *Paul M Harari*

It is often said that we learn more from our toxicities and failures than our successes. This is a relevant message from the article by Machtay et al. entitled, "Factors Associated with Severe Late Toxicity After Concurrent Chemoradiation for Locally Advanced Head and Neck Cancer: An RTOG Analysis".

Despite modest incremental advances in overall outcome for head and neck (H&N) cancer patients over several decades, the literature is characterized by numerous reports describing "promising steps forward, valuable new treatment techniques and gratifying improvements in tumor control". Such is the optimistic prism through which we view our specialty, and there is no question that promising new developments emerge every few years. Nevertheless, robust and detailed reports that rigorously characterize treatment failures and long-term toxicities in H&N cancer are considerably less common. This is the backdrop for the Machtay article, which describes severe late toxicities for advanced H&N cancer patients receiving concurrent chemoradiation (CRT).

Drawing from patients treated with concurrent CRT in three well-annotated RTOG clinical trials between 1991–2001, Machtay identified 230 patients assessable for late toxicity analysis. From this cohort, 99 patients (43%) manifested severe late toxicity, defined as grade 3 or higher, present > 180 days after the start of radiation, and related to dysfunction of the larynx and/or pharynx. Patients with severe laryngo-pharyngeal dysfunction from cancer before the start of treatment were excluded. This is a central finding from the Machtay study, namely that in excess of 40% of advanced H&N patients treated with concurrent CRT were scored with significant toxicities more than 6 months following treatment. Significant variables associated with the development of severe late toxicity included older age, more advanced T-stage, larynx/pharynx primary tumor site, and the use of neck dissection after CRT. Overall, increasing age was the most significant pretreatment factor associated with the development of severe late toxicity.

The Machtay report illuminates an important theme and provides a powerful reminder for H&N oncologists to remain conscious of organ function and quality of life following treatment. Although true that a cured H&N cancer patient (with toxicity) is preferable to death from cancer, there can be severe late toxicities that are indeed debilitating. We would all prefer to limit these severe late toxicities to the very lowest possible levels. Several decades of clinical research in non-operative treatment strategies for H&N cancer have focused largely on intensification of radiation and chemotherapy. The refinement of altered radiation fractionation schedules, sequential and concurrent CRT regimens, and the selective incorporation of neck dissection for patients with advanced neck disease means that many patients receive all three major treatment modalities for their H&N cancer. This approach can sometimes prove highly toxic if each specialist is intent on delivering their strongest independent punch without careful consideration of the overall treatment package.

Are we simply near the ceiling of normal tissue tolerance with current CRT treatment regimens for H&N cancer? The use of 70 Gy in 35 fractions of 2 Gy is well known to be a robust, successful, and moderately toxic cancer therapy regimen that requires delivery expertise regarding field design, dose homogeneity, target definition, and nursing care for each patient throughout their treatment course. The addition of concurrent chemotherapy for advanced H&N cancer patients has modestly pushed up survival rates (on the order of 5–8%) but at the expense of significantly increased acute toxicities, and in some cases, consequential late toxicities. Swallow function is often compromised in this setting, with the use of prolonged feeding tubes for a subset of patients. Indeed, the use of prophylactic gastric feeding tubes has increased exponentially during the last decade with the common use of concurrent CRT. Perhaps we are pushing normal tissue tolerance "over the edge" for some patients in the concurrent CRT era? The patients in the Machtay review come from the two-dimensional treatment era of H&N radiation just prior to the rapid uptake of intensity modulated radiation therapy (IMRT) techniques. More normal tissues can be selectively spared from high dose with IMRT, but the learning curve for H&N IMRT is steep, and many patients are treated by practitioners with modest expertise and case load experience for this high complexity cancer therapy.

As identified in the major H&N treatment meta-analyses in which patients 70 years and older do not appear to benefit from altered fractionation or from the addition of chemotherapy to radiation, the Machtay study identifies increasing age as the single most important pretreatment factor associated with the development of severe late toxicity. These data raise significant questions about whether aggressive CRT regimens are truly justified and ultimately beneficial for many of our older H&N cancer patients.

The Machtay article provides much more to the H&N literature than a simple review of late toxicities in a cohort of H&N cancer clinical trials. It provides a wakeup call to H&N cancer specialists to look carefully at treatment successes and failures over time. Continuing to simply increase the intensity of our therapy approaches will exact a toxicity price that can compromise the ultimate treatment outcome that practitioners and cancer patients ultimately strive to achieve.

With the recent advent of the HPV era in H&N cancer, increasing attention is being given to methods of therapy de-intensification for selected patients. This is relatively new in H&N oncology where several decades of systematic increase in treatment intensity has been the hallmark of clinical trials. Much akin to pediatric oncology in which concerted efforts to maintain cure rates while diminishing long-term toxicities have been at the forefront, so too can a more judicious approach of therapies to H&N cancer patients be applied in the coming years. Optimizing treatment regimens that incorporate conformal radiation techniques, selective use of chemotherapy or molecular-targeted therapies, application of transoral surgery techniques to reduce normal tissue damage and enable reduction in adjuvant therapies are actively emerging. Thoughtful consideration of patient age and performance status will help ensure that we personalize treatment approaches and objectives. Harmonizing the interaction of H&N specialists on behalf of each cancer patient has never been more critical for the future.

Chapter 19

Quality of Life

QUALITY OF LIFE IN PATIENTS WITH HEAD AND NECK CANCER
Lessons Learned from 549 Prospectively Evaluated Patients

Ernest A Weymuller, Bevan Yueh, Frederic WB Deleyiannis, et al.

Objectives: To summarize our quality-of-life (QOL) research findings for patients with head and neck cancer, to suggest areas for future productive QOL research, and to discuss how to undertake QOL studies in a costeffective manner.

Design: Review of previously published analyses of advanced larynx cancer, advanced oropharynx cancer, and neck-dissection cases and current data from the complete set of patients.

Patients: From January 1, 1993, through December 31, 1998, data on 549 patients were entered in our head and neck database. Of these patients, 364 met additional criteria for histologic findings (squamous cell carcinoma) and the restriction of their cancer to 4 major anatomical sites (oral, oropharynx, hypopharynx, or larynx). Of these, 339 patients were more than 1 year beyond initial treatment. Complete baseline TNM staging and QOL data were obtained for 260 these patients of whom 210 presented with an untreated first primary tumor (index cases) to the University of Washington, Seattle.

Intervention: Pretreatment QOL was assessed with an interviewer-supervised self-administered questionnaire. Subsequent self-administered tests were completed at 3, 6, 12, 24, and 36 months. Other data collected on each patient included cancer site, stage, treatment, histologic findings, type of surgical reconstruction, and current disease and vital status.

Results/Conclusions: It is difficult to achieve "statistically significant" results in a single-institution setting. The "composite" QOL score may not be a sufficiently sensitive tool. Analysis of separate domains may be more effective.

Weymuller EA, Yueh B, Deleyiannis FWB, et al. Quality of life in patients with head and neck cancer: lessons learned from 549 prospectively evaluated patients. Arch Otolaryngol Head Neck Surg. 2000;126:329-335; discussion 335-336.

Commentary by: *Randall P Morton*

It is instructive to reflect on this "Lessons Learned..." paper, a landmark publication from the University of Washington (UW) Department of Otolaryngology-Head and Neck Surgery. After more than a decade, the essential points contained within this report on quality of life (QOL) in head and neck cancer patients remain highly relevant, and indeed, serve as a signpost for future work in the area of patient-based outcomes in the management of head and neck cancer. One sense of the impact and importance of this paper comes from a glance at the high number of citations that this work has attracted in a relatively short period of time.

The publication might be considered as a culmination of many years of hard labor, working with data acquired from hundreds of head and neck cancer patients being treated in Seattle. The authors actually include a synopsis of previous published studies on subsets of the data from this study. That effectively provides an internal context for the work, as well as a commentary on the evolution of the UW QOL dataset.

To put "Lessons Learned..." into a broader context, we should appreciate that QOL-related outcomes in cancer patients only started to appear in the 1970s; in 1977, the term "quality of life" became a "key word" in the United States National Library of Medicine MEDLINE computer search program. The interest and activity in QOL research in head and neck cancer grew with a steady flow of cross-sectional studies of QOL in head and neck cancer patients in the 1980s. In 1993, Dr Weymuller's group at UW published a lucid exposition of QOL assessment for head and neck cancer patients. It was only the fourth longitudinal study of QOL to have been published up to that time, but it set the scene for most head and neck surgical oncologists interested in this field, and formed the basis for the database from which the "Lessons Learned..." paper was generated.

Around the time that this latter paper was published, the experience alone represented a significant addition to the QOL literature, but the breadth of the analysis and the quality of the recommendations makes this report a "must read", not only for aspiring researchers of QOL in head and neck cancer patients but also for practitioners wanting to monitor their patients' QOL in the clinical setting.

Some valuable insights regarding the use of the popular UW QOL instrument emerge from the authors' synopsis of the previous studies. They point out (a) that a composite QOL score may not be as sensitive to important changes as specific domain scores, (b) that inclusion of a global QOL score provides a valuable contrast to the disease-specific domains, and (c) that patients may adapt to their new health status such that the scores of specific disability and dysfunction are not necessarily perceived by the patients as being important. These principles are clinically very significant and are clearly spelled out in this paper.

While the above dynamics relating to QOL outcomes may appear to be clearly understood nowadays, at the time of publication many researchers seemed not to fully appreciate these issues. Weymuller et al.'s paper was a major contribution toward bringing these aspects to the fore, helping to raise awareness among QOL researchers. Indeed, the pedigree of the UW team lent credibility to these issues, ensuring that others paid close attention and started to incorporate the principles into their own work.

From an original 549 patients, only 66% had squamous carcinoma arising from the four major sites (oral, oro-pharynx, hypopharynx, and larynx). The term *"Head and Neck Cancer"* applies to a very heterogeneous group of tumors, but the "Big Four" are the sites that impact most forcefully on patients' QOL. Weymuller et al. confined their attention to the major tumor sites, thereby reducing the potential for misleading and irrelevant data "outliers". This message seems to have resonated, as in recent years QOL studies directed to other sites (salivary, skin, sino-nasal, thyroid) have started to appear.

The UW team assigned considerable resource and energy to recruiting and tracking the patients attending the department. Even so, it took the authors 5 years to gather QOL data on 210 patients that had been followed for 12 months or more, and only 50 patients (24%) had QOL data spanning 2 years. The message here is that we need to be clear and focused on what it is we want to know, so that energy is not spent in unnecessary data collection. With this, the authors build a powerful case for multi-institution trials if QOL is to be an endpoint for study.

So it is that the "Lessons Learned..." paper endows a critical understanding of the nature of QOL with crucial advice for institutions aiming to conduct QOL studies. There is of course plenty of advice for those wishing to pursue single-institution studies of QOL outcomes. Headline lessons such as "Eliminate Exhaustive Data Collection". "Obtain Long Term Funding", and "Direct Data Entry" provide sound, pithy, and essential advice. It is always helpful to not have to repeat the painful process of trial-and-error that others have already endured. This paper provides a wealth of information to save the reader from taking unnecessary steps or making unfortunate mistakes.

Dr Weymuller has led the way the past 2 decades, following up on his early work with several studies and commentaries, in the area of QOL in head and neck cancer. The incorporation of QOL data into regular clinical practice has not yet become common practice; rather, QOL remains largely in the research domain. Further research using the principles espoused in this landmark "Lessons Learned ..." paper will result in time with QOL outcomes being used and understood as readily as data related to survival.

STUDIES IN THE QUALITY OF LIFE OF HEAD AND NECK CANCER PATIENTS: RESULTS OF A TWO-YEAR LONGITUDINAL STUDY AND A COMPARATIVE CROSS-SECTIONAL CROSS-CULTURAL SURVEY

Randall P Morton

Objectives: To examine quality-of-life (QL) changes that occur over time among patients treated for head and neck cancer and to compare QL outcomes in two geographically separate and culturally distinct populations.

Study Design: A prospective, observational longitudinal study was made of QL changes over time in head and neck cancer patients, and a matched-pairs cross-sectional study was conducted for comparison of QL outcomes between groups of head and neck cancer patients from two different sociocultural environments.

Methods: Patients attending a tertiary head and neck cancer center in Auckland, New Zealand, were interviewed using a validated questionnaire before treatment and at 3, 12, and 24 months after treatment. Changes over time were assessed according to gender, site and stage of primary tumor, and type of treatment received. A second group of patients from Toronto, Ontario, Canada, were matched to the first group for age, gender, site and stage of tumor, and time since treatment and interviewed using the same questionnaire. The group comparison was followed by a matched-pairs analysis for the 12-month follow-up interval.

Results: In the longitudinal study, combined modality treatment resulted in greater physical and somatic dysfunction than single modality treatment. Patients learned to cope well with dysfunction and disability and with adjusting their lifestyle so that overall QL was not related to treatment received. Even so, pain scores and measures of psychological distress were related to overall QL. Otherwise there was no consistent correlation between specific symptoms and QL. An illustration of patients' adaptation to dysfunction was evident in scores for perceived difficulty swallowing, which decrease despite the ongoing need for a soft or liquid diet. In the comparative study, significantly different global QL scores were evident in the two clinical groups studied, despite similar social, somatic, and physical functioning. There was also a significant but inconstant difference in emotional functioning. Although the clinical groups received significantly different treatment regiments, the observed differences in global QL were independent of treatment received.

Conclusions: Patients with head and neck cancer generally managed well despite disability and dysfunction after treatment. Patients' expectations, emotional responses, and desired outcomes seemed to be determined by sociocultural factors, causing different patient groups to view their overall QL outcome somewhat differently.

Morton RP. Studies in the quality of life of head and neck cancer patients: results of a two-year longitudinal study and a comparative cross-sectional cross-cultural study, Laryngoscope. 2003;113:1091-1103.

Commentary by: *Ernest A Weymuller*

I am pleased to offer a reflection on this major contribution by my friend and colleague, Dr Randall Morton, who has been actively involved in quality of life (QL) research for three decades. It is important for readers of the "new generation" to understand that just 20 years ago the notion of investigating quality of life in the head and neck cancer patient population was largely dismissed as unnecessary and essentially impossible. Those of us who began QL studies in that era gained comfort from the wisdom of Lord Kelvin who once opined that one could not understand a phenomenon if one could not measure it.

Accordingly, in the first bloom of head and neck QL investigation a number of instruments were designed and validated (including the one developed by Dr Morton and used in this study). They became established and were used for a variety of purposes. In the subsequent years, studies emerged that improved the definition of the disabilities caused by the disease and by the various treatments that have been used. As experience with QL studies evolved, more sophisticated issues emerged, including the question raised by Dr Morton, e.g. are there significantly different expectations between cultures and how might those differences affect the QL response to head and neck cancer and its treatment?

The paper initially presents the results of a 2-year longitudinal QL survey of patients with head and neck cancer (Group A, Auckland, New Zealand). The QL outcomes for this group are quite similar to those reported in other studies. T and N status are strongly associated with overall quality of life, dysphasia, and pain. Quality of life is worst at 3 months after treatment and gradually improves at 12 and 24 months. The dominant long-term factors associated with a reduction in quality of life are pain, dysphagia, and eating out socially.

Having established this foundation, Dr Morton moves to the novel and creative aspect of the paper in which Group A is used as a comparator for a cross-sectional QL assessment of a matched set of head and neck cancer patients treated in a different country (Group B, Toronto, Canada). The main finding of this segment is that the global QL was worse in Group B and that psychological distress (GHQ-12) was a major component of that difference. As stated by Dr Morton, "*It is the authors view that, having lived and worked in each of the centers involved in the present study, patients in Toronto (Group B) had greater demands and higher expectations than those in Auckland (Group A)*".

Commentary: Dr Morton opens with an elegantly concise statement that quality of life "*encompasses an extensive range of physical and psychological characteristics that describe one's ability to function and derive satisfaction in doing so*". Being sensitive to that complexity, the study utilizes a spectrum of investigative instruments to gain a broad portrayal of the patient groups:

1. A validated institutional questionnaire that includes head and neck specific issues, such as dysphagia, pain, speech difficulty, dyspnea and diet, as well as questions regarding occupation, social functioning, family support, and occupation.

2. Additionally, patients completed a General Health Questionnaire (GHQ) and a Life Satisfaction Scale (LS).

As might be expected, even though Group A and Group B are matched for age, gender, primary site, T stage, N stage, and overall stage, there were notable dissimilarities. There was a predominance of combined therapy (including surgery) in Group A, while Group B was treated most often with definitive radiotherapy (p < 0.0005).

Using a correlation matrix for overall quality of life at 12 and 24 months, the variables with the highest correlation coefficients were the clinical groups (A or B) themselves and psychological distress. In the detailed discussion of the results Dr Morton presents data to support his conclusion that even though the patients received quite different treatment, *"the effect of the different treatments received was that each group had a slightly different pattern of symptoms; Group B had generally more head and neck pain, more xerostomia, and more difficulty swallowing than Group A. It is tempting to ascribe the observed QL differences between the groups to the effects of high-dose radiotherapy. However the observed differences in variables of the symptoms domain did not have a prominent effect on determining QL in either Group A or Group B. This is consistent with the finding from the earlier longitudinal study analysis, in which treatment-related symptoms differed according to the treatment received but did not impact overall patient related QL in any consistent manner".*

Typical of QL studies, there may be more than one conclusion or interpretation. Since ablative surgery was performed in 70% of Group A and 24% of Group B, an alternative interpretation of the QL outcomes would be to place emphasis on the differences in treatment offered to the two groups. As is true for most QL studies, Dr Morton indicates, *"larger longitudinal studies stratified according to site and stage are needed".*

Another important issue highlighted by Dr Morton relates to the timing of QL analysis. Before and immediately after treatment the dominant issues affecting quality of life are dysphasia, pain and psychological distress, but by 24 months significant physical symptoms are less numerous, although head and neck pain, difficulty breathing, and the inability to socialize remain the important factors correlated with overall quality of life. Also noted by Dr Morton (and others), head and neck cancer survivors (2 year) generally have a good quality of life in spite of their disabilities, perhaps because they *"learn to value their survival in the face of handicap and disability".*

The major thrust of this study is to amplify our sensitivity to the cultural differences among the patients we treat. This issue is exemplified by a QL project in Africa, which identified the profound impact of tracheotomy in that patient population. In Kenya, where illiteracy is endemic, patients cannot rely on written language for communication and the loss of speech via tracheotomy is a particularly devastating event in terms of quality of life. By comparison, in the "developed world", swallowing has a greater QL impact than aphasia, while in Kenya the normal diet is composed of soft foods and the QL impact of treatment on swallowing is less profound. As emphasized by Dr Morton, sensitivity to such cultural issues during treatment selection is of great importance to each individual patient, especially since we have yet to prove a significant survival difference between the major treatment options.

In closing, I want to express my deep admiration of Dr Morton for having garnered the sabbatical support that allowed him to spend 6 months in Toronto to pursue this seminal AL study and for his masterful analysis and leadership in QL research. Our decades long discussion of these and other issues has been a delightful and stimulating highlight of my career.